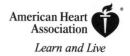

American Heart Association

Learn and Live

The AHA Clinical Series

SERIES EDITOR ELLIOTT ANTMAN

Antiplatelet Therapy In Ischemic Heart Disease

To my family Caroline, Jack, Sam and Lucy

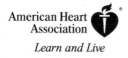

American Heart
Association
Learn and Live

The AHA Clinical Series

SERIES EDITOR ELLIOTT ANTMAN

Antiplatelet Therapy In Ischemic Heart Disease

EDITED BY

Stephen D. Wiviott, MD
Cardiovascular Division
Brigham and Women's Hospital
Assistant Professor of Medicine
Harvard Medical School
Investigator, TIMI Study Group
Boston, MA

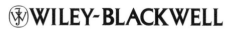

A John Wiley & Sons, Ltd., Publication

This edition first published 2009, © 2009 American Heart Association
American Heart Association National Center, 7272 Greenville Avenue, Dallas, TX 75231, USA
For further information on the American Heart Association:
www.americanheart.org

Blackwell Publishing was acquired by John Wiley & Sons in February 2007.
Blackwell's publishing program has been merged with Wiley's global Scientific,
Technical and Medical business to form Wiley-Blackwell.

Registered office: John Wiley & Sons Ltd, The Atrium, Southern Gate, Chichester, West Sussex, PO19 8SQ, UK
Editorial offices: 9600 Garsington Road, Oxford, OX4 2DQ, UK
    The Atrium, Southern Gate, Chichester, West Sussex, PO19 8SQ, UK
    111 River Street, Hoboken, NJ 07030-5774, USA

For details of our global editorial offices, for customer services and for information about how to
apply for permission to reuse the copyright material in this book please see our website at
www.wiley.com/wiley-blackwell

Library of Congress Cataloging-in-Publication Data
Antiplatelet therapy in ischemic heart disease / edited by Stephen D. Wiviott.
   p. ; cm.—(AHA clinical series)
  Includes bibliographical references.
  ISBN 978-1-4051-7626-2
  1. Coronary heart disease—Chemotherapy. 2. Blood platelets—Aggregation. I. Wiviott, Stephen D.
II. American Heart Association. III. Series.
  [DNLM: 1. Myocardial Ischemia—drug therapy. 2. Platelet Aggregation Inhibitors—therapeutic use.
3. Myocardial Ischemia—blood. QV 180 A634 2009]
  RC685.C6A69 2009
  616.1'23061—dc22
                                                       2008037317

ISBN: 9781405176262
A catalogue record for this book is available from the British Library.

Set in Palatino 9/12 by Charon Tec Ltd (A Macmillan Company), Chennai, India
(www.macmillansolutions.com)
Printed and bound in Malaysia by Vivar Printing Sdn Bhd

1 2009

Contents

Contributors

Editor

Stephen D. Wiviott, MD
Cardiovascular Division, Brigham and Women's Hospital
Assistant Professor of Medicine, Harvard Medical School
Investigator, TIMI Study Group
Boston, MA

Contributors

Boris Aleil, MD
INSERM U311 Unit – Etablissement Français du Sang–Alsace (EFS-Alsace)
Strasbourg
France

Peter B. Berger, MD
Associate Chief Research Officer
Director, Center for Clinical Studies
Geisinger Health Systems
Danville, PA, USA

Deepak L. Bhatt, MD, FACC, FAHA
Chief of Cardiology, VA Boston Healthcare System
Director, Integrated Interventional Cardiovascular Program at Brigham and
Women's Hospital and the VA Boston Healthcare System
Senior Investigator, TIMI Study Group
Boston, MA
USA

James C. Blankenship, MD
Director, Cardiac Catheterization Laboratories
Geisinger Medical Center
Danville, PA
USA

Anne Burdess, BSc (Hons), MBCHB, MRCS
Clinical Research Fellow
Department of Clinical and Surgical Sciences
University of Edinburgh
Edinburgh
UK

John F. Canales, MD
Cardiology Department
Texas Heart Institute
Baylor College of Medicine
St. Luke's Episcopal Hospital
Houston, Tx
USA

Wai-Hong Chen, MBBS, FACC, FAHA
Division of Cardiology, Department of Medicine
The University of Hong Kong
Queen Mary Hospital
Hong Kong, China

Nina Chetty Raju, MBBS, FRACP, FRCPA
Clinical Research Fellow
Thrombosis Service, Hamilton General Hospital
Department of Medicine McMaster University
Ontario, Canada

Marc Cohen, MD, FACC
Director, Division of Cardiology
Newark Beth Israel Medical Center
Newark, NJ
USA

Jean-Philippe Collet, MD, PhD
INSERM U856 Unit – Institut de Cardiologie
Centre Hospitalier Universitaire Pitié-Salpêtrière
Paris
France

Alanna Coolong, MD, MSc
Instructor of Medicine
Brigham and Women's Hopsital
Harvard Medical School
Boston, MA
USA

Dr Nicholas L. Cruden, PhD, MRCP
Clinical Lecturer in Cardiology
University of Edinburgh
Edinburgh
UK

Steven P. Dunn, PharmD
Department of Pharmacy Services and Division of Cardiology
Linda and Jack Gill Heart Institute
University of Kentucky
Lexington, KY, USA

John W. Eikelboom, MBBS, MSc, FRACP, FRCPA
Associate Professor
Thrombosis Service, Hamilton General Hospital
Population Health Research Institute
Department of Medicine, McMaster University
Ontario, Canada

James J. Ferguson, MD
Cardiology Research
St. Luke's Episcopal Hospital
Houston, TX
USA

Keith A. Fox, BSC (Hons), FRCP, FESC
BHF Professor of Cardiology
Uinveristy of Edinburgh
Edinburgh
UK

A.L. Frelinger, III, PhD
Associate Director, Center for Platelet Function Studies
Associate Professor of Pediatrics and Molecular Genetics & Microbiology
University of Massachusetts Medical School
Worcester, MA
USA

Christian Gachet, MD
INSERM U311 Unit – Etablissement Français du Sang–Alsace (EFS-Alsace)
Strasbourg
France

Nisheeth Goel, MD
Interventional Cardiology Fellow
Texas Heart Institute/Baylor College of Medicine
St. Luke's Episcopal Hospital
Houston, TX, USA

Larry B. Goldstein, MD, FAAN, FAHA
Department of Medicine (Neurology)
Center for Cerebrovascular Disease
Center for Clinical Health Policy Research
Duke University and Durham VA Medical Center
Durham, NC
USA

Heather L. Gornik, MD, MHS
Medical Director, Non-Invasive Vascular Laboratory
Department of Cardiovascular Medicine
Assistant Professor of Medicine
Cleveland Clinic
Lerner College of Medicine
Cleveland, OH
USA

Paul A. Gurbel, MD
Sinai Center for Thrombosis Research
Sinai Hospital
Baltimore, MD, USA

Christian W. Hamm, MD
Medical Director
Director of Cardiology
Kerckhoff Heart Center
Bad Nauheim
Germany

Esther S. Kim, MD, MPH
Associate Staff Physician
Department of Cardiovascular Medicine
Cleveland Clinic
Cleveland, OH
USA

Laura Mauri, MD, MSc
Assistant Professor of Medicine
Harvard Medical School
Director of Clinical Biometrics
Brigham and Women's Hospital
Boston, MA
USA

Nicolai Mejevoi, MD, PhD
Fellow, Division of Cardiology
Newark Beth Israel Medical Center
Newark, NJ
USA

Alan D. Michelson, MD
Director, Center for Platelet Function Studies
Professor of Pediatrics, Medicine, and Pathology
University of Massachusetts Medical School
Worcester, MA
USA

Gilles Montalescot, MD
INSERM U856 Unit – Institut de Cardiologie,
Centre Hospitalier Universitaire Pitié-Salpêtrière
Paris
France

Kamran I. Muhammad, MD
Fellow in Cardiovascular Medicine
Cleveland Clinic
Cleveland, OH, USA

Michelle O'Donoghue, MD
Cardiovascular Division
Department of Medicine
Massachusetts General Hospital
Boston, MA, USA

Marc S. Sabatine, MD, MPH
Cardiovascular Division
TIMI Study Group
Department of Medicine
Brigham and Women's Hospital
Boston, MA, USA

Daniel I. Simon, MD
Harrington-McLanghlin Heart & Vascular Institute
University Hospitals Case Medical Center
Case Western Reserve University School of Medicine
Cleveland, OH, USA

Steven R. Steinhubl, MD
Associate Professor of Medicine
Division of Cardiology
Linda and Jack Gill Heart Institute
University of Kentucky
Lexington, KY, USA

Robert F. Storey, BSc, BM, MRCP, DM
Cardiovascular Research Unit
School of Medicine and Biomedical Sciences
University of Sheffield, UK

Thomas A. Suarez, MD
Sinai Center for Thrombosis Research
Sinai Hospital
Baltimore, MD, USA

Udaya S. Tantry, PhD
Laboratory Director
Sinai Center for Thrombosis Research
Sinai Hospital
Baltimore, MD, USA

Anjum Tanwir, MD
Fellow, Division of Cardiology
Newark Beth Israel Medical Center
Newark, NJ, USA

Preface

Platelet activation and aggregation play key roles in the pathogenesis of atherosclerotic vascular disease. It is perhaps not surprising, then, that platelet function inhibitors have assumed a central role in the prevention of ischemic complications of these conditions including myocardial infarction, stroke, and limb ischemia and a major place in support of vascular procedures. In part because of the central role of these processes, there has been a growing identification of key pharmacologic targets and agents designed to alter these targets in hopes of improving clinical outcomes. This book is therefore designed to assist the clinician, clinical and basic scientist, student, and allied health personnel in navigating this rapidly growing field.

The book is divided into five sections. First, concepts in platelet physiology, function, and measurement are introduced to provide a basic understanding of platelet biology and biometrics and serve as the foundation on which the rest of the text is built. The next two sections introduce the pharmacology of key oral and intravenous antiplatelet agents that are available to the clinician or in late stages of clinical development. These sections provide an understanding of mechanisms of action of these agents and their pharmacology leading to the sections on the clinical use of antiplatelet agents. The fourth section summarizes the use of antiplatelet therapy by atherosclerotic disease states including coronary artery disease (unstable angina and non-ST-elevation myocardial infarction, ST-elevation myocardial infarction, and chronic coronary artery disease), peripheral vascular disease, and cerebrovascular disease. The fifth section, addresses "special circumstances" encountered by the clinician, the interaction between and management of antiplatelet agents in the settings of cardiac surgery, non-cardiac surgery, and percutaneous coronary intervention with stenting.

This book was made possible by an outstanding group of authors, all leaders in their fields, and their generous contributions are greatly appreciated.

I would like to thank Dr. Elliott Antman, editor of this book series, who first taught me how manage patients with ischemic vascular disease when I was a house officer, and later has served as an extremely generous research mentor. I would also like to thank Dr. Eugene Braunwald, the consummate physician scientist, for giving me an opportunity, and for giving all of us in academic medicine something to aspire to.

Stephen D. Wiviott, MD

Foreword

The strategic driving force behind the American Heart Association's mission of reducing disability and death from cardiovascular diseases and stroke is to change practice by providing information and solutions to healthcare professionals. The pillars of this strategy are Knowledge Discovery, Knowledge Processing, and Knowledge Transfer. The books in the AHA Clinical Series, of which *Antiplatelet Therapy In Ischemic Heart Disease* is included, focus on high-interest, cutting-edge topics in cardiovascular medicine. This book series is a critical tool that supports the AHA mission of promoting healthy behavior and improved care of patients. Cardiology is a rapidly changing field and practitioners need data to guide their clinical decision-making. The AHA Clinical series, serves this need by providing the latest information on the physiology, diagnosis, and management of a broad spectrum of conditions encountered in daily practice.

Rose Marie Robertson, MD, FAHA
Chief Science Officer, American Heart Association

Elliott Antman, MD, FAHA
Director, Samuel A. Levine Cardiac Unit,
Brigham and Women's Hospital

PART I

Concepts in Platelet Physiology, Function, and Measurement

Chapter 1

Platelet physiology and the role of the platelet in ischemic heart disease

Robert F. Storey

Blood platelets – equipped for action

The platelet, a tiny anucleate blood cell 2–4 μm in diameter, has major and diverse roles in health and disease and underlying this is a complex structure that supports a wide range of functional responses [1]. Approximately 1×10^{11} new platelets are released each day into the circulation from bone marrow where they are formed by fragmentation from megakaryocytes [2,3]. Thrombopoietin is the most important cytokine regulating platelet production and some disease states, such as inflammatory conditions, can increase thrombopoietin levels and platelet production [3]. This is of relevance when considering the rate of recovery of haemostatic function (and susceptibility to thrombosis) following exposure to irreversible platelet inhibitors such as aspirin and thienopyridines.

Platelets in the resting state are smooth, discoid cells possessing an open canalicular system and an exterior glycocalyx [1]. Ca^{2+} is sequestered in intracellular stores and released into the cytoplasm upon activation of the platelet by agonists, where it plays a major part in mediating platelet responses to activation [4]. Contained within the platelet cytoplasm are three types of granule, namely α-granules, dense granules and lysosomes [5]. α-Granules are the most abundant granules and contain a large number of proteins, many of which play a role in regulating the balance of thrombosis and fibrinolysis, such as α_2-antiplasmin and plasminogen activator inhibitor-1 (PAI-1) [6]. The membranes of α-granules also contain proteins that are expressed on the cell surface following platelet activation, including glycoprotein (GP) IIb/IIIa

Antiplatelet Therapy in Ischemic Heart Disease, 1st edition. Edited by Stephen D. Wiviott.
© 2009 American Heart Association, ISBN: 9-781-4051-7626-2

($\alpha_{IIb}\beta_3$) and P-selectin (CD62P). Dense granules contain concentrated stores of ADP, ATP, pyrophosphate, ionized calcium and 5HT, and release of the contents of dense granules contributes to platelet activation and hemostasis [5,7]. Lysosomes contain numerous acid hydrolases and these are secreted by platelets only in response to strong agonist stimulation. Platelet activation leads to fusion of granules with the open canalicular system and release of granule contents [8].

Platelets possess a cytoskeleton which determines cell shape and consists mainly of microtubules and microfilaments [5]. Reorganization of the platelet cytoskeleton during platelet activation leads to a change in cell shape, with the platelets becoming spherical and extending finger-like projections known as pseudopodia. Activation of platelets also leads to a reorganization of components of the plasma membrane that leads to the assembly of prothrombinase complex on the platelet surface, catalyzing thrombin generation and coagulation [9].

Figure 1.1 provides an overview of mechanisms for platelet activation and associated responses which will be covered in subsequent sections.

The platelet glycoprotein IIb/IIIa complex

The GPIIb/IIIa complex is an adhesion receptor belonging to the integrin gene superfamily and, like other integrins, is a heterodimer composed of an α (α_{IIb}) and a β (β_3) transmembrane subunit [10]. Approximately 40,000 to 80,000 GPIIb/IIIa complexes are present on the surface of each resting platelet and this number can rapidly increase following activation by strong agonists due to exposure of internal receptors normally present within the open canalicular system and α-granule membranes [10]. Activation of platelets induces conformational changes in GPIIb/IIIa so that it can bind fibrinogen, vWF or fibronectin, whereas in the resting state GPIIb/IIIa binds fibrinogen only weakly so as to allow uptake into α-granules [11]. Fibrinogen molecules possess two binding regions for GPIIb/IIIa and act as bivalent ligands, forming cross-bridges between activated platelets and leading to aggregation of activated platelets. In this way, GPIIb/IIIa mediates the so-called "final common pathway" of platelet aggregation, regardless of the stimulatory agent(s) [12]. The cytoplasmic domains of both IIb and IIIa play an important role in this "inside-out" signaling and also mediate "outside-in" signaling, whereby ligand binding to GPIIb/IIIa leads to cytoskeletal reorganization and other post-ligand binding events that amplify platelet activation [13,14]. This explains why therapeutic concentrations of GPIIb/IIIa antagonists inhibit platelet dense granule secretion and platelet procoagulant responses as well as platelet aggregation [15,16], although, through less well understood mechanisms, low concentrations of GPIIb/IIIa antagonists potentiate α-granule release and soluble CD40L release [17,18].

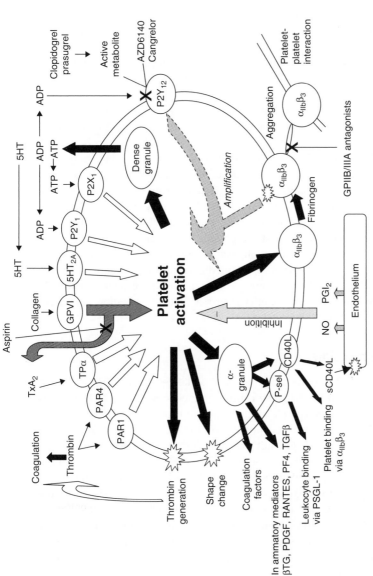

Fig. 1.1 Overview of platelet activation mechanisms and associated functional responses. Numerous agonists including thrombin, TXA$_2$, collagen, 5HT, ADP and ATP bind to platelet surface receptors to initiate platelet activation and subsequent activation of GPIIb/IIIa ($\alpha_{IIb}\beta_3$) mediates platelet aggregation. Collagen binding to GPVI induces TXA$_2$ formation and release. Dense granules release 5HT, ADP and ATP which amplify platelet activation, with activation of P2Y$_{12}$ by ADP playing a major role in amplification. α-Granule release promotes thrombus formation and associated inflammatory responses. Microparticle formation and assembly of tenase and prothrombinase on the platelet surface promote thrombin generation. Nitric oxide (NO) and prostacyclin (PGI$_2$) released by intact endothelium inhibit platelet activation. Adapted from Ref. [27] with permission.

Platelet adhesion and initiation of thrombus formation

The presence on the platelet surface of various receptors that bind to adhesive ligands underlies the ability of platelets to adhere to subendothelial components that are exposed upon injury and breaching of the vascular endothelium, a process that represents the first step in the hemostatic response of platelets [19]. Plasma von Willebrand factor (VWF) can bind to subendothelial components such as collagen, and platelets, via GPIbα in the GPIb-IX-V receptor complex, bind rapidly to immobilized VWF, providing a mechanism for platelet adhesion at high shear rates [19]. $\alpha_2\beta_1$ and GPVI play pivotal roles in the binding of platelets to collagen in the subendothelial matrix, with GPVI playing a dominant role in the subsequent activation of platelets by collagen [19,20]. Initially, weak adhesion is stabilized through integrin activation and binding of VWF to GPIIb/IIIa as well as collagen to $\alpha_2\beta_1$ [20]. Signaling through GPIb–IX–V, GPVI and GPIIb/IIIa leads to powerful activation of platelets and the release of soluble agonists via the following mechanisms: (1) release of dense granule contents containing the soluble agonists ADP, ATP and 5HT; (2) activation of phospholipase A_2 and the formation and release of thromboxane A_2; and (3) platelet procoagulant activity leading to generation of thrombin (Figure 1.1). These soluble agonists bind to platelet receptors that are linked to G proteins and mediate further platelet activation and recruitment of other platelets into platelet aggregates.

Platelet P2 receptors

There are three P2 receptor subtypes on the platelet surface, $P2X_1$, $P2Y_1$ and $P2Y_{12}$ [21]. $P2X_1$ is a ligand-gated cation channel activated by ATP and plays a role in platelet shape change and collagen-induced platelet activation [21]. $P2Y_1$ and $P2Y_{12}$ are G-protein coupled receptors activated by ADP. The $P2Y_1$ receptor is linked to Gq and initiates ADP-induced platelet activation, this activation being then sustained and amplified via $P2Y_{12}$, which is coupled to Gi [21–24]. $P2Y_{12}$ also plays a major role in sustaining and amplifying the responses to numerous agonists since other agonists induce dense granule release and ADP released from dense granules then binds to the P2Y receptors. In addition to sustaining and amplifying platelet aggregation, $P2Y_{12}$ activation amplifies granule secretion and platelet procoagulant activity [24–26]. This is the basis for the importance of $P2Y_{12}$ in platelet function and the growing therapeutic success of antagonists that target this receptor [27].

In a similar fashion to ADP's action via the $P2Y_{12}$ receptor, epinephrine (adrenaline) and norepinephrine (noradrenaline) can also amplify platelet activation via α_{2A} adrenergic receptors but the observation that this requires supraphysiological concentrations of epinephrine and norepinephrine renders the pathophysiological significance of this pathway uncertain [28].

Platelet protease-activated receptors (PARs) and thrombin

PAR1 and PAR4 are expressed on human platelets with PAR1 likely playing the more important role, since it is activated at low thrombin concentrations whereas PAR4 requires higher thrombin concentrations in order to contribute to thrombin-induced platelet responses [29]. Thrombin cleaves the N-terminal exodomain on the PARs leading to a tethered peptide ligand that activates the receptor, a process that can be mimicked by thrombin receptor-activating peptides or TRAPs [29]. Whereas the $P2Y_1$ receptor is linked only to Gq, PAR1 is linked to both Gq and G12/13 and mediates strong platelet activation as manifest by the extent of granule secretion and procoagulant activity induced by PAR1 activation [29–31]. $P2Y_{12}$ activation plays a key role in promoting these responses [24,26,32]. GPIbα may serve as a cofactor at the platelet surface, supporting PAR cleavage by thrombin [29,33]. The presence of PAR1 on other cell types involved in inflammatory responses provides a rationale for targeting this receptor in order to treat thrombotic diseases and associated inflammation [29].

The arachidonic acid pathway and thromboxane A_2

A group of phospholipases, collectively termed phospholipase A_2 (PLA_2), hydrolyse membrane phospholipids, such as phosphatidylcholine and phosphatidylserine, to produce arachidonic acid [34,35]. Arachidonic acid is rapidly converted by cyclooxygenase (COX) to prostaglandin G_2, which is then converted by peroxidase to prostaglandin H_2 (PGH_2) [34,36]. PGH_2 is then rapidly converted by thromboxane synthase to thromboxane A_2 (TXA_2). PGH_2 and TXA_2 are highly labile, potent platelet agonists that can diffuse across the plasma membrane and bind to specific G-protein coupled platelet receptors [30,34,37]. Studies of aspirin (acetylsalicylic acid), which acetylates and irreversibly inhibits COX, demonstrate the role of the arachidonic acid pathway in platelet responses to stimulation by different agonists. Aspirin abolishes platelet macroaggregation induced by arachidonic acid and substantially reduces platelet aggregation induced by low concentrations of collagen [38,39]. It also inhibits the "secondary wave" of macroaggregation induced by ADP, adrenaline and platelet-activating factor in citrated platelet-rich plasma but has little or no effect on platelet aggregation induced by these agonists in media containing physiological levels of divalent cations, indicating a restricted role for the arachidonic acid pathway in platelet activation under physiological conditions [24,40–43]. This explains why effective inhibition of COX by aspirin leaves many aspects of platelet function relatively intact.

Receptor pathways that inhibit platelet activation

The vascular endothelium presents an antithrombotic surface, in part related to the release by intact endothelium of nitric oxide (NO) and prostacyclin

(PGI$_2$), both of which act on platelet pathways that suppress platelet activation as well as having vasodilatory effects [44]. NO activates platelet guanylyl cyclase, raising platelet cyclic GMP levels and inhibiting agonist-induced rises in cytoplasmic calcium levels [45,46]. Platelet-derived NO also appears to limit thrombus formation and synthetic NO donors may have substantial antithrombotic effects [46,47]. Glutathione peroxidase potentiates inhibition of platelets by NO donors and inherited deficiency of the plasma isoform of this enzyme can lead to childhood ischemic stroke [46].

Endothelial COX-1 and prostaglandin G/H synthase-2 (PGHS-2; known as COX-2) mediate the production of PGI$_2$, which activates IP receptors on platelets and, via coupling to Gs, mediates an increase in platelet cyclic AMP, which in turn inhibits platelet activation [48,49]. The inhibition of these endothelial COX enzymes by traditional non-steroidal anti-inflammatory drugs (NSAIDs) and newer selective COX-2 inhibitors, and subsequent impairment of endothelial PGI$_2$ release, underlies the adverse cardiovascular effects of these drugs [49].

Another COX metabolite, PGE$_2$, has contradictory actions on platelets but, acting at low concentration via EP3 receptors, may enhance platelet responses by opposing increases in cyclic AMP [50]. It is suggested that release of PGE$_2$ from inflamed vessel wall, such as atherosclerotic plaque, may counteract the inhibitory effects of PGI$_2$ and contribute to arterial thrombosis [50,51].

Adenosine has an inhibitory effect on platelet function, acting via A$_{2A}$ receptors and increasing cyclic AMP levels [52]. It is proposed that plasma levels of adenosine increase sufficiently during ischemia or hypoxia to activate these receptors [52]. Adenosine and other A$_{2A}$ receptor agonists have antithrombotic effects in animal models of thrombosis [53]. The antiplatelet drug dipyridamole acts by inhibiting adenosine uptake by blood cells, thereby increasing exposure of platelets to adenosine, as well as by inhibiting platelet cyclic GMP-dependent phosphodiesterase [54].

Platelet procoagulant activity

In their resting state, platelets have asymmetric distribution of aminophospholipids in the surface membrane bilayer with enzymes acting to keep these aminophospholipids (predominantly phosphatidylserine and phosphatidylethanolamine) in the inner layer [55]. Platelet activation is associated with an increase in the cytoplasmic ionized calcium concentration that inhibits the activity of these enzymes and also activates the enzyme scramblase that causes redistribution of the aminophospholipids to the outer layer where they are able to support the assembly of tenase and prothrombinase complexes and subsequent generation of thrombin in plasma. Microparticles are also shed under the action of calpain and these also have procoagulant properties. These processes are triggered by platelet GPVI receptor binding to collagen and play an important role in thrombin generation and arterial thrombogenesis [56].

Thrombin-induced activation of platelets further promotes platelet procoagulant activity, and $P2Y_{12}$ receptor activation and GPIIb/IIIa receptor outside-in signaling play important roles in amplifying this process, such that antagonists of these receptors inhibit platelet procoagulant responses [16,24,32,57–59].

Inflammatory responses of platelets

α-Granule secretion consequent to platelet activation leads to a number of processes that are considered pro-inflammatory. CD40L and P-selectin are translocated to the platelet surface as a result of fusing of the α-granule membrane with the surface membrane and are then gradually shed into the surrounding medium in their soluble forms. Soluble CD40L (sCD40L) induces cytokine production in vascular cells and may play a role in atherogenesis and restenosis, as well as promoting thrombosis by stabilizing platelet aggregates [60,61]. P-selectin binds to its counter-receptor on leukocytes, PSGL-1, helping to recruit leukocytes and monocyte-derived microparticles into thrombus, and the ensuing cross-talk between platelets, leukocytes and the microparticles promotes thrombogenesis and inflammatory responses [62,63]. Release of the chemokine RANTES by platelets, in conjunction with P-selectin, supports the binding of monocytes to inflamed endothelium and contributes to intimal hyperplasia in murine models [64,65]. β-thromboglobulin, platelet-derived growth factor and platelet factor 4 are other platelet α-granule contents that also contribute to inflammatory responses [6].

Nucleotides released from platelet dense granules may also have pro-inflammatory effects: both ADP and ATP can activate leukocytes whilst ATP acts on P2X receptors on vascular smooth muscle cell (VSMC) and may contribute to VSMC proliferation and migration [66,67]. These nucleotides also act on endothelial cells to promote nitric oxide and prostacyclin release [66].

The role of the platelet in coronary atherothrombosis

Atherothrombosis refers to the process whereby progression of atherosclerosis leads to plaque rupture or erosion, which induces arterial thrombus formation and, in some instances, clinical sequelae such as coronary artery thrombosis causing acute coronary syndromes or sudden cardiac death [68,69]. Coronary arterial plaques that have a thin fibrous cap overlying a lipid-rich core and abundance of inflammatory cells are particularly prone to rupture and are termed "vulnerable" or "high-risk" plaques [68,70]. Exposure of collagen, vWF and fibronectin following endothelial disruption leads to platelet adhesion and activation, as described in the previous section but, furthermore, the exposed lipid-rich core of high-risk plaque is highly thrombogenic, containing abundant tissue factor that initiates the coagulation cascade culminating in thrombin formation, which then leads to platelet activation and fibrin deposition [68,69]. The central role of thrombin in the thrombosis that ensues following plaque disruption explains why anticoagulants such as heparins, direct thrombin inhibitors and factor Xa inhibitors have beneficial effects in the management of acute coronary syndromes [71–73] in addition to antiplatelet agents that target pathways that are involved in the platelet responses to thrombin and collagen, as described above. As well as exposure of tissue factor in the vessel wall, there is a circulating pool of tissue factor in blood that becomes concentrated at the site of vessel wall injury and contributes to thrombus formation [74]. Platelets, leukocytes and endothelial cells can express tissue factor, which may then be borne on circulating microparticles derived from these cells [75].

The formation of non-occlusive, platelet-rich thrombi over the sites of atherosclerotic plaque erosion or rupture with subsequent release of inflammatory mediators from platelet α-granules and platelet-leukocyte interactions may contribute to the progression of atherosclerotic lesions [76]. Such mural thrombi in coronary arteries may not be immediately associated with any clinical manifestations but instead contribute to the progressive narrowing of the arterial lumen that eventually leads to myocardial ischemia under conditions of increased myocardial oxygen demand and the associated symptom of angina pectoris. Platelets may also contribute to the vascular smooth muscle cell proliferation that leads to restenosis following percutaneous coronary intervention [77].

Conclusion

The rich variety of characteristics of platelets equips them for their role in hemostasis and physiological responses to vascular injury. Except in exceptional circumstances, it is only when the vessel wall becomes diseased that these physiological responses tend to be exaggerated and lead to thrombotic occlusion of the vessel lumen and excessive inflammation of the vessel wall. This explains why the platelet plays such an important role in the various manifestations of ischemic heart disease. Advances in the knowledge of platelet physiology have led to the development of antithrombotic therapies for managing ischemic heart disease and continue to inform the development of novel strategies.

References

1 White JG. Anatomy and structural organization of the platelet. In: Colman RW, Hirsh J, Marder VJ, Salzman EW, eds. *Hemostasis and Thrombosis: Basic Principles and Clinical Practice*, 3rd edn. J.B. Lippincott Company, Philadelphia, 1994: 397–413.

2 Chang Y, Bluteau D, Deb Il I N, Vainchenker W. From hemopoietic stem cells to platelets. *J Thromb Haemost* 2007; **5** (Suppl. 1): 318–327.

3 Deutsch VR, Tomer A. Megakaryocyte development and platelet production. *Br J Haematol* 2006; **134**: 453–466.

4 Rosado JA, Sage SO. A role for the actin cytoskeleton in the initiation and maintenance of store-mediated calcium entry in human platelets. *Trends Pharmacol Sci* 2000; **10**: 327–332.

5 Lind SE. Platelet morphology. In: Loscalzo J, Schafer AI, eds. *Thrombosis and Hemorrhage*. Blackwell Scientific Publications, Boston, 1994: 201–218.

6 Harrison P, Cramer EM. Platelet alpha-granules. *Blood Rev* 1993; **7**: 52–62.

7 McNicol A, Israels SJ. Platelet dense granules: structure, function and implications for haemostasis. *Thromb Res* 1999; **95**: 1–18.

8 White JG, Krumwiede M. Further studies of the secretory pathway in thrombin-stimulated human platelets. *Blood* 1987; **69**: 1196–1203.

9 Walsh PN. Platelet-coagulant protein interactions. In: Colman RW, Hirsh J, Marder VJ, Salzman EW, eds. *Hemostasis and Thrombosis: Basic Principles and Clinical Practice*, 3rd edn. J.B. Lippincott Company, Philadelphia 1994: 629–651.

10 Shattil SJ. Function and regulation of the B3 integrins in hemostasis and vascular biology. *Thromb Haemost* 1995; **74**: 149–155.

11 Clemetson KJ. Platelet activation: signal transduction via membrane receptors. *Thromb Haemost* 1995; **74**: 111–116.

12 Charo IF, Kieffer N, Phillips DR. Platelet membrane glycoproteins. In: Colman RW, Hirsh J, Marder VJ, Salzman EW, eds. *Hemostasis and Thrombosis: Basic Principles and Clinical Practice*, 3rd edn. Philadelphia: Lippincott Company 1994: 603–628.

13 Levy-Toledano S, Gallet C, Nadal F, Bryckaert M, Maclouf J, Rosa J-P. Phosphorylation and dephosphorylation mechanisms in platelet function: a tightly regulated balance. *Thromb Haemost* 1997; **78**: 226–233.

14 Shattil SJ, Gao J, Kashiwagi H. Not just another pretty face: regulation of platelet function at the cytoplasmic face of integrin $\alpha_{IIb}\beta_3$. *Thromb Haemost* 1997; **78**: 220–225.

15 Storey RF. The platelet $P2Y_{12}$ receptor as a therapeutic target in cardiovascular disease. *Platelets* 2001; **12**: 197–209.

16 Judge HM, Buckland RJ, Holgate CE, Storey RF. Glycoprotein IIb/IIIa and $P2Y_{12}$ receptor antagonists yield additive inhibition of platelet aggregation, granule secretion, soluble CD40L release and procoagulant responses. *Platelets* 2005; **16**: 398–407.

17 Schneider DJ, Taatjes DJ, Sobel BE. Paradoxical inhibition of fibrinogen binding and potentiation of alpha-granule release by specific types of inhibitors of glycoprotein IIb-IIIa. *Cardiovascular Research* 2000; **45**: 437–446.

18 Nannizzi-Alaimo L, Alves VL, Phillips DR. Inhibitory effects of glycoprotein IIb/IIIa antagonists and aspirin on the release of soluble CD40 ligand during platelet stimulation. *Circulation* 2003; **107**: 1123–1128.

19 Ruggeri ZM, Mendolicchio GL. Adhesion mechanisms in platelet function. *Circ Res* 2007; **100**: 1673–1685.

20 Watson SP, Auger JM, McCarty OJT, Pearce AC. GPVI and integrin $\alpha IIb\beta3$ signaling in platelets. *J Thromb Haemost* 2005; **3**: 1752–1762.

21 Hechler B, Cattaneo M, Gachet C. The P2 receptors in platelet function. *Sem Thromb Haemost* 2005; **31**: 150–161.

22 Jin J, Kunapuli SP. Coactivation of two different G protein-coupled receptors is essential for ADP-induced platelet aggregation. *Proc Natl Acad Sci USA* 1998; **95**: 8070–8074.

23 Hechler B, Leon C, Vial C, Vigne P, Frelin C, Cazenave JP, et al. The P2Y1 receptor is necessary for adenosine-5'-diphosphate-induced platelet aggregation. *Blood* 1998; **92**: 152–159.

24 Storey RF, Sanderson HM, White AE, May JA, Cameron KE, Heptinstall S. The central role of the P_{2T} receptor in amplification of human platelet activation, aggregation, secretion and procoagulant activity. *Br J Haematol* 2000; **110**: 925–934.

25 Cattaneo M, Lombardi R, Zighetti ML, Gachet C, Ohlmann P, Cazenave J-P, *et al.* Deficiency of (33P)2MeS-ADP binding sites on platelets with secretion defect, normal granule stores and normal thromboxane A2 production: evidence that ADP potentiates platelet secretion independently of the formation of large platelet aggregates and thromboxane A2 production. *Thromb Haemost* 1997; **77**: 986–990.

26 Trumel C, Payrastre B, Plantavid M, Hechler B, Vial C, Presek P, *et al.* A key role of adenosine diphosphate in the irreversible platelet aggregation induced by the PAR-1 activating peptide through the late activation of phosphoinositide 3-kinase. *Blood* 1999; **94**: 4156–4165.

27 Storey RF. Biology and pharmacology of the platelet $P2Y_{12}$ receptor. Curr Pharm Design 2006; **12**: 1255–1259.

28 Colman RW, Cook JJ, Niewiarowski S. Mechanisms of platelet aggregation. In: Colman RW, Hirsh J, Marder VJ, Salzman EW, eds. *Hemostasis and Thrombosis: Basic Principles and Clinical Practice*, 3rd edn. Lippincott Company, Philadelphia 1994: 508–523.

29 Coughlin SR. Protease-activated receptors in hemostasis, thrombosis and vascular biology. *J Thromb Haemost* 2005; **3**: 1800–1814.

30 Offermanns S, Laugwitz K, Spicher K, Schultz G. G Proteins of the G_{12} family are activated via thromboxane A_2 and thrombin receptors in human platelets. *Proc Natl Acad Sci* USA 1994; **91**: 504–508.

31 Offermanns S, Toombs CF, Hu Y-H, Simon MI. Defective platelet activation in $G\alpha_q$-deficient mice. *Nature* 1997; **389**: 183–186.

32 Dorsam RT, Tuluc M, Kunapuli SP. Role of protease-activated and ADP receptor subtypes in thrombin generation on human platelets. *J Thromb Haemost* 2004; **2**: 804–812.

33 Celikel R, McClintock RA, Roberts JR, Mendolicchio GL, Ware J, Varughese KI, *et al.* Modulation of alpha-thrombin function by distinct interactions with platelet glycoprotein Ibalpha. *Science* 2003; **301**: 218–221.

34 Moncada S, Vane JR. Arachidonic acid metabolites and the interactions between platelets and blood vessel walls. *New Engl J Med* 1979; **300**: 1142–1147.

35 Rittenhouse-Simmons S. Differential activation of platelet phospholipases by thrombin and ionophore A23187. *J Biol Chem* 1981; **256**: 4153–4155.

36 Lagarde M. Metabolism of fatty acids by platelets and the functions of various metabolites in mediating platelet function. *Prog Lipid Res* 1988; **27**: 135–152.

37 Brass LF, Hoxie JA, Manning DR. Signaling through G proteins and G protein-coupled receptors during platelet activation. *Thromb Haemost* 1993; **70**: 217–223.

38 Kuster LJ, Frolich JC. Platelet aggregation and thromboxane release induced by arachidonic acid, collagen, ADP and platelet-activating factor following low dose acetylsalicylic acid in man. *Prostaglandins* 1986; **32**: 415–423.

39 Berglund U, Wallentin L. Persistent inhibition of platelet function during long-term treatment with 75 mg acetylsalicylic acid daily in men with unstable coronary artery disease. *Eur Heart J* 1991; **12**: 428–433.

40 Heptinstall S, Mulley GP. Adenosine diphosphate-induced platelet aggregation and release reaction in heparinized platelet rich plasma and the influence of added citrate. *Br J Haematol* 1977; **36**: 565–571.

41 Heptinstall S, Taylor PM. The effects of citrate and extracellular calcium ions on the platelet release reaction induced by adenosine diphosphate and collagen. *Thromb Haemost* 1979; **42**: 778–793.

42 Lages B, Weiss HJ. Dependence of human platelet functional responses on divalent cations: aggregation and secretion in heparin- and hirudin-anticoagulated platelet-rich plasma and the effects of chelating agents. *Thromb Haemost* 1981; **45**: 173–179.

43 Packham MA, Bryant NL, Guccione MA, Kinlough-Rathbone RL, Mustard JF. Effect of concentration of Ca^{2+} in the suspending medium on the responses of human and rabbit platelets to aggregating agents. *Thromb Haemost* 1989; **62**: 968–976.

44 Cines DB, Pollak ES, Buck CA, Loscalzo J, Zimmerman GA, McEver RP, *et al.* Endothelial cells in physiology and in the pathophysiology of vascular disorders. *Blood* 1998; **91**: 3527–3561.

45 Mendelsohn ME, O'Neill S, George D, Loscalzo J. Inhibition of fibrinogen binding to human platelets by S-nitroso-N-acetylcysteine. *J Biol Chem* 1990; **265**: 19028–19034.

46 Loscalzo J. Nitric oxide insufficiency, platelet activation, and arterial thrombosis. *Circ Res* 2001; **88**: 756–762.

47 Vilahur G, Segales E, Salas E, Badimon L. Effects of a novel platelet nitric oxide donor (LA816), aspirin, clopidogrel, and combined therapy in inhibiting flow- and lesion-dependent thrombosis in the porcine ex vivo model. *Circulation* 2004; **110**: 1686–1693.

48 Boie Y, Rushmore TH, Darmon-Goodwin A, Grygorczyk R, Slipetz DM, Metters KM, *et al.* Cloning and expression of a cDNA for the human prostanoid IP receptor. *J Biol Chem* 1994; **269**: 12173–12178.

49 Grosser T, Fries S, FitzGerald GA. Biological basis for the cardiovascular consequences of COX-2 inhibition: therapeutic challenges and opportunities. *J Clin Invest* 2006; **116**: 4–15.

50 Fabre J-E, Nguyen M, Athirakul K, Coggins K, McNeish JD, Austin S, *et al.* Activation of the murine EP3 receptor for PGE2 inhibits cAMP production and promotes platelet aggregation. *J Clin Invest* 2001; **107**: 603–610.

51 Gross S, Tilly P, Hentsch D, Vonesch J-L, Fabre J-E. Vascular wall-produced prostaglandin E2 exacerbates arterial thrombosis and atherothrombosis through platelet EP3 receptors. *J Exp Med* 2007; **204**: 311–320.

52 Gessi S, Varani K, Merighi S, Ongini E, Borea PA. A2A adenosine receptors in human peripheral blood cells. *Br J Pharmacol* 2000; **129**: 2–11.

53 Linden MD, Barnard MR, Frelinger AL, Michelson AD, Przyklenk K. Effect of adenosine A2 receptor stimulation on platelet activation-aggregation: Differences between canine and human models. *Thromb Res* 2008; **121**: 689–698.

54 Schaper W. Dipyridamole, an underestimated vascular protective drug. *Cardiovasc Drug Ther* 2005; **19**: 357–363.

55 Solum NO. Procoagulant expression in platelets and defects leading to clinical disorders. *Arterioscler Thromb Vasc Biol* 1999; **19**: 2841–2846.

56 Siljander P, Farndale RW, Feijge MAH, Comfurius P, Kos S, Bevers EM, *et al.* Platelet adhesion enhances the glycoprotein VI-dependent procoagulant response: involvement of p38 MAP kinase and calpain. *Arterioscler Thromb Vasc Biol* 2001; **21**: 618–627.

57 Keularts IM, Beguin S, de Zwaan C, Hemker HC. Treatment with a GPIIb/IIIa antagonist inhibits thrombin generation in platelet rich plasma from patients. *Thromb Haemost* 1998; **80**: 370–371.

58 Ramstrom S, Ranby M, Lindahl TL. Effects of inhibition of P2Y$_1$ and P2Y$_{12}$ on whole blood clotting, coagulum elasticity and fibrinolysis resistance studied with free oscillation rheometry. *Thromb Res* 2003; **109**: 315–322.

59 Keuren JF, Wielders SJH, Ulrichts H, Hackeng T, Heemskerk JWM, Deckmyn H, *et al.* Synergistic effect of thrombin on collagen-induced platelet procoagulant activity is mediated through protease-activated receptor-1. *Arterioscler Thromb Vasc Biol* 2005; **25**: 1499–1505.

60 Henn V, Slupsky JR, Grafe M, Anagnostopoulos I, Forster R, Muller-Berghaus G, *et al.* CD40 ligand on activated platelets triggers an inflammatory reaction of endothelial cells. *Nature* 1998; **391**: 591–594.

61 Andre P, Nannizzi-Alaimo L, Prasad SK, Phillips DR. Platelet-derived CD40L: the switch-hitting player of cardiovascular disease. *Circulation* 2002; **106**: 896–899.

62 Furie B, Furie BC, Flaumenhaft R. A journey with platelet P-selectin: the molecular basis of granule secretion, signalling and cell adhesion. *Thromb Haemost* 2001; **86**: 214–221.

63 Andre P. P-selectin in haemostasis. *Br J Haematol* 2004; **126**: 298–306.

64 von Hundelshausen P, Weber KSC, Huo Y, Proudfoot AEI, Nelson PJ, Ley K, *et al.* RANTES deposition by platelets triggers monocyte arrest on inflamed and atherosclerotic endothelium. *Circulation* 2001; **103**: 1772–1777.

65 Schober A, Manka D, von Hundelshausen P, Huo Y, Hanrath P, Sarembock IJ, *et al.* Deposition of platelet RANTES triggering monocyte recruitment requires P-selectin and is involved in neointima formation after arterial injury. *Circulation* 2002; **106**: 1523–1529.

66 Kunapuli SP, Daniel JL. P2 receptor subtypes in the cardiovascular system. *Biochem J* 1998; **336**: 513–523.

67 Erlinge D. Extracellular ATP: a growth factor for vascular smooth muscle cells. *Gen Pharmacol* 1998; **31**: 1–8.

68 Viles-Gonzalez JF, Fuster V, Badimon JJ. Atherothrombosis: A widespread disease with unpredictable and life-threatening consequences. *Eur Heart J* 2004; **25**: 1197–1207.

69 Ruggeri ZM. Platelets in atherothrombosis. *Nature Medicine* 2002; **8**: 1227–1234.

70 Robbie L, Libby P. Inflammation and atherothrombosis. *Ann N Y Acad Sci* 2001; **947**: 167–180.

71 Wallentin L. Prevention of cardiovascular events after acute coronary syndrome. *Semin Vasc Med* 2005; **5**: 293–300.

72 Antman EM, Cohen M. Newer antithrombin agents in acute coronary syndromes. *Am Heart J* 1999; **138**: S563–569.

73 Oasis-6 Trial Group. Effects of fondaparinux on mortality and reinfarction in patients with acute ST-segment elevation myocardial infarction: The OASIS-6 randomized trial. *JAMA* 2006; **295**: 1519–1530.

74 Balasubramanian V, Grabowski E, Bini A, Nemerson Y. Platelets, circulating tissue factor, and fibrin colocalize in ex vivo thrombi: real-time fluorescence images of thrombus formation and propagation under defined flow conditions. *Blood* 2002; **100**: 2787–2792.

75 Mackman N, Tilley RE, Key NS. Role of the extrinsic pathway of blood coagulation in hemostasis and thrombosis. *Arterioscler Thromb Vasc Biol* 2007; **27**: 1687–1693.

76 Libby P. Changing concepts of atherogenesis. *J Int Med* 2000; **247**: 349–358.

77 Weber A-A, Schror K. The significance of platelet-derived growth factors for proliferation of vascular smooth muscle cells. *Platelets* 1999; **10**: 77–96.

Chapter 2

Laboratory assessment of platelet function and the effects of antiplatelet agents

Alan D. Michelson and A.L. Frelinger, III

Introduction

Because platelets have a central role in ischemic heart disease [1,2] (as discussed in detail in Chapter 1 of this book), antiplatelet therapy has been demonstrated to be beneficial in this clinical setting [3,4]. However, there is variability between patients in the response of their platelets to antiplatelet therapy [5]. There is therefore increasing interest in the use of platelet function tests to monitor the effects of antiplatelet drugs in ischemic heart disease, with the goal of guiding antiplatelet therapy to the optimal dose for prevention or treatment of thrombosis while minimizing hemorrhagic side effects [5]. These platelet function tests are frequently used for the measurement of "aspirin resistance" or "clopidogrel resistance" [5–7]. The clinical relevance of "resistance", also referred to as response variability, is discussed in detail in Chapters 4 and 6 of this book. The present chapter reviews the laboratory assessment of platelet function and the effects of antiplatelet agents. Tables 2.1–2.3 summarize laboratory methods that can potentially be used to guide the clinical use of antiplatelet drugs in ischemic heart disease.

The bleeding time

The bleeding time, the first test of platelet function, was developed in the early 1900s [8]. The basis of the test is the timed, platelet-dependent cessation of bleeding from a standardized *in vivo* wound. Although the bleeding time is therefore a physiologically relevant test, it has many disadvantages: non-specificity (e.g. affected by von Willebrand factor), insensitivity, high interoperator variability

Antiplatelet Therapy in Ischemic Heart Disease, 1st edition. Edited by Stephen D. Wiviott.
© 2009 American Heart Association, ISBN: 9-781-4051-7626-2

Table 2.1 Methods for the laboratory assessment of platelet function.

Test	Basis	Advantages	Disadvantages
Turbidometric aggregometry	Platelet aggregation	Historical gold standard	High sample volume Sample preparation Time consuming
Impedance aggregometry	Platelet aggregation	Whole blood assay	High sample volume Sample preparation Time consuming
VerifyNow®	Platelet aggregation	Simple, rapid Point-of-care (no pipetting required) Low sample volume Whole blood assay	Limited hematocrit & platelet count range
Plateletworks®	Platelet aggregation	Minimal sample preparation Whole blood assay	Not well studied
TEG® Platelet Mapping™ system	Platelet contribution to clot strength	Whole blood assay Clot information	Limited studies Requires pipetting
Impact® cone-and-plate(let) analyzer	Shear induced platelet adhesion	Simple, rapid Point-of-care Low sample volume No sample preparation Whole blood assay Shear-dependent	Instrument not widely available Requires pipeting

Assay	Principle	Features	Limitations
PFA-100®	*In vitro* cessation of high shear blood flow by platelet plug	Simple, rapid Point-of-care Low sample volume No sample preparation Whole blood assay Shear-dependent	Dependent on VWF & hematocrit Requires pipetting Does not correlate well with clopidogrel therapy
VASP phosphorylation state (flow cytometry)	Activation-dependent signaling	Dependent on thienopyridine target, $P2Y_{12}$ Low sample volume Whole blood assay Blood samples can be mailed at RT to core lab	Sample preparation Requires flow cytometer and experienced technician
Platelet surface P-selectin, activated GP IIb/IIIa, leukocyte-platelet aggregates (flow cytometry)	Activation-dependent changes in platelet surface	Low sample volume Whole blood assays Fixed samples can be mailed to core lab	Sample preparation Requires flow cytometer and experienced technician
Serum thromboxane B_2 (ELISA)	Activation-dependent release from platelets	Directly dependent on aspirin target, COX-1	Indirect measure Not platelet-specific
Urinary 11-dehydro thromboxane B_2/creatinine ratio	Stable urinary metabolite of thromboxane B_2	Directly dependent on aspirin target, COX-1	Indirect measure Not platelet-specific

Table 2.2 Platelet function tests for the monitoring of response to aspirin

Thromboxane as the end point:
- Serum thromboxane B_2
- Urinary 11-dehydro thromboxane B_2

Arachidonic acid as the stimulus:
- VerifyNow® Aspirin assay
- Platelet aggregation (turbidometric)
- Platelet aggregation (impedance)
- Platelet surface P-selectin, platelet surface activated GP IIb/IIIa, leukocyte-platelet aggregates (flow cytometry)
- Plateletworks®
- TEG® PlateletMapping system™
- Impact® cone and plate(let) analyzer

Other
- PFA-100®

Reproduced with permission from Michelson *et al. Eur Heart J* 2006; **8**: G53–G58[41].

Table 2.3 Platelet function tests for the monitoring of response to clopidogrel

P2Y$_{12}$ signaling-dependent
- Vasodilator stimulated phosphoprotein (VASP) phosphorylation state

ADP as the stimulus
- VerifyNow® P2Y$_{12}$ assay
- Platelet aggregation (turbidometric)
- Platelet aggregation (impedance)
- Platelet surface P-selectin, platelet surface activated GP IIb/IIIa, leukocyte-platelet aggregates (flow cytometry)
- Plateletworks®
- TEG® PlateletMapping™ system
- Impact® cone and plate(let) analyzer

Reproduced with permission from Michelson *et al. Eur Heart J* 2006; **8**: G53–G58[41].

and frequent scar formation [8]. The bleeding time is therefore no longer recommended as a clinical test of platelet function.

Platelet aggregometry

Although a number of other platelet function tests were developed subsequent to the bleeding time, platelet aggregometry, as described in 1962 by Born,

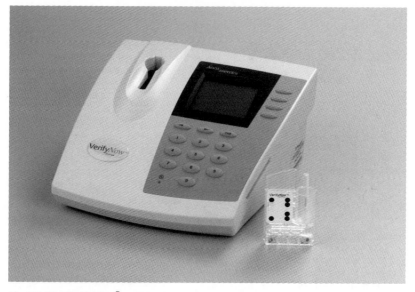

Fig. 2.1 The VerifyNow® system.

became the *de facto* "gold standard" [9]. In this test, platelet-to-platelet aggregation in response to an agonist is measured in platelet-rich plasma by turbidometry or, as described subsequently, in whole blood by electrical impedance. The fundamental advantage of platelet aggregometry is that it measures, albeit in an *in vitro* system, the most important function of platelets – their aggregation with each other in a glycoprotein (GP) IIb/IIIa (integrin αIIbβ3)-dependent manner.

Turbidometric platelet aggregation has been the platelet function test most often used in clinical trials. Several studies have reported that platelet aggregometry can predict major adverse cardiac events (MACE), although the number of MACE in all these studies was low [10–12]. There are major disadvantages to platelet aggregometry as a clinical test of platelet function, including high sample volume, requirement for sample preparation, length of assay time, requirement of a skilled technician and expense [9].

VerifyNow®

VerifyNow® (Accumetrics, San Diego, CA) (Figure 2.1), formerly known as the Ultegra rapid platelet function analyzer (RPFA), is a point-of-care test that is FDA-approved to measure the aspirin- or thienopyridine-induced defects in platelet function [13]. VerifyNow® uses the same principle, and therefore has the same fundamental advantage, as platelet aggregometry, that is it measures a key function of platelets – their aggregation with each other in a GP IIb/IIIa-dependent manner. Fibrinogen-coated beads are included in the VerifyNow®

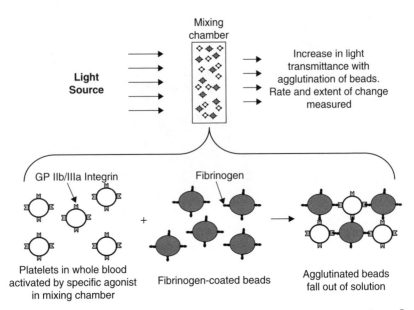

Mixing chamber

Light Source

Increase in light transmittance with agglutination of beads. Rate and extent of change measured

GP IIb/IIIa Integrin

Fibrinogen

+

Platelets in whole blood activated by specific agonist in mixing chamber

Fibrinogen-coated beads

Agglutinated beads fall out of solution

Fig. 2.2 Diagram representing how platelet function is determined with the VerifyNow® system. The mixing chamber contains a platelet agonist (thrombin receptor activating peptide [iso-TRAP], arachidonic acid or ADP) and fibrinogen-coated beads. After anticoagulated whole blood is added to the mixing chamber, the platelets become activated. The activated GP IIb/IIIa receptors on the platelets bind via the fibrinogen on the beads and cause agglutination of the platelets and the beads. Light transmittance through the chamber is measured and increases as the agglutinated platelets and beads fall out of solution. Direct pharmacologic blockade of GP IIb/IIIa receptors with a GP IIb/IIIa antagonist, or the prevention of their expression by the inhibition of arachidonic acid- or ADP-induced platelet activation, diminishes agglutination in proportion to the degree of platelet inhibition achieved.

system to augment the GP IIb/IIIa-dependent signal (Figure 2.2). There is a direct relationship between the results of testing with the VerifyNow® GP IIb/IIIa Assay and both platelet aggregometry and GP IIb/IIIa receptor occupancy [13]. Advantages of the VerifyNow® system include point-of-care, simplicity, rapidity (results in 5 min), low sample volume, no sample preparation (including no pipetting) and a whole blood system.

There are three currently-available VerifyNow® assays: the GP IIb/IIIa Assay (sensitive to GP IIb/IIIa antagonists), the Aspirin Assay (sensitive to aspirin), and the $P2Y_{12}$ Assay (sensitive to thienopyridines) [13]. In the VerifyNow® Aspirin Assay, arachidonic acid is used as the agonist. This assay is aspirin-specific because arachidonic acid-induced platelet aggregation requires the activity of COX-1 – which is specifically blocked by aspirin [4]. In the Verify Now® $P2Y_{12}$ Assay, adenosine diphosphate (ADP) is used as the agonist. ADP

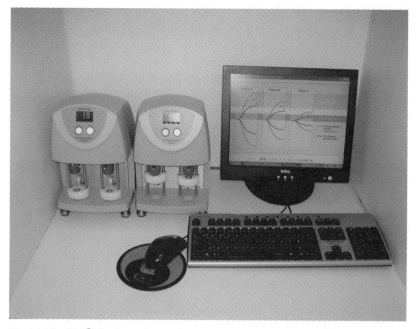

Fig. 2.3 The TEG® PlateletMapping™ system.

stimulates platelet aggregation via its two platelet receptors: $P2Y_1$ and $P2Y_{12}$ [14]. While the agonist utilized in the VerifyNow® $P2Y_{12}$ Assay is ADP 20μM, a second agent, prostaglandin E_1 (PGE_1) 22nM is also added in order to suppress intracellular free calcium levels and thereby to reduce the platelet activation contribution from ADP binding to its $P2Y_1$ receptor.

A lower level of platelet inhibition, as determined by VerifyNow® GP IIb/IIIa Assay, is associated with the incidence of MACE in patients treated with a GP IIb/IIIa antagonist (abciximab) [15]. In aspirin-treated patients before percutaneous coronary intervention (PCI), the level of platelet function (or "aspirin resistance"), as determined by the VerifyNow® Aspirin Assay, is associated with the incidence of post-PCI myonecrosis [16].

TEG® PlateletMapping System™

The thromboelastograph (TEG) was invented more than 50 years ago, but has recently been updated as the TEG® PlateletMapping™ System (Haemoscope, Niles, IL) (Figure 2.3). As blood clots in a rotating sample cup, the cup motion is transmitted by the strengthening clot to a suspended pin. In the PlateletMapping™ System, a weak clot is generated in heparinized blood by the addition of reptilase and factor XIII. By adding a platelet agonist (arachidonic acid or ADP) the clot strength is greatly enhanced, allowing this test to be sensitive to inhibition of platelet function [17]. Advantages of the TEG® PlateletMapping™ system include that it is a point-of-care (although, unlike the VerifyNow® device, pipetting is required), whole blood assay that also provides information on clot formation and clot lysis. Although small studies suggest that results of the TEG® PlateletMapping™ system are associated with MACE [18], additional studies need to be performed to determine its possible role in monitoring antiplatelet therapy.

Impact® cone and plate(let) analyzer

In the Impact® cone and plate(let) analyzer (Diamed, Cressier, Switzerland) (Figure 2.4), whole blood is exposed to uniform shear by the spinning of a

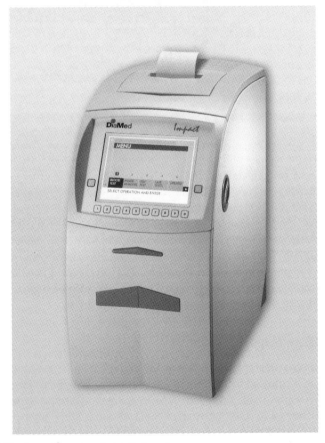

Fig. 2.4 The Impact® cone and plate(let) analyzer.

cone in a standardized cup [19]. After automated staining, platelet adhesion to the cup is evaluated by image analysis software. Advantages of the Impact® include: point-of-care (although, unlike the VerifyNow® device, pipetting of the blood sample is required), simplicity, rapidity, low sample volume, physiologically relevant high shear, and a whole blood system. The assay has been used to monitor GP IIb/IIIa antagonist therapy. The *ex vivo* addition of arachidonic acid or ADP enable the Impact to be used to monitor aspirin or thienopyridines, respectively [19]. However, additional studies need to be performed to determine the possible role of the Impact® in the monitoring of antiplatelet therapy.

PFA-100®

The platelet function analyzer 100 (PFA-100® assay, Dade Behring, Newark, DE) (Figure 2.5) draws an anticoagulated blood sample under high shear conditions through a 150 μm diameter, collagen-coated aperture in the presence of ADP or epinephrine [20]. The time taken for a clot to occlude the aperture is reported as the closure time (CT). Advantages of the PFA-100® include simplicity, rapidity, low sample volume, physiologically relevant high shear, no sample preparation (although pipetting of the blood sample is required) and a whole blood system.

The PFA-100® CT may be an independent predictor of the extent of myocardial damage in ST-elevation myocardial infarction (MI), as measured by markers of myonecrosis, and may help in the risk stratification of these patients [21]. In patients undergoing PCI, baseline platelet reactivity, as measured by the PFA-100® CT, predicts the angiographic success of the procedure, the degree of ST-segment resolution, the extent of myocardial necrosis, and the

One	Two	Three
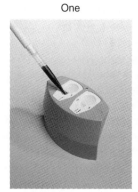	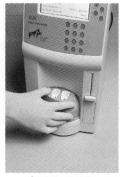	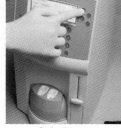
Pipet 800 μl blood	*Insert cassette*	*Start the test*

Fig. 2.5 The PFA-100®.

short- and mid-term clinical outcomes [22]. In patients with stable angina, the PFA-100® CT may help to predict the presence or absence of coronary artery stenoses at angiography [23].

The PFA-100® collagen–epinephrine CT is associated with the stability of coronary artery disease, and may reflect plaque instability, an ongoing thrombotic state and/or reduced responsiveness to aspirin [24]. Although it is conceptually less specific for aspirin resistance than the other assays listed in Table 2.2 (all of which are directly dependent on the aspirin-sensitive arachidonic acid/COX-1/thromboxane A_2 metabolic pathway), the PFA-100® has been widely used in clinical studies of aspirin resistance [20]. Furthermore, aspirin non-responder status in patients with recurrent cerebral ischemic attacks has been reported to predict MACE [25]. The PFA-100® has also been used to monitor GP IIb/IIIa antagonists, and failure to observe non-closure in the PFA-100® may be associated with an increased incidence of subsequent MACE [26]. However, the PFA-100® is not recommended for monitoring clopidogrel therapy [20,27].

Whole blood flow cytometry

As in the VerifyNow® $P2Y_{12}$ Assay, the combination of ADP and PGE_1 is used in the flow cytometric-based VASP assay (BioCytex, Marseilles, France) (Figure 2.6) [28]. Under these conditions, the phosphorylation of VASP (identified by a monoclonal antibody specific for the phosphorylated form of VASP) is directly proportional to the degree of inhibition of the $P2Y_{12}$ receptor [29]. The major advantage of the VASP assay is its direct dependence on the target of thienopyridines, the $P2Y_{12}$ receptor (Figure 2.6). Comparison of the VASP assay with ADP-induced turbidometric platelet aggregation demonstrated that the level of thienopyridine-induced inhibition is higher in the VASP assay, presumably because platelet aggregation can still occur via ADP stimulation of $P2Y_1$ in the presence of a thienopyridine [28]. Patients with a poorer platelet response to clopidogrel, as determined by the VASP assay, have been reported to have a higher incidence of subacute stent thrombosis [30].

Platelet surface P-selectin and/or the activated conformation of platelet surface GP IIb/IIIa (reported by monoclonal antibody PAC1) can also be measured by whole blood flow cytometry [31]. Flow cytometric analysis of platelet activation markers before PCI can predict an increased risk of acute and subacute ischemic events after PCI [32–35]. Circulating leukocyte–platelet aggregates (Figure 2.7), especially monocyte–platelet aggregates, are a particularly sensitive marker of *in vivo* platelet activation [36]. Circulating leukocyte–platelet aggregates, as measured by whole blood flow cytometry, increase after PCI [36] with a greater magnitude in patients experiencing late clinical events [37]. Furthermore, circulating monocyte–platelet aggregates are an early marker of acute MI [38].

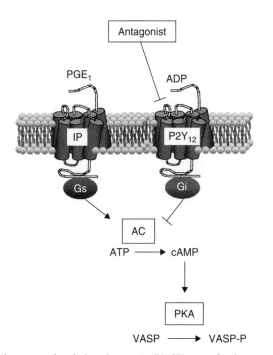

Fig. 2.6 Vasodilator-stimulated phosphoprotein (VASP) assay for the measurement of $P2Y_{12}$ antagonism. Prostaglandin E_1 (PGE_1) binds to its IP receptor on the platelet surface and signals through a G stimulatory (Gs) protein and adenylyl cyclase (AC) to convert ATP to cyclic AMP (cAMP), and then through protein kinase A (PKA) to convert VASP to phosphorylated VASP (VASP-P). ADP binds to its $P2Y_{12}$ receptor on the platelet surface and signals through a G inhibitory (Gi) protein to inhibit PGE_1-induced signaling through AC. $P2Y_{12}$ antagonists, for example the active metabolite of clopidogrel, inhibit this ADP-induced effect. Therefore, in the presence of both PGE_1 and ADP, VASP-P is directly proportional to the degree of $P2Y_{12}$ antagonism. VASP-P is measured by whole blood flow cytometry, using permeabilization and a monoclonal antibody specific for the phosphorylated form of VASP. Figure modified from Ref. [40].

Whole blood flow cytometry has a number of advantages as a test of platelet function [31,39]. Platelets are analyzed in their physiological milieu of whole blood and only tiny volumes of blood are required. Whole blood flow cytometry has particular advantages in clinical trials. Samples can be simply prepared at a local site with no required expertise, and then mailed to a core laboratory. The local site does not need access to an aggregometer or other platelet function analyzer or local expertise. This may result in better quality control, because all assays are performed in a single, experienced core laboratory. For the VASP assay, citrated whole blood can be mailed at room temperature and the sample is stable for 72h before analysis at the core laboratory.

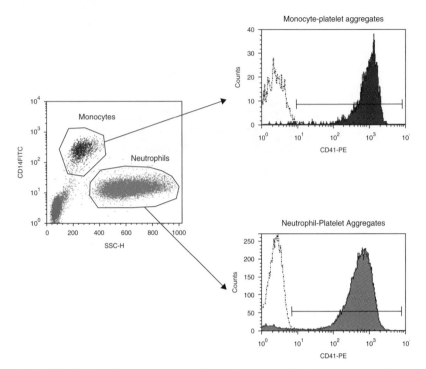

Fig. 2.7 Whole blood flow cytometric analysis of monocyte–platelet aggregates and neutrophil–platelet aggregates after activation with thrombin receptor activating peptide (TRAP) 20 μM. Monocytes (light grey) and neutrophils (dark grey) were identified by their characteristic light scatter properties and the binding of FITC-conjugated CD14-specific monoclonal antibody TUK4 (left panel). Platelet-positive monocytes (i.e. monocyte–platelet aggregates) were identified by the binding of the phycoerythrin (PE)-conjugated αIIb (CD41)-specific monoclonal antibody 5B12 in the monocyte region (upper right panel). Platelet-positive neutrophils (i.e. neutrophil–platelet aggregates) were identified by the binding of the PE-conjugated αIIb (CD41)-specific monoclonal antibody 5B12 in the neutrophil region (lower right panel). SSC-H, side scatter height. Reproduced from Ref. [31] with permission.

For analysis of leukocyte–platelet aggregates, citrated, fixed whole blood can be mailed on ice and the sample is stable for 72 h before analysis at the core laboratory.

Summary

Because of the variability between patients in the response of their platelets to antiplatelet therapy, there is increasing interest in the use of platelet function tests to monitor the effects of antiplatelet drugs, with the ultimate goal of guiding antiplatelet therapy to the optimal dose for the prevention or treatment of thrombosis while minimizing hemorrhagic side effects. Aspirin "resistance" or response variability can be assessed by assays that use thromboxane as the end point or arachidonic acid as the stimulus (Table 2.2). Thienopyridine "resistance" or response variability can be assessed by a $P2Y_{12}$ signaling-dependent assay (VASP phosphorylation state) or by using ADP as the stimulus (although ADP activates platelets via two receptors, $P2Y_1$ and $P2Y_{12}$, only the latter is blocked by thienopyridines [40]) (Table 2.3).

Turbidometric platelet aggregation remains the gold standard platelet function test, in part because most large clinical trials of antiplatelet agents have used this end point. However, turbidometric platelet aggregation has many disadvantages, for example expense and the requirements for a high sample volume, a skilled technician and sample preparation. Whole blood flow cytometry has particular advantages in clinical trials because samples can be simply prepared at a local site (with no required expertise and without the need for a platelet aggregometer or other platelet function analyzer at the local site), and then mailed to a core laboratory with good quality control.

True point-of-care assays, e.g. VerifyNow®, overcome the disadvantages of turbidometric platelet aggregation and show great promise for clinical utility in patients with coronary artery disease who are treated with antiplatelet agents. In patients treated with antiplatelet drugs, the degree of platelet inhibition, as determined by VerifyNow® and several other new platelet function assays, has been shown to predict MACE.[5;41] Nevertheless, no published studies address the clinical effectiveness of altering therapy based on a laboratory finding of aspirin or clopidogrel "resistance" or hyporesponsiveness.[6;41]

References

1 Michelson AD. *Platelets*, 2nd edn. Elsevier/Academic Press, San Diego, 2007.
2 Ruggeri ZM. Platelets in atherothrombosis. *Nature Medicine* 2002; **8**: 1227–1234.
3 Antithrombotic Trialists' Collaboration. Collaborative meta-analysis of randomised trials of antiplatelet therapy for prevention of death, myocardial infarction, and stroke in high risk patients. *BMJ* 2002; **324**: 71–86.
4 Patrono C, Coller B, FitzGerald GA, Hirsh J, Roth G. Platelet-active drugs: the relationships among dose, effectiveness, and side effects. *Chest* 2004; **126**: 234S–264S.
5 Michelson AD. Platelet function testing in cardiovascular diseases. *Circulation* 2004; **110**: e489–e493.
6 Michelson AD, Cattaneo M, Eikelboom JW *et al.* Aspirin resistance: position paper of the Working Group on Aspirin Resistance. *J Thromb Haemost* 2005; **3**:1309–1311.
7 Cattaneo M. Aspirin and clopidogrel: efficacy, safety and the issue of drug resistance. *Arterioscler Thromb Vasc Biol* 2004; **24**: 1980–1987.
8 Lind SE, Kurkjian CD. The bleeding time. In: Michelson AD, ed. *Platelets*, 2nd edn. Elsevier/Academic Press, San Diego, 2007; 485–493.

9 Jennings LK, White MM. Platelet aggregation. In: Michelson AD, ed. *Platelets*, 2nd edn. Elsevier/Academic Press, San Diego, 2007: 495–508.

10 Gum PA, Kottke-Marchant K, Welsh PA, White J, Topol EJ. A prospective, blinded determination of the natural history of aspirin resistance among stable patients with cardiovascular disease. *J Am Coll Cardiol* 2003; **41**: 961–965.

11 Mueller MR, Salat A, Stangl P *et al.* Variable platelet response to low-dose ASA and the risk of limb deterioration in patients submitted to peripheral arterial angioplasty. *Thromb Haemost* 1997; **78**: 1003–1007.

12 Matetzky S, Shenkman B, Guetta V *et al.* Clopidogrel resistance is associated with increased risk of recurrent atherothrombotic events in patients with acute myocardial infarction. *Circulation* 2004; **109**: 3171–3175.

13 Steinhubl SR. The Verify Now system. In: Michelson AD, ed. *Platelets*, 2nd edn. Elsevier/Academic Press, San Diego, 2007; 509–518.

14 Cattaneo M. The platelet P2 receptors. In: Michelson AD, ed. *Platelets*, 2nd edn. Elsevier/Academic Press, San Diego, 2007; 201–220.

15 Steinhubl SR, Talley JD, Braden GA *et al.* Point-of-care measured platelet inhibition correlates with a reduced risk of an adverse cardiac event after percutaneous coronary intervention: results of the GOLD (AU-Assessing Ultegra) multicenter study. *Circulation* 2001; **103**: 2572–2578.

16 Chen WH, Lee PY, Ng W, Tse HF, Lau CP. Aspirin resistance is associated with a high incidence of myonecrosis after non-urgent percutaneous coronary intervention despite clopidogrel pretreatment. *J Am Coll Cardiol* 2004; **43**: 1122–1126.

17 Harrison P, Keeling D. Clinical tests of platelet function. In: Michelson AD, ed. *Platelets*, 2nd edn. Elsevier/Academic Press, San Diego, 2007; 445–474.

18 Bliden KP, DiChiara J, Tantry US *et al.* Increased risk in patients with high platelet aggregation receiving chronic clopidogrel therapy undergoing percutaneous coronary intervention: is the current antiplatelet therapy adequate? *J Am Coll Cardiol* 2007; **49**: 657–666.

19 Varon D, Savion N. Impact cone and plate(let) analyzer. In: Michelson AD, ed. *Platelets*, 2nd edn. Elsevier/Academic Press, San Diego, 2007; 535–544.

20 Francis JL. The platelet function analyzer (PFA)-100. In: Michelson AD, ed. *Platelets*, 2nd edn. Elsevier/Academic Press, San Diego, 2007; 519–534.

21 Frossard M, Fuchs I, Leitner JM *et al.* Platelet function predicts myocardial damage in patients with acute myocardial infarction. *Circulation* 2004; **110**: 1392–1397.

22 Campo G, Valgimigli M, Gemmati D *et al.* Value of platelet reactivity in predicting response to treatment and clinical outcome in patients undergoing primary coronary intervention: insights into the STRATEGY Study. *J Am Coll Cardiol* 2006; **48**: 2178–2185.

23 Lanza GA, Sestito A, Iacovella S *et al.* Relation between platelet response to exercise and coronary angiographic findings in patients with effort angina. *Circulation* 2003; **107**: 1378–1382.

24 Linden MD, Furman MI, Frelinger III AL *et al.* Indices of platelet activation and the stability of coronary artery disease. *J Thromb Haemost* 2007; **5**: 761–765.

25 Grundmann K, Jaschonek K, Kleine B, Dichgans J, Topka H. Aspirin non-responder status in patients with recurrent cerebral ischemic attacks. *J Neurol* 2003; **250**: 63–66.

26 Madan M, Berkowitz SD, Christie DJ *et al.* Determination of platelet aggregation inhibition during percutaneous coronary intervention with the platelet function analyzer PFA-100. *Am Heart J* 2002; **144**: 151–158.

27 Hayward CP, Harrison P, Cattaneo M *et al.* Platelet function analyzer (PFA)-100 closure time in the evaluation of platelet disorders and platelet function. *J Thromb Haemost* 2006; **4**: 312–319.

28 Aleil B, Ravanat C, Cazenave JP *et al.* Flow cytometric analysis of intraplatelet VASP phosphorylation for the detection of clopidogrel resistance in patients with ischemic cardiovascular diseases. *J Thromb Haemost* 2005; **3**: 85–92.

29 Schwarz UR, Geiger J, Walter U, Eigenthaler M. Flow cytometry analysis of intracellular VASP phosphorylation for the assessment of activating and inhibitory signal transduction pathways in human platelets – definition and detection of ticlopidine/clopidogrel effects. *Thromb Haemost* 1999; **82**: 1145–1152.

30 Gurbel PA, Bliden KP, Samara W *et al.* Clopidogrel effect on platelet reactivity in patients with stent thrombosis. Results of the CREST study. *J Am Coll Cardiol* 2005; **46**: 1827–1832.

31 Michelson AD, Linden MD, Barnard MR, Furman MI, Frelinger AL, III. Flow cytometry. In: Michelson AD, ed. *Platelets*, 2nd edn. Elsevier/Academic Press, San Diego, 2007: 545–564.

32 Tschoepe D, Schultheiss HP, Kolarov P *et al.* Platelet membrane activation markers are predictive for increased risk of acute ischemic events after PTCA. *Circulation* 1993; **88**: 37–42.

33 Gawaz M, Neumann FJ, Ott I *et al.* Role of activation-dependent platelet membrane glycoproteins in development of subacute occlusive coronary stent thrombosis. *Coron Artery Dis* 1997; **8**: 121–128.

34 Kabbani SS, Watkins MW, Ashikaga T *et al.* Platelet reactivity characterized prospectively: a determinant of outcome 90 days after percutaneous coronary intervention. *Circulation* 2001; **104**: 181–186.

35 Kabbani SS, Watkins MW, Ashikaga T *et al.* Usefulness of platelet reactivity before percutaneous coronary intervention in determining cardiac risk one year later. *Am J Cardiol* 2003; **91**: 876–878.

36 Michelson AD, Barnard MR, Krueger LA, Valeri CR, Furman MI. Circulating monocyte-platelet aggregates are a more sensitive marker of in vivo platelet activation than platelet surface P-selectin: studies in baboons, human coronary intervention, and human acute myocardial infarction. *Circulation* 2001; **104**: 1533–1537.

37 Mickelson JK, Lakkis NM, Villarreal-Levy G, Hughes BJ, Smith CW. Leukocyte activation with platelet adhesion after coronary angioplasty: a mechanism for recurrent disease? *J Am Coll Cardiol* 1996; **28**: 345–353.

38 Furman MI, Barnard MR, Krueger LA *et al.* Circulating monocyte-platelet aggregates are an early marker of acute myocardial infarction. *J Am Coll Cardiol* 2001; **38**: 1002–1006.

39 Michelson AD. Flow cytometry: a clinical test of platelet function. *Blood* 1996; **87**: 4925–4936.

40 Cattaneo M. ADP receptor antagonists. In: Michelson AD, ed. *Platelets*, 2nd edn. Elsevier/Academic Press, San Diego, 2007; 1127–1144.

41. Michelson AD, Frelinger AL, Furman MI. Resistance to antiplatelet drugs. *Eur Heart J* 2006; **8**: G53–G58.

PART II

Pharmacology of Oral Antiplatelet Agents

Chapter 3

Cyclooxygenase inhibitors

Nina Chetty Raju and John W. Eikelboom

Introduction

The first cyclooxygenase (COX) inhibitor, acetyl salicylic acid (ASA), is widely used, inexpensive, and highly effective for the treatment of patients with cardiovascular disease, reducing the risk of vascular death by about 15% and serious non-fatal vascular events by about 30% during long-term therapy [1]. More recently introduced COX inhibitors are used primarily for their anti-inflammatory effects and some may paradoxically increase the risk of cardiovascular events [2,3].

This chapter reviews the pharmacology of COX inhibitors. We focus primarily on ASA, which is the prototype COX inhibitor and the single most widely used pharmaceutical agent worldwide.

Historical development of COX inhibitors

We salute the future, but we honour the past on which the future rests

Lester B Pearson

Scientists have long recognized that plants containing salicylic acid have medicinal properties. One of the world's oldest preserved medical texts, the Ebers Papyrus, described the analgesic properties of dried myrtle leaves in 1500 BC [4,5]. Salicylate in the form of willow bark was used as an analgesic during the time of Hippocrates [4,6,7]. Johann Buchner isolated salicylic acid as the active ingredient of willow bark in 1828 [4], and in 1897 Felix Hoffman with the Bayer Company in Germany synthesized the acetylated form of salicylic acid to treat his father who could not tolerate the gastric irritation associated with salicylic acid [4,5]. With this development, the trademark name "Aspirin" was born and over-the-counter sales of aspirin followed 12 years later. However, it was not until the 1960s that ASA was demonstrated to prolong the bleeding time and inhibit platelet aggregation [8]. In 1971 Sir John Vane described the effect of ASA and non-steroidal anti-inflammatory drugs (NSAIDs) on inhibiting prostaglandin synthesis [9]. Subsequently, the

Antiplatelet Therapy in Ischemic Heart Disease, 1st edition. Edited by Stephen D. Wiviott.
© 2009 American Heart Association, ISBN: 9-781-4051-7626-2

crystal structure of COX was elucidated [10] and the structural basis of ASA [11] and NSAID [12] inhibition of COX was described.

COX physiology

The molecular biology, structure, function and tissue expression of the two major COX isoforms are summarized in Table 3.1.

Structure

The two main COX isoforms, COX-1 and COX-2, have a 63% homology in their amino acid sequence [13]. The enzyme consists of three independent folding units, namely an epidermal growth factor-like domain, a membrane-binding motif and an enzymatic domain [10]. It integrates into a single layer of the lipid membrane bilayer with the active site at the apex of

Table 3.1 Comparison of the two isoforms of cyclooxygenase (adapted with permission from Ref. [28])

Property	COX-1 (PGH$_2$ synthase 1)	COX-2 (PGH$_2$ synthase 2)
Molecular mass	72 kDa (599 amino acids)	72 kDa (604 amino acids)
Chromosome	9	1
DNA	22 kb	8.3 kb
mRNA	2.8 kb	4.5 kb
Regulation	Predominantly constitutive (most tissues) but can be induced 2–4 × by hormones, growth factors and inflammation	Predominantly inducible 10–20 × (by bacterial lipopolysaccharides, phorbol esters, cytokines, growth factors, laminar shear stress)
		Constitutive in some organs (brain, kidney, testes, tracheal epithelium, bones, female reproductive system)
ASA binding site in humans	Serine 529	Serine 516
		Larger active site

a long hydrophobic channel [10]. The active site of COX-2 is larger and more accommodating than the COX-1 active site [14].

Function and tissue expression

COX plays a key role in arachidonic acid (AA) metabolism. AA is released from the cell membrane phospholipids by phospholipase A_2 in response to chemical, mechanical, hormonal, infectious, inflammatory and mitogenic stimuli [15,16]. COX oxidizes AA to form prostaglandin (PG)G_2 and PGH_2. PGH_2 is further catalyzed by specific synthases to form the prostaglandins, D_2, E_2, $F_{2\alpha}$ and I_2 (prostacyclin) and thromboxane A_2 (TXA_2) [7,17,18] (Figure 3.1), all of which mediate specific cellular functions (Table 3.2).

COX-1 (also referred to as prostaglandin H synthase 1) is constitutively expressed in most cells and has a primary "housekeeping" function, resulting in the production of homeostatic prostanoids that are responsible for normal cell function, including gastric protection and platelet function [7].

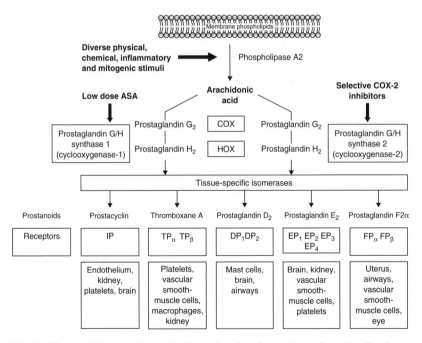

Fig. 3.1 The arachidonic acid cascade. Reproduced with permission from *New Eng J Med* [15].

COX-2 (PGH synthase 2) is upregulated in response to inflammatory stimuli and growth factors, resulting in the production of prostanoids that are involved in the response to tissue injury [19] (Table 3.2). Newly budded platelets express both isoforms of the COX enzyme but mature platelets express only COX-1 [17,20]. Vascular endothelial cells express both isoforms of COX.

Platelets process PGH_2 to form TXA_2, which interacts with its membrane receptor to activate platelets, resulting in irreversible platelet aggregation.

Table 3.2 The location and function of the various prostanoids

Prostanoid	Receptor	Site of concentration of receptor	Function(s) of prostanoid
Thromboxane A_2	$TP\alpha$ $TP\beta$	Platelets, vascular smooth muscle cells, macrophages, kidney	Promote platelet aggregation, vasoconstriction, proliferation of smooth muscle cells, pro-atherogenic
Prostacyclin	IP	Platelets, renal cortex, endothelium, brain	Inhibit platelet aggregation, vasodilatation, inhibit vascular smooth muscle proliferation, antiatherogenic
Prostaglandin E_2	EP_1, EP_2, EP_3, EP_4	Platelets, vascular smooth muscle cells, renal medulla, brain, gastric mucosa, osteoblasts, seminal vesicles, fetal membranes, uterus	Salt and water excretion, gastric cytoprotection, bone formation and resorption, parturition, labor, menstruation, fertilization, ovulation, etc.
Prostaglandin D_2	DP_1, DP_2	Brain, airways, mast cells	Pulmonary vasoconstriction
Prostaglandin $F_{2\alpha}$	$FP\alpha$ $FP\beta$	Vascular smooth muscle cells, airways, eye, fetal membranes, uterus	Pulmonary vasoconstriction, parturition, labor, menstruation

TXA$_2$ also causes potent vasoconstriction and proliferation of vascular smooth muscle cells [21]. The vascular endothelium processes PGH$_2$ to form prostacyclin, which inhibits platelet aggregation and the proliferation of vascular smooth muscle cells, causes vasodilatation, protects the myocardium against oxidant stress and is antiatherogenic [21]. Prostacyclin is the most potent inhibitor of platelet aggregation *in vivo* [16].

COX variants
Several variants of cyclooxygenase 1 (COX-3, PCOX-1a, PCOX-1b) have recently been characterized [22,23]. COX-3 is sensitive to inhibition by paracetamol [23].

COX inhibitors

COX inhibitors are a heterogeneous group of drugs that inhibit COX with varying selectivity and reversibility. They can be classified into four main groups:
1 ASA, an irreversible inhibitor of COX that primarily inhibits COX-1 at low doses and inhibits both COX-1 and COX-2 at higher doses.
2 Traditional (non-COX selective) NSAIDs, which reversibly inhibit both COX-1 and COX-2 to varying degrees.
3 Selective COX-2 inhibitors, developed specifically to avoid the COX-2 mediated adverse gastric effects of traditional NSAIDs whilst retaining potent anti-inflammatory effects.
4 Other COX inhibitors.

Acetyl salicylic acid
Structure
Salicylic acid consists of carboxylic acid (benzene ring with one organic acid group) with an alcohol group on the para position of the benzene ring. This undergoes acetylation to produce ASA (Figure 3.2).

Pharmacokinetics
Acetyl salicylic acid is available as several formulations including uncoated or soluble ASA, enteric-coated ASA, soluble granules and a sustained-release microencapsulated form [24].

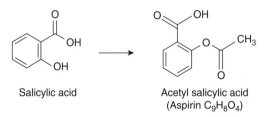

Salicylic acid　　　　　Acetyl salicylic acid
　　　　　　　　　　　(Aspirin C$_9$H$_8$O$_4$)

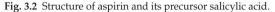

Fig. 3.2 Structure of aspirin and its precursor salicylic acid.

Following oral ingestion, ASA is absorbed by passive diffusion in the stomach and proximal small bowel. ASA can also be absorbed through the skin and rectal mucosa. Soluble ASA achieves peak plasma levels within 30 to 40 minutes of oral ingestion while enteric-coated ASA does not reach peak levels until 3–4 hours after oral ingestion [21]. If an immediate antiplatelet effect is required, soluble ASA should be used or the enteric-coated ASA preparation should be chewed [21].

The oral bioavailability of soluble ASA is 40–50% and that of enteric-coated ASA is lower [21,25]. Drug concentrations in the portal circulation are much higher than in the systemic circulation because ASA undergoes extensive first-pass metabolism in the liver by hepatic esterases [21]. However, the antiplatelet effect of ASA is not dependent on systemic bioavailability because circulating platelets are exposed to ASA in the portal circulation. The higher plasma concentration of ASA in the portal circulation compared with the systemic circulation [21] results in preferential inhibition of platelet TXA_2 with relative sparing of endothelial prostacyclin synthesis in the systemic circulation. The prostacyclin-sparing effect of low-dose ASA is no longer evident when higher doses of ASA are used.

ASA has a half life of 15 to 20 minutes [21] but requires only once daily dosing to inhibit platelet function because it irreversibly inhibits platelet COX-1 and platelets are unable to synthesize additional COX-1 because they do not have a nucleus. Thus, the platelet-inhibitory effect of ASA lasts for the life of the platelet (5 to 10 days) [21].

Salicylic acid is eliminated primarily by hepatic metabolism and some is also excreted unchanged in the urine. Urinary excretion of salicylate increases with dose and alkalinization of the urine [26]. Salicylic acid can also be removed by hemodialysis.

Pharmacodynamics

ASA irreversibly inhibits the initial committed step of prostanoid biosynthesis by preventing the conversion of AA to PGG_2 by COX-1 and COX-2. ASA initially binds an arginine 120 residue, a common docking site for all NSAIDs, after which it acetylates a COX serine residue [21]. In the human COX-1 enzyme, serine is acetylated at position 529 whereas in COX-2 this occurs at position 516 [21]. Acetylation of the serine residue by ASA stops AA from accessing the catalytic site of the COX [11] and prevents formation of the downstream prostanoids. AA is able to bypass ASA bound to COX-2 due to structural differences between the isoforms that cause COX-2 to have a more capacious active site, but is converted to 15-R-hydroxyeicosatetraenoic acid instead of PGH_2 [7]. The inhibition of COX-1 by ASA is saturable to a dose of 0.5mg/kg/day which means that low-dose aspirin is able to inhibit platelet aggregation to the same extent as higher doses [28,29]. ASA is 170 times less potent in inhibiting COX-2 than COX-1 and much larger doses are required to achieve an anti-inflammatory effect [27].

The relation between inhibition of platelet TXA_2 generation and inhibition of TXA_2-mediated platelet aggregation is non-linear; more than 95% of platelet TXA_2 generation must be inhibited to fully inhibit thromboxane-dependent platelet function [28]. A residual 10% capacity to generate TXA_2 is adequate to fully sustain thromboxane-dependent platelet aggregation [28]. This has implications for the use of reversible COX inhibitors as antiplatelet agents; high drug levels must be sustained to adequately inhibit thromboxane A_2 generation.

Acetyl salicylic acid's effects on preventing cardiovascular disease are believed to be mediated primarily by its inhibition of platelet COX-1 but anti-thrombotic effects unrelated to inhibition of COX have also been proposed [27,28]. Suggested mechanisms include reduced thrombin generation, enhanced fibrinolysis and dose-dependent inhibition of platelet function [27,28].

Adverse effects

ASA is an effective treatment for preventing pathological thrombosis but also inhibits physiological processes. One of its most important adverse effects is gastrointestinal (GI) toxicity. Other important adverse effects include hyper-sensitivity and bleeding (a target-related effect), including intracranial bleed-ing. Low-dose ASA does not adversely influence hypertension and renal dysfunction [21,28], and does not interfere with the effect of ACE inhibitors [7].

GI toxicity

COX-1 is the dominant isoform in the gastric mucosa and its inhibition by ASA suppresses production of PGE_2, which has a cytoprotective role in the stomach. Minor GI symptoms are common in patients taking aspirin and can be reduced by administering the drug with food. Up to 70% of patients taking ASA have occult GI blood loss, which may result in iron deficiency with long-term use. The incidence of serious GI bleeds in patients on low-dose ASA is twice that in patients on placebo but the absolute incidence is low [21,30], with an estimated excess of one to two major bleeds per 1000 middle aged patients treated for a year. Thus 500 to 1000 patients would need to be treated with low-dose ASA for 1 year to cause one to two major GI bleeds [31].

The mechanisms that contribute to the increased risk of GI bleeding with ASA are twofold: the first is the inhibition of TXA_2-mediated platelet aggrega-tion and the second is the loss of gastric mucosal protection mediated by PGE_2 [28]. Inhibition of platelet aggregation is dose-independent at doses above $0.5\,mg/kg/day$ but GI mucosal injury is dose-dependent and higher doses of ASA increase the risk of major GI bleeding by 4–10 fold [21]. When used to prevent cardiovascular disease, ASA should be given in the lowest proven effective dose to minimize the risk of bleeding [28]. Increasing age increases the risk of GI symptoms during ASA use, while a history of GI bleeding or peptic ulcer disease, *H. pylori* infection, concomitant warfarin therapy, NSAIDs or steroid use increase the risk of bleeding [31].

Enteric coated and buffered forms of ASA do not reduce the risk of a GI bleed compared with soluble aspirin but may reduce minor symptoms of gastric irritation [28,31].

Intracranial bleeding
There is a small absolute increase (<1/1000 patients per year in high-risk trials) in risk of intracranial hemorrhage in patients taking ASA [28].

ASA hypersensitivity
ASA can cause an acquired non-allergic hypersensitivity, manifest in the airways as asthma, rhinosinusitis and nasal polyps; and manifest in the tissues as urticaria, angioedema and anaphylaxis. The prevalence of ASA hypersensitivity is variable, ranging from 1 to 40%, with the higher rates reported in patients with personal or family history of atopy, asthma or rhinitis and nasal polyps [32]. The mechanism is thought to be related to inhibition of COX-1 causing reduced PGE_2 production, which results in loss of inhibition of proinflammatory mediators [32]. There also is unopposed lipooxygenase activity with increased synthesis of leukotrienes, reduction in mast cell stability, and increased release of histamine and tryptase, all of which contribute to the airway hyper-reactivity [32]. Virtually all patients with ASA hypersensitivity can be successfully desensitized.

Non-selective NSAIDs
Structure
Non-selective NSAIDs are derived from a variety of structural classes. Some of the more commonly used NSAIDs include diclofenac and ketolorac (heteroaryl acetic acids), naproxen and ibuprofen (arylpropionic acids), indomethacin (indole and indene acetic acids) and piroxicam (enolic acids) [33].

Mechanism of action
Most non-selective NSAIDs rapidly and reversibly inhibit COX by competing with arachidonic acid for the enzyme's active site. Indomethacin causes a slow, time-dependent inhibition of COX-1 and COX-2 [34]. Inhibition of platelet TXA_2 synthesis by traditional NSAIDs is intermittent and incomplete, which contrasts with the irreversible and permanent inhibition of platelet TXA_2 synthesis by ASA. There also are differences in the extent to which individual agents inhibit COX-1 versus COX-2 (Figure 3.3) [17], which is reflected in their side-effect profiles. NSAIDs with greater COX-2 inhibitory action have fewer GI and renal side effects than NSAIDs that primarily inhibit COX-1.

Adverse effects of non-selective NSAIDs
The most important adverse effects of NSAIDs result from inhibition of COX in the GI mucosa and kidneys.

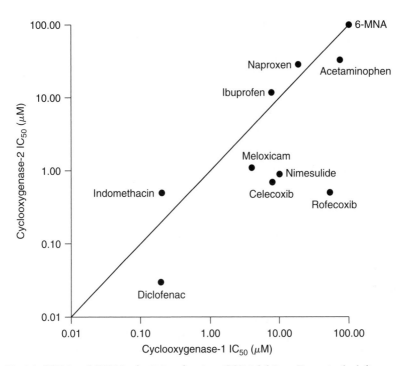

Fig. 3.3 COX-1 and COX-2 selectivity of various COX-inhibitors. Drugs to the left of the line preferentially inhibit COX-1 and those on the right have more potent COX-2 activity. 6-MNA (6-methoxy-2-naphthylacetic acid) is the active metabolite of nabumetone. Reproduced with permission from *New Eng J Med* [15].

Gastrointestinal effects

NSAIDs are associated with a two to seven-fold increase in serious GI events compared with controls [35] and NSAIDs with preferential COX-1 activity show the most gastric toxicity. Concomitant use of ASA with NSAIDs significantly increases the risk of bleeding and the risk factors for GI bleeding with ASA also extend to NSAIDs.

Two-thirds of regular users of NSAIDs have subclinical small bowel enteropathy, a spectrum of inflammation and increased intestinal permeability that results in hypoalbuminemia and iron deficiency [36]. This can be attributed to NSAID-related direct damage to enterocyte mitochondria [36].

Renal effects

In the kidneys, COX-2 is found in the cortical macula densa and medullary interstitial cells [37] while COX-1 is found in the collecting ducts and thin loops of Henle. The renal vasculature contains both COX isoforms. The vasodilator prostaglandins are essential to maintain adequate renal perfusion in the presence of volume depletion. Inhibition of this response by COX inhibitors leads to the nephrotoxicity of NSAIDs, exhibited by decreased urinary sodium excretion and glomerular filtration rate (GFR), and a multitude of other renal effects including acute renal failure, papillary necrosis and interstitial nephritis [37]. Up to 5% of patients treated with non-selective NSAIDs may develop renal toxicity [38].

The renal side effects of NSAIDs are dose-dependent and include peripheral edema, elevation of blood pressure, and interference with antihypertensive medications [37]. These effects can potentially translate to increased cardiovascular events in patients treated with traditional NSAIDs.

Hypersensitivity
NSAIDs demonstrate 100% cross-reactivity in patients with ASA hypersensitivity. The mechanism is identical to that of ASA and is abolished by ASA desensitization [32].

Selective COX 2 inhibitors
Structure
The development of COX-2 inhibitors followed the discovery of the COX-2 isoenzyme in the 1990s. The prototype COX-2 inhibitors are celecoxib and rofecoxib, which belong to the diarylheterocycle structural class [33] and have sulfur containing groups in place of the carboxyl group of NSAIDs [13]. Other drugs in this group include etoricoxib, parecoxib and valdecoxib. Lumiracoxib is the most recent addition and differs from the others in that it is a phenyl acetic acid derivative. Parecoxib is a prodrug of valdecoxib and is available in intravenous form.

Mechanism of action
The sulfur-containing phenyl rings of COX-2 inhibitors bind the side pocket of the COX catalytic channel of COX-2 causing a slow, time-dependent inhibition of COX-2 [34]. They interact only weakly with the active site of COX-1 and thus have little COX-1 inhibitory activity.

Adverse effects
The development of COX-2 inhibitors was prompted by the need to reduce the gastrointestinal complications of the non-selective NSAIDs. However, new unexpected toxicities have emerged, restricting the use of these drugs.

Gastrointestinal toxicity
COX-2 inhibitors cause fewer GI symptoms, symptomatic and endoscopic ulcers, and possibly serious GI complications than traditional NSAIDs [39]. Co-treatment with aspirin eliminates the GI advantage of COX-2 inhibitors [7].

Cardiovascular toxicity
COX-2 inhibitors have been associated with increased rates of myocardial infarction [3,40]. Postulated mechanisms include reduced prostacyclin synthesis, elevated blood pressure, abnormal vascular remodeling, inhibition of protective mechanisms against ischemia–reperfusion injury, and inhibition of lipoxin A_4 production, which has a wide range of anti-inflammatory effects [41]. The relationship between COX-2 inhibition and prostacyclin inhibition appears linear [19], and marked suppression of COX-2 (70–80%) may significantly reduce the cardioprotective effect of prostacyclin.

Renal effects
COX-2 inhibitors have a similar renal risk profile to non-selective NSAIDs.

Other
COX-2 inhibitors show no cross-reactivity with ASA-sensitive asthma but reactions have rarely been reported. Thus, caution is required in patients with a history of ASA allergy [32].

Other drugs with COX inhibitory activity
COX inhibitors that do not fit any other category include acetaminophen (paracetamol), Dipyrone and COX-inhibiting nitric oxide donors (CINODs).

CINODS are a new class of drugs designed to minimize the toxicity of NSAIDs. They consist of the parent COX inhibitor with a nitroxybutyl or nitrosothiol moiety, which allow the COX-inhibiting anti-inflammatory activity to be retained whilst nitric oxide donation reduces gastrointestinal, renal and cardiovascular toxicity [38,42]. CINODS prevent platelet activation *in vitro* and exhibit antithrombotic activity *in vivo* [38]. Several CINODS are in various stages of clinical development but whether they have a beneficial role in the management of cardiovascular disease is yet to be established.

Conclusion

The unique pharmacological properties of low-dose ASA have given it a preeminent role as an antiplatelet drug for the prevention of cardiovascular disease in high risk patients. The most important adverse effect of ASA is upper GI bleeding, which can be reduced by using the lowest dose that has been proven to be effective for the prevention of cardiovascular disease. Traditional non-COX-selective NSAIDs and selective COX-2 inhibitors have little or no clinically significant antiplatelet activity. Both these classes of COX inhibitors may paradoxically increase the risk of cardiovascular disease through their effects on the vasculature and kidneys and perhaps via other less well-defined mechanisms. The ability of CINODs to release nitric oxide may confer a more favorable side-effect profile than other COX inhibitors but this remains to be established.

Acknowledgements

NCR is the recipient of a Young Investigator Scholarship from the Haematology Society of Australia and New Zealand. JWE holds a Tier II Canada Research Chair in Cardiovascular Medicine from the Canadian Institutes of Health Research.

References

1 Antithrombotic Trialists' Collaboration. Collaborative meta-analysis of randomized trials of antiplatelet therapy for prevention of death, myocardial infarction, and stroke in high risk patients. *BMJ* 2002; **324**: 71–86.

2 Bombardier C, Laine L, Reicin A, *et al*. Comparison of upper gastrointestinal toxicity of rofecoxib and naproxen in patients with rheumatoid arthritis *New Eng J Med* 2000; **343**: 1520–1528.

3 Kearney PM, Baigent C, Godwin J, *et al*. Do selective cyclo-oxygenase 2 inhibitors and traditional non-steroidal anti-inflammatory drugs increase the risk of athero-thrombosis? Meta-analysis of randomized trials. *BMJ* 2006; **332**: 1302–1308.

4 Hawkey CJ. COX-2 chronology. *Gut* 2005; **54**: 1509–1514.

5 http://www.aspirin.com/world_of_aspirin_en.html#

6 Vane JR, Botting RM. Mechanism of action of nonsteroidal anti-inflammatory drugs. *Am J Med* 1998; **104**: 2S–8S.

7 Awtry EH, Loscalzo J. Cardiovascular drugs. *Circulation* 2000; **101**: 1206.

8 Weiss HJ. The discovery of the antiplatelet effect of aspirin: a personal reminiscence. *J Thromb Haemost* 2003; **1**: 1869–1875.

9 Vane J. Towards a better aspirin. *Nature* 1994; **367**: 215–216.

10 Picot D, Loll PJ, Garavito RM. The Xray crystal structure of the membrane protein prostaglandin H2 synthase 1. *Nature* 1994; **367**: 243–249.

11 Loll PJ, Picot D, Garavito RM. The structural basis of ASA activity inferred from the crystal structure of inactivated prostaglandin H2 synthase. *Nat Struct Biol* 1995; **2**: 637–643.

12 Loll PJ, Picot D, Ekabo O, Garavito RM. Synthesis and use of iodinated nonsteroidal anti-inflammatory drug analogues as crystallographic probes of the prostaglandin H_2 synthase cyclooxygenase active site. *Biochemistry* 1996; **35**: 7330–7340.

13 Botting RM. Inhibitors of cyclooxygenases:mechanisms, selectivity and uses. *J Physiol Pharmacol* 2006; **57** (Supp. 5): 113–124.

14 Vane JR, Botting RM. The mechanism of action of ASA. *Thromb Res* 2003; **110**: 255–258.

15 Fitzgerald G, Patrono C. The coxibs, selective inhibitors of cycooxygenase-2. *New Eng J Med* 2001; **345**: 433–442.

16 Miller S. Prostaglandins in health and disease, an overview. *Semin Arthritis Rheum* 2006; **36**: 37–49.

17 Patrono C The PGH-synthase system and isozyme-selective inhibition. *J Cardiovasc Pharm* 2006; **47** (Suppl. 1): S1–6.

18 Capone ML, Tyacconelli S, Di Francesco L, *et al*. Pharmacodynamic of cyclooxygenase inhibitors in humans. *Prostag Other Lipid Med* 2007; **82**: 85–94.

19 Smith WL, Garavito RM, DeWitt DL. Prostaglandin endoperoxide H synthases (cyclo-oxgenases)-1 and -2. *J Biol Chem* 1996; **271**: 33157–33160.

20 Rocca B, Secchiero P, Ciabattoni G, *et al*. Cyclooxygenase 2 expression is induced during human megakaryopoiesis and characterizes newly formed platelets. *Proc Natl Acad Sci USA* 2002; **99**: 7634–7639.

21 Patrono C, Garcia Rodriguez LA, Landolfi R, Baigent C. Low dose ASA for the prevention of atherothrombosis. *New Eng J Med* 2005; **353**: 2373–2383.

22 Botting R. COX-1 and COX-3 inhibitors. *Thromb Res* 2003; **110**: 269–272.

23 Simmons DL. Variants of cyclooxygenase-1 and their roles in medicine. *Thromb Res* 2003; **110**: 265–268.

24 Bayer Health Care. Aspirin. Available at http://www.aspirin.com/products_en.html Accessed June 18, 2007.

25 Pedersen AK, Fitzgerald GA. Dose related kinetics of ASA: presystemic acetylation of platelet cyclooxygenase. *New Eng J Med* 1984; **311**: 1206–1211.

26 MacPherson CR, Milne MD, Evans BM. The excretion of Salicylate. *Br J Pharmacol* 1955; **10**: 484–489.

27 Undas A, Brummel-Ziedins KE, Mann KG. Antithrombotic properties of aspirin and resistance to aspirin: beyond strictly antiplatelet actions. *Blood* 2006; **109**: 2285–2292.

28 Patrono C, Coler B, Fitzgerald GA, Hirsh J, Roth G. Platelet active drugs: the relationships between dose, effectiveness , and side effects: The seventh ACCP Conference on Antithrombotic and Thrombolytic Therapy. *Chest* 2004; **126** (Suppl.); 234S–264S.

29 Campbell C, Smyth S, Montalescot, Steinhubl S. Aspirin dose for the prevention of cardiovascular disease. *JAMA* 2007; **297**: 2018–2024.

30 Patrono C, Coller B, Dalen JE *et al*. Platelet-active drugs: the relationships among dose, effectiveness and side effects. *Chest* 2001; **119** (Suppl.): 39S–63S.

31 Laine L. Review article: gastrointestinal bleeding with low-dose ASA-what's the risk? *Aliment Pharm Therap* 2006; **24**: 896–908.

32 Stevenson DD, Szczeklik A. Clinical and pathologic perspectives on ASA sensitivity and asthma. *Curr Rev Allergy Clin Immunol* 2006; **118**: 773–786.

33 Warner TD, Mitchell JA. Cyclooxygenases: new forms, new inhibitors, and lessons from the clinic *FASEB J* 2004; **18**: 790–804.

34 Kurumbail RG, Stevens AM, Gierse JK *et al*. Structural basis for selective inhibition of cyclooxygenase 2 by anti-inflammatory agents. *Nature* 1996; **384**: 644–648.

35 Schaffer D, Florin T, Eagle C *et al*. Risk of serious NSAID-related gastrointestinal events during longterm exposure: a systematic review. *Med J Aust* 2006; **185**: 501–506.

36 Fortun PJ, Hawkey CJ. Nonsteroidal anti-inflammatory drugs and the small intestine. *Curr Opin Gastroentol* 2007; **23**: 134–141.

37 Gambaro G, Perazella MA. Adverse renal effects of anti-inflammatory agents: evaluation of selective and nonselective cyclooxygenase inhibitors. *J Int Med* 2003; **253**: 643–652.

38 Muscara MN, Wallace JL. COX-inhibiting nitric oxide donors (CINODs): potential benefits on cardiovascular and renal function. *Cardiovasc Hematol Agents Med Chem* 2006; **4**: 155–164.

39 Hooper L, Brown TJ, Elliott R, *et al*. The Effectiveness of 5 strategies for the prevention of GI toxicity by NSAIDs: systematic review. *BMJ* 2004; **329**: 948–958.

40 Andersohn F, Suissa S, Garbe E. Use of first and second generation cyclooxygenase 2 selective nonsteroidal anti-inflammatory drugs and risk of acute myocardial infarction. *Circulation* 2006; **113**: 1950.

41 Salinas G, Rangasetty UC, Uretsky BF, Birnbaum Y. The cycloxygenase 2 (COX-2) story: it's time to explain, not inflame. *Cardiovasc Pharmacol Ther* 2007; **12**: 98–111.

42 Stefano F, Distrutti E. Cyclo-oxygenase (COX) inhibiting nitric oxide donating (CINODs) drugs: a review of their current status. *Curr Top Medicin Chem* 2007; **7**: 277–282.

Chapter 4

Aspirin response variability and resistance

Wai-Hong Chen and Daniel I. Simon

Introduction

Aspirin is the most commonly used oral antiplatelet drug for preventing ischemic events of atherothrombotic disease. Aspirin inhibits platelet cyclooxygenase-1 (COX-1) by irreversible acetylation of a serine residue at position 529, which prevents the conversion of arachidonic acid to thromboxane A_2 (TXA_2) [1]. The antithrombotic effect of aspirin is resultant from the decreased production of TXA_2, a potent vasoconstrictor and platelet agonist. The Antithrombotic Trialists' Collaboration reported that aspirin therapy was associated with 15% reduction in vascular mortality, 34% reduction in myocardial infarction, and 25% reduction in stroke among high-risk patients with atherothrombotic disease [2]. Aspirin has also been shown to reduce the acute ischemic complications of coronary angioplasty [3–5].

While the benefits of aspirin are widely accepted, cardiovascular events may still occur in patients treated with aspirin. It has been estimated that 10% to 20% of aspirin-treated patients may experience recurrent thrombotic events during long-term follow-up [6], suggesting that the antiplatelet effects of aspirin may not be equivalent in all patients. In addition to these clinical observations, measurements of platelet aggregation, platelet activation and bleeding time have indeed confirmed a wide variability in patients' responses to aspirin therapy [7–9]. It is based on this constellation of clinical and laboratory evidence of a diminished or absent response to aspirin treatment in some individuals, that the concept of "aspirin resistance" has emerged.

Antiplatelet Therapy in Ischemic Heart Disease, 1st edition. Edited by Stephen D. Wiviott
© 2009 American Heart Association, ISBN: 9-781-4051-7626-2

Definition(s) of aspirin resistance

Aspirin resistance may be defined as the inability of aspirin to produce an anticipated effect on one or more *in vitro* tests of platelet function, mainly platelet aggregation, and has been referred to as laboratory aspirin resistance. A clinical definition of aspirin resistance is the failure of the drug to prevent an atherothrombotic event despite prescription of aspirin. This phenomenon has also been described as aspirin treatment failure. Laboratory definitions of aspirin resistance have involved either detecting the failure of aspirin's pharmacological effect, or the failure of aspirin to prevent inhibition of platelet aggregation (Table 4.1). Aspirin resistance, defined by its pharmacological action, is persistent production of TXA_2 despite therapy, measured by the presence of TXA_2 metabolites in serum or urine. In contrast, persistent platelet aggregation despite aspirin treatment defines failure of aspirin-mediated platelet inhibition, and this may occur via non-TX mediated pathways of platelet activation. It has been suggested that aspirin resistance is a misleading term since, in some situations, aspirin successfully inhibits TX synthesis but platelet aggregation persists. The term aspirin "non-response" encompasses the failure of aspirin to both inhibit TX synthesis and reduce platelet aggregation [10].

Table 4.1 Laboratory tests for measuring the antiplatelet effects of aspirin

Test	Advantages	Disadvantages
Bleeding time	*In vivo* test; physiological	Non-specific; operator dependent; insensitive
Aspirin Works® Test (urinary 11-dehydrothromboxane B2)	Cyclooxygenase-1 dependent; correlation with clinical outcomes	Not platelet specific; indirect measure; dependent on renal function; uncertain reproducibility
Light transmission aggregometry	Gold standard; correlation with clinical outcomes	Time consuming; expensive; poor reproducibility
Platelet Function Analyzer-100®	Simple; rapid; correlation with clinical outcomes	Dependent on von Willebrand factor and hematocrit; no instrument adjustment
VerifyNow Aspirin™	Simple; rapid; point-of-care; correlation with clinical outcomes	No instrument adjustment

Mechanisms of aspirin resistance

Although much is currently known about the effects of aspirin on platelets, the mechanisms for aspirin resistance have not been fully elucidated. It is likely that clinical, pharmacological, biological and genetic factors are contributing to the variable platelet response to aspirin (Figure 4.1) [11–13]. Patient non-compliance to prescribed therapy [14] and reduced gastrointestinal absorption [15] are simple causes for aspirin resistance/failure. Cigarette smoking has been shown to increase platelet thrombus formation in aspirin-treated patients with coronary artery disease [16]. Intake of non-steroidal anti-inflammatory drugs can interfere with the binding of aspirin to COX-1 [17] but the clinical significance is uncertain [18,19]. The issue of whether a higher aspirin dose is associated with a greater platelet inhibitory response remains uncertain, and is influenced by the assay used and the platelet agonist tested [20–28]. Reduction in the platelet inhibitory effect during long-term treatment (or tolerance) has been observed [29] but the mechanisms remain unknown. Increased platelet turnover, as seen after coronary artery bypass graft surgery, can lead to inadequate suppression of platelet COX-1 because of an increased proportion of platelets not exposed to aspirin [30]. Alternative pathways of TXA_2 production by COX-2 from platelets [31] and endothelial cells [32] have been proposed as factors in aspirin resistance. Persistent platelet activation despite aspirin inhibition of TXA_2 may be a reflection of the redundancy of platelet activation pathways from adenosine diphosphate (ADP), collagen and other agonists [28,33,34].

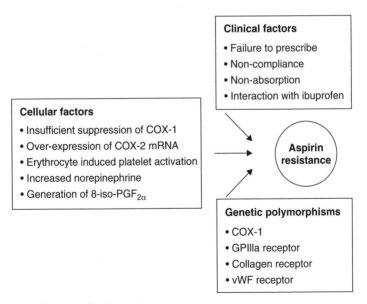

Fig. 4.1 Mechanisms of aspirin resistance.

Genetics play an important role in determining the laboratory response to antiplatelet drugs. Polymorphisms involving COX-1 [35], COX-2 [36], platelet glycoprotein receptors [37–39] and ADP receptor gene $P2Y_{12}$ [40] have all been reported to affect platelet response to aspirin. Finally, polygenic heritable factors have been shown to affect interindividual variability to aspirin response more strongly than traditional risk factors (hypertension, diabetes, hypercholesterolemia, cigarette smoking, obesity), particularly in pathways indirectly related to COX-1 [41].

Prevalence of aspirin resistance

As the antiplatelet effects of aspirin may not be uniform among all patients and over time, the exact prevalence of aspirin resistance remains uncertain. In previous studies, it has been reported to range from 5% to 60% of the population [7–10,26,45]. Variability in aspirin-mediated platelet inhibition was noted not only in patients with cerebrovascular disease, coronary artery disease or presenting for coronary artery bypass surgery, but also in normal subjects [7,8,22,26,42,43]. The absence of standardized diagnostic criteria and a single validated method of identifying aspirin-resistant individuals, as well as the lack of precise biological mechanisms for this phenomenon, have led to a wide range of population estimates.

Clinical relevance of aspirin resistance

Several recent studies linking laboratory measures of aspirin resistance to adverse clinical outcomes have been reported and prospective series are summarized in Figure 4.2. Grotemeyer et al. [7] determined aspirin responsiveness in 180 stroke patients 12 hours after an oral intake of 500 mg aspirin. Patients with a platelet reactivity index ≤1.25 were categorized as aspirin responders while those with an index >1.25 were defined as secondary aspirin non-responders (i.e. aspirin-resistant). All patients were prescribed aspirin 500 mg three times daily and were followed for 24 months. Stroke, myocardial infarction (MI) or vascular death were major outcome measures. The incidence of aspirin resistance was 33%. Complete follow-up was obtained in 174 patients (96%). Major events were noted in 29 patients: five (4.4%) in the aspirin responder group versus 24 (40%) in the aspirin-resistant group (p < 0.0001).

In a retrospective analysis using the Platelet Function Analyzer (PFA)-100®, Grundmann et al. [44] reported from a cross-sectional study that, in 53 patients treated with aspirin for secondary prevention of transient ischemic attack (TIA) or stroke, the rate of aspirin resistance was significantly higher (12/35; 34%) in those with recurrent cerebrovascular events as compared to those without recurrence (0/18; 0%) (p = 0.0006).

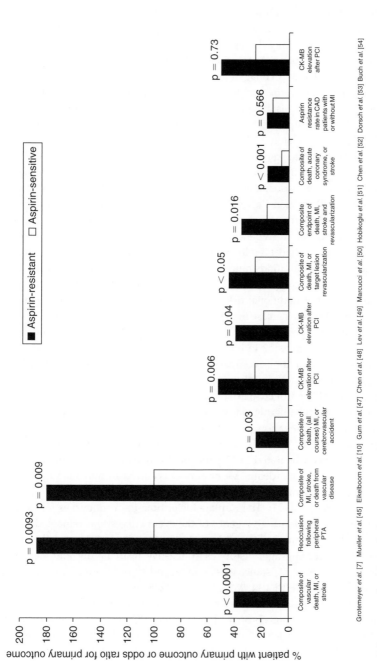

Fig. 4.2 Summary of studies relating aspirin resistance and clinical outcomes.

Mueller *et al.* [45] studied 100 patients with intermittent claudication undergoing elective percutaneous balloon angioplasty. Aspirin was prescribed at a dose of 100 mg daily. Using corrected whole blood aggregometry they defined a normal response to aspirin as at least 20% reduction in platelet function with both ADP and collagen as agonists. Fluctuations in aspirin responsiveness among the studied population were noted on serial monitoring. The incidence of aspirin resistance was ~60% at each time point of measurement. At 52-week follow-up, eight patients in the aspirin resistance group were noted to have reocclusion at the angioplasty site, compared with none of the patients with a normal response to aspirin (87% increase in risk, p = 0.0093).

Eikelboom *et al.* [10] performed a nested case–control study on 976 aspirin-treated patients, with documented or at high-risk of cardiovascular disease, from the Heart Protection Prevention Evaluation (HOPE) trial. Aspirin responsiveness was divided into quartiles by urinary 11-dehydrothromboxane B_2 levels, a marker of *in vivo* TX generation. After 5 years of follow-up, those patients in the upper quartile had 1.8-fold increase in risk for the composite of MI, stroke or cardiovascular death (odds ratio [OR] 1.8; 95% confidence intervals [CI] 1.2 to 2.7; p = 0.009) when compared to those in the lower quartile, and the association was independent of traditional risk factors. There was a twofold increase in the risk of MI and 3.5-fold increase in the risk of cardiovascular death as well.

In a 4-year retrospective cohort study among 129 post-MI patients, Andersen *et al.* [46] noted a tendency to higher incidence of adverse vascular events in aspirin-resistant patients as compared with sensitive patients (36% vs. 24%), although the difference did not reach statistical significance (p = 0.28).

Gum *et al.* [47] enrolled 326 stable patients with cardiovascular disease treated with aspirin (325 mg daily for ≥7 days) and defined aspirin resistance as a mean aggregation of ≥70% with 10 μM ADP and a mean aggregation of ≥20% with 0.5 mg/ml arachidonic acid by optical platelet aggregation. Aspirin resistance was noted in 17 patients (5.2%). After a mean follow-up of 1.8 years, major events (death, MI or stroke) occurred in four (24%) patients in the aspirin-resistant group, compared with 30 (10%) patients in the aspirin-sensitive group (p = 0.03). The Kaplan–Meier time-to-event curves for event-free survival showed late divergence of the event curves that remained to be explained. Multivariate analysis demonstrated that, in addition to other risk factors, like increasing age, history of congestive heart failure and elevated platelet count, aspirin resistance was an independent predictor of adverse outcomes (hazard ratio [HR] 4.14, 95% CI 1.42 to 12.06, p = 0.009).

Chen *et al.* [48] examined aspirin responsiveness in patients undergoing elective percutaneous coronary intervention (PCI) treated with aspirin at 80–300 mg daily for at least 7 days, in combination with a clopidogrel loading dose of 300 mg at least 12 hours before intervention, and procedural anticoagulation using heparin. Using a point-of-care device for arachadonic acid induced platelet aggregation*, 29 (19.2%) out of the 151 enrolled patients were found to be aspirin-resistant, as defined by an aspirin reaction unit (ARU) ≥550. Patients with aspirin resistance were at increased risk of myocardial necrosis (OR 2.9; 95% CI 1.2 to 6.9; p = 0.015) determined by creatine kinase–myocardial band (CK–MB) elevation, when compared with aspirin-sensitive patients (ARU <550). In an elective PCI population (n = 150), Lev *et al.* [49] tested for both aspirin and clopidogrel responsiveness in patients receiving aspirin 81–325 mg daily for ≥1 week and clopidogrel at 300 mg loading-dose on completion of the PCI, and 75 mg daily thereafter. Bivalirudin was used for procedural anticoagulation to reduce the confounding effect of heparin on platelet activation. Blood samples were taken at baseline and 20 to 24 hours after clopidogrel loading. Adopting the criteria by Gum *et al.* [47] and Chen *et al.* [48], they defined aspirin resistance as the presence of at least two of the followings: (1) 0.5 mg/ml arachidonic acid-induced platelet aggregation ≥20%; (2) 5 μmol/L ADP-induced platelet aggregation ≥70%; and (3) ARU ≥550 by a point-of-care device for arachadonic acid induced platelet aggregation*. Clopidogrel resistance was defined as baseline minus post-treatment aggregation ≤10% in response to both 5 and 20 μmol/L ADP. The rates of aspirin and clopidogrel resistance were 12.7% and 24%, respectively. Clopidogrel resistance was noted in nine (47.4%) of the aspirin-resistant patients and 27 (20.6%) of aspirin-sensitive patients. Similar to the study results of Chen *et al.*, a significant increase in the incidence of CK–MB elevation was observed in aspirin-resistant patients, when compared with aspirin-sensitive patients (38.9% vs. 18.3%; p = 0.04). Dual drug-resistant patients were also more likely than dual drug-sensitive patients to have CK–MB elevations (44.4% vs. 15.8%; p = 0.05).

Marcucci *et al.* [50] prospectively evaluated 146 patients with acute MI undergoing primary PCI receiving oral 300 mg loading dose of clopidogrel and intravenous 500 mg aspirin, followed by 75 mg daily of clopidogrel and 100 mg daily of aspirin. Unfractionated heparin was used for procedural anticoagulation and platelet glycoprotein IIb/IIIa inhibitor use was an exclusion. They noted aspirin resistance in 28% using the point-of-care device aperture closure device for platelet function measurement**. At 1 year, cardiac death, new acute MI or target lesion revascularization occurred in 43.9% of aspirin-resistant patients and 24.8% of aspirin-sensitive patients, respectively (p < 0.05). Aspirin resistance was shown to be an independent risk factor for adverse coronary events (HR 2.9; 95% CI 1.1 to 9.2, p <0.05). Similar results were observed in the prospective study by Hobikoglu *et al.* [51] on 140 patients with acute coronary syndromes and aspirin responsiveness measured by a point-of-care device aperture closure device for platelet function measurement**. The composite

---

* VerifyNow Aspirin™ assay device
** PFA-100 assay®.

endpoint of death, MI, stroke and revascularization at 20 months was present in 35% of patients with aspirin resistance and 16% of patients without aspirin resistance (HR 2.46; 95% CI 1.18 to 5.13, p = 0.016). Multivariate analysis revealed aspirin resistance to be an independent predictor for long-term adverse events (HR 3.03; 95% CI 1.06 to 8.62, p = 0.038).

After reporting the prevalence and predictors of aspirin resistance among 468 stable patients with CAD using a point-of-care device for arachadonic acid induced platelet aggregation* [26], Chen *et al.* followed this cohort prospectively and noted that after a mean follow-up of 379 ± 200 days, patients with aspirin resistance (n = 128; 27.4%) were at increased risk of the composite outcome of cardiovascular death, MI, unstable angina requiring hospitalization, stroke and TIA compared with patients who were aspirin-sensitive (15.6% vs. 5.3%, HR 3.12, 95% CI 1.65 to 5.91, p < 0.001) [52]. Cox proportional hazard regression modeling identified aspirin resistance, diabetes, prior MI and a low hemoglobin to be independently associated with major adverse long-term outcomes (HR for aspirin resistance 2.46, 95% CI 1.27 to 4.76, p = 0.007).

Studies failing to show an association between aspirin resistance and clinical outcomes have also been reported. In a case–control study of 100 stable CAD patients on aspirin therapy, Dorsch *et al.* [53] studied aspirin responsiveness using a point-of-care device for arachadonic acid induced platelet aggregation*. The prevalence of aspirin resistance was 16% among patients with documented history of MI (cases) and 12% in those with no history of MI (OR 1.40; 95% CI 0.45 to 4.37, p = 0.566). In another study on patients undergoing elective PCI, Buch *et al.* [54] recruited 330 patients receiving aspirin ≥1 week and clopidogrel pretreatment at 300 mg or 600 mg ≥6 hours before PCI. Aspirin and clopidogrel responsiveness were both measured using a point-of-care device for arachadonic acid induced platelet aggregation* and Ultegra Rapid Platelet Function Assay-P2Y$_{12}$, Accumetrics, respectively. Aspirin resistance was detected in 3.7% of the patients. There were no differences in the incidence of post-PCI CK–MB or troponin I elevation between the aspirin-resistant and non-aspirin-resistant groups (50% vs. 24.6%; p = 0.26 and 50% vs. 53.8%; p = 0.73, respectively).

The major issue regarding the studies published to date is whether the data show a correlation between aspirin response and clinical outcomes. These limitations include the small numbers of subjects, study designs inadequate for controlling confounding variables and a non-uniform definition of antiplatelet resistance. In studies of aspirin, the dosage varied and treatment compliance was not verified.

---

* VerifyNow Aspirin™ assay device

Conclusions and future directions

Numerous studies have documented interindividual variability in platelet inhibitory responsiveness to aspirin. There is a growing body of evidence demonstrating that hypo- or non-responsiveness to aspirin in the laboratory (i.e. resistance) is associated with adverse clinical events in diverse populations of patients with atherosclerotic disease in both stable and unstable phases as well as in the postpercutaneous coronary and postperipheral intervention setting.

Widespread clinical application of the concept of aspirin resistance will require additional studies on larger populations that define antiplatelet resistance in a standardized manner using assays with consistent and reproducible results. These measures should correlate the measurements with clinical outcomes, and provide for strategies of modifying antiplatelet regimens to improve outcome (e.g. increasing dose of antiplatelet agent, adding or substituting a second antiplatelet agent). Prospective randomized trials are underway. The ASCET (ASpirin non-responsiveness and Clopidogrel Endpoint Trial) is recruiting stable patients with angiographically documented coronary artery disease to evaluate whether switching to clopidogrel will be superior to continued aspirin therapy in improving clinical outcomes among aspirin-resistant patients [55]. Surrogate efficacy markers are used with antihypertensive (blood pressure), antihyperlipidemic (LDL cholesterol), and anticoagulant (protime INR) agents. Therefore, it seems reasonable and probable that in vitro measures of platelet inhibitory responses will someday play an integral role in the management of cardiovascular patients requiring antiplatelet agents.

References

1 Loll PJ, Picot D, Garavito RM. The structural basis of aspirin activity inferred from the crystal structure of inactivated prostaglandin H_2 synthase. *Nat Struct Biol* 1995; **2**: 637–643.

2 Antithrombotic Trialists' Collaboration. Collaborative meta-analysis of randomised trials of antiplatelet therapy for prevention of death, myocardial infarction, and stroke in high risk patients. *BMJ* 2002; **324**: 71–86.

3 Barnathan ES, Schwartz JS, Taylor L, *et al.* Aspirin and dipyridamole in the prevention of acute coronary thrombosis complicating coronary angioplasty. *Circulation* 1987; **76**: 125–134.

4 Schwartz L, Bourassa MG, Lesperance J, *et al.* Aspirin and dipyridamole in the prevention of restenosis after percutaneous transluminal coronary angioplasty. *New Engl J Med* 1988; **318**: 1714–1719.

5 Lembo NJ, Black AJR, Roubin GS, *et al.* Effect of pre-treatment with aspirin versus aspirin plus dipyridamole on frequency and type of acute complications of percutaneous transluminal coronary angioplasty. *Am J Cardiol* 1990; **65**: 422–426.

6 Patrono C, Coller B, FitzGerald GA, Hirsh J, Roth G. Platelet-active drugs: the relationships among dose, effectiveness, and side effects. *Chest* 2004; **126**: 234S–264S.

7 Grotemeyer KH, Scharafinski HW, Husstedt IW. Two-year follow-up of aspirin responder and aspirin non-responder: a pilot-study including 180 post-stroke patients. *Thromb Res* 1993; **71**: 397–403.

8 Pappas JM, Westengard JC, Bull BS. Population variability in the effect of aspirin on platelet function. Implications for clinical trials and therapy. *Arch Pathol Lab Med* 1994; **118**: 801–804.

9 Gum PA, Kottke-Marchant K, Poggio ED, *et al*. Profile and prevalence of aspirin resistance in patients with cardiovascular disease. *Am J Cardiol* 2001; **88**: 230–235.

10 Eikelboom JW, Hirsh J, Weitz JI, Johnston M, Yi Q, Yusuf S. Aspirin-resistant thromboxane biosynthesis and the risk of myocardial infarction, stroke, or cardiovascular death in patients at high risk for cardiovascular events. *Circulation* 2002; **105**: 1650–1655.

11 Mason PJ, Jacobs AK, Freedman JF. Aspirin resistance and atherothrombotic disease. *J Am Coll Cardiol* 2005; **46**: 986–993.

12 Hankey GJ, Eikelboom JW. Aspirin resistance. *Lancet* 2006; **367**: 606–617.

13 Wang TH, Bhatt DL, Topol EJ. Aspirin and clopidogrel resistance: an emerging clinical entity. *Eur Heart J* 2006; **27**: 647–654.

14 Schwartz KA, Schwartz DE, Ghosheh K, *et al*. Compliance as a critical consideration in patients who appear to be resistant to aspirin after healing of myocardial infarction. *Am J Cardiol* 2005; **95**: 973–975.

15 Gonzalez-Conejero R, Rivera J, Corral J, *et al*. Biological assessment of aspirin efficacy on healthy individuals: heterogeneous response or aspirin failure? *Stroke* 2005; **36**: 276–280.

16 Hung J, Lam JYT, Lacoste L, *et al*. Cigarette smoking acutely increases platelet thrombus formation in patients with coronary artery disease taking aspirin. *Circulation* 1995; **92**: 2432–2436.

17 Catella-Lawson F, Reilly MP, Kapoor SC, *et al*. Cyclooxygenase inhibitors and the antiplatelet effects of aspirin. *New Engl J Med* 2001; **345**: 1809–1817.

18 MacDonald TM, Wei L. Effect of ibuprofen on cardioprotective effect of aspirin. *Lancet* 2003; **361**: 573–574.

19 Curtis JP, Krumholz HM. The case for an adverse interaction between aspirin and non-steroidal anti-inflammatory drugs: is it time to believe the hype? *J Am Coll Cardiol* 2004; **43**: 991–993.

20 Caterina RD, Giannessi D, Boem A, *et al*. Equal antiplatelet effects of aspirin 50 or 324 mg/day in patients after acute myocardial infarction. *Thromb Haemost* 1985; **54**: 528–532.

21 Tohgi H, Konno S, Tamura K, *et al*. Effects of low-to-high doses of aspirin on platelet aggregability and metabolites of thromboxane A2 and prostacyclin. *Stroke* 1992; **23**: 1400–1403.

22 Helgason CM, Bolin KM, Hoff JA, *et al*. Development of aspirin resistance in persons with previous ischemic stroke. *Stroke* 1994; **25**: 2331–2336.

23 Dabaghi SF, Kamat SG, Payne J, *et al*. Effects of low-dose aspirin on in vitro platelet aggregation in the early minutes after ingestion in normal subjects. *Am J Cardiol* 1994; **74**: 720–723.

24 Feng D, McKenna C, Murillo J, *et al*. Effect of aspirin dosage and enteric coating on platelet reactivity. *Am J Cardiol* 1997; **80**: 189–193.

25 Hart RG, Leonard AD, Talbert RL, *et al.* Aspirin dosage and thromboxane synthesis in patients with vascular disease. *Pharmacotherapy* 2003; **23**: 579–584.

26 Lee PY, Chen WH, Ng W, *et al.* Low-dose aspirin increases aspirin resistance in patients with coronary artery disease. *Am J Med* 2005; **118**: 723–727.

27 Mehta SS, Silver RJ, Aaronson A, *et al.* Comparison of aspirin resistance in type 1 versus type 2 diabetes mellitus. *Am J Cardiol* 2006; **97**: 567–570.

28 Frelinger AL, Furman MI, Linden MD, *et al.* Residual arachidonic acid-induced platelet activation via an adenosine diphosphate-dependent but cyclooxygenase-1- and cyclooxygenase-2-independent pathway: a 700-patient study of aspirin resistance. *Circulation* 2006; **113**: 2888–2896.

29 Pulcinelli FM, Pignatelli P, Celestini A, *et al.* Inhibition of platelet aggregation by aspirin progressively decreases in long-term treated patients. *J Am Coll Cardiol* 2004; **43**: 979–984.

30 Zimmermann N, Wenk A, Kim U, *et al.* Functional and biochemical evaluation of platelet aspirin resistance after coronary artery bypass surgery. *Circulation* 2003; **108**: 542–547.

31 Weber AA, Zimmermann KC, Meyer-Kirchrath J, Schror K. Cyclooxygenase-2 in human platelets as a possible factor in aspirin resistance. *Lancet* 1999; **353**: 900.

32 Karim S, Habib A, Levy-Toledano S, Maclouf J. Cyclooxygenase-1 and -2 of endothelial cells utilize exogenous or endogenous arachidonic acid for transcellular production of thromboxane. *J Biol Chem* 1996; **271**: 12042–12048.

33 Kawasaki T, Ozeki Y, Igawa T, Kambayashi J. Increased platelet sensitivity to collagen in individuals resistant to low-dose aspirin. *Stroke* 2000; **31**: 591–595.

34 Macchi L, Christiaens L, Brabant S, *et al.* Resistance to aspirin in vitro is associated with increased platelet sensitivity to adenosine diphosphate. *Thromb Res* 2002; **107**: 45–49.

35 Halushka M, Walker LP, Halushka PV. Genetic variation in cyclooxygenase 1: effects on response to aspirin. *Clin Pharmacol Ther* 2003; **73**: 122–130.

36 Cipollone F, Toniato E, Martinotti S, *et al.* A polymorphism in the cyclooxygenase 2 gene as an inherited protective factor against myocardial infarction and stroke. *JAMA* 2004; **291**: 2221–2228.

37 Michelson AD, Furman MI, Goldschmidt-Clermont P, *et al.* Platelet GP IIIa Pl(A) polymorphisms display different sensitivities to agonists. *Circulation* 2000; **101**: 1013–1018.

38 Undas A, Brummel K, Musial J, Mann KG, Szczeklik A. Pl(A2) polymorphism of beta(3) integrins is associated with enhanced thrombin generation and impaired antithrombotic action of aspirin at the site of microvascular injury. *Circulation* 2001; **104**: 2666–2672.

39 Macchi L, Christiaens L, Brabant S, *et al.* Resistance in vitro to low-dose aspirin is associated with platelet PlA1 (GP IIIa) polymorphism but not with C807T(GP Ia/IIa) and C-5T Kozak (GP Ibalpha) polymorphisms. *J Am Coll Cardiol* 2003; **42**: 1115–1119.

40 Jefferson BK, Foster JH, McCarthy JJ, *et al.* Aspirin resistance and a single gene. *Am J Cardiol* 2005; **95**: 805–808.

41 Faraday N, Yanek LR, Mathias R, *et al.* Heritability of platelet responsiveness to aspirin in activation pathways directly and indirectly related to cyclooxygenase-1. *Circulation* 2007; **115**: 2490–2496.

42 Gum PA, Kottke-Marchant K, Poggio ED, *et al*. Profile and prevalence of aspirin resistance in patients with cardiovascular disease. *Am J Cardiol* 2001; **88**: 230–235.

43 Wang JC, Aucoin-Barry D, Manuelian D, *et al*. Incidence of aspirin nonresponsiveness using the Ultegra Rapid Platelet Function Assay-ASA. *Am J Cardiol* 2003; **92**: 1492–1494.

44 Grundmann K, Jaschonek K, Kleine B, Dichgans J, Topka H. Aspirin non-responder status in patients with recurrent cerebral ischemic attacks. *J Neurol* 2003; **250**: 63–66.

45 Mueller MR, Salat A, Stangl P, *et al*. Variable platelet response to low-dose ASA and the risk of limb deterioration in patients submitted to peripheral arterial angioplasty. *Thromb Haemost* 1997; **78**: 1003–1007.

46 Andersen K, Hurlen M, Arnesen H, Seljeflot I. Aspirin non-responsiveness as measured by PFA-100 in patients with coronary artery disease. *Thromb Res* 2002; **108**: 37–42.

47 Gum PA, Kottke-Marchant K, Welsh PA, White J, Topol EJ. A prospective, blinded determination of the natural history of aspirin resistance among stable patients with cardiovascular disease. *J Am Coll Cardiol* 2003; **41**: 961–965.

48 Chen WH, Lee PY, Ng W, Tse HF, Lau CP. Aspirin resistance is associated with a high incidence of myonecrosis after non-urgent percutaneous coronary intervention despite clopidogrel pretreatment. *J Am Coll Cardiol* 2004; **43**: 1122–1126.

49 Lev EI, Patel RT, Maresh KJ, *et al*. Aspirin and clopidogrel drug response in patients undergoing percutaneous coronary intervention: the role of dual drug resistance. *J Am Coll Cardiol* 2006; **47**: 27–33.

50 Marcucci R, Paniccia R, Antonucci E, *et al*. Usefulness of aspirin resistance after percutaneous coronary intervention for acute myocardial infarction in predicting one-year major adverse coronary events. *Am J Cardiol* 2006; **98**: 1156–1159.

51 Hobikoglu GF, Norgaz T, Aksu H, *et al*. The effect of acetylsalicylic acid resistance on prognosis of patients who have developed acute coronary syndrome during acetylsalicylic acid therapy. *Can J Cardiol* 2007; **23**: 207–208.

52 Chen WH, Cheng X, Lee PY, *et al*. Aspirin resistance and adverse clinical events in patients with coronary artery Disease. *Am J Med* 2007; **120**: 631–635.

53 Dorsch MP, Lee JS, Lynch DR, *et al*. Aspirin resistance in patients with stable coronary artery disease with and without a history of myocardial infarction. *Ann Pharmacother* 2007; **41**: 737–741.

54 Buch AN, Singh S, Javaid A, *et al*. Measuring aspirin resistance, clopidogrel responsiveness, and postprocedural markers of myonecrosis in patients undergoing percutaneous coronary intervention. *Am J Cardiol* 2007; **99**: 1518–1522.

55 Pettersen AA, Seljeflot I, Abdelnoor M, Arnesen H. Unstable angina, stroke, myocardial infarction and death in aspirin non-responders. A prospective, randomized trial. The ASCET (ASpirin non-responsiveness and Clopidogrel Endpoint Trial) design. *Scand Cardiovasc J* 2004; **38**: 353–356.

Chapter 5

P2Y$_{12}$ inhibitors: Thienopyridines and direct oral inhibitors

Jean-Philippe Collet, Boris Aleil, Christian Gachet and
Gilles Montalescot

Introduction

Among the multiple mediators of platelet activation, adenosine diphosphate (ADP) has key effects on both physiological hemostasis and thrombosis. After platelet activation, ADP is released from platelet intracellular storage granules to further activate platelets through binding to several receptors on the platelet membrane. The thienopyridines derivatives are metabolized in the liver to compounds which covalently bind to ADP P2Y$_{12}$ receptor leading to an irreversible inhibition.

Ticlopidine is the first-generation thienopyridine, which, in combination with aspirin, has shown to be beneficial and superior to oral anticoagulants in preventing thrombotic complications after coronary stenting. Clopidogrel, a second-generation thienopyridine with similar efficacy, has largely replaced ticlopidine due to its better tolerability profiles and is the antiplatelet treatment of choice for prevention of stent thrombosis. The spectrum of clinical benefit of clopidogrel includes percutaneous coronary intervention (PCI) and unstable coronary artery disease irrespective of management strategy. New competitors are emerging and agents in development are being evaluated in large-scale, randomized clinical trials. Prasugrel is a novel, orally active, third-generation thienopyridine with greater *in vivo* antiplatelet potency compared to clopidogrel, reflecting more efficient *in vivo* generation of active metabolites. AZD6140 is a reversible, non-thienopyridine, oral P2Y$_{12}$ receptor antagonist. It has been shown to provide greater and more consistent inhibition of platelet

Antiplatelet Therapy in Ischemic Heart Disease, 1st edition. Edited by Stephen D. Wiviott.
© 2009 American Heart Association, ISBN: 9-781-4051-7626-2

aggregation than clopidogrel. This chapter reviews the different oral $P2Y_{12}$ receptor antagonists.

The $P2Y_{12}$ receptor: A complex target?

ADP is a central mediator of platelet activation and plays a crucial role in the physiological process of hemostasis and in the development and extension of arterial thrombosis [1,2]. Adenine nucleotides are present in very high concentrations inside platelet dense granules and are released when platelets are exposed to thrombin, collagen or thromboxane A_2 (TXA_2) [3]. Two G protein-coupled receptors, $P2Y_1$ and $P2Y_{12}$, mediate the effects of ADP on platelets. Platelets also express a non-selective cation channel, the $P2X_1$ receptor, triggered by ATP. Each of these receptors has a selective role during platelet activation, which has implications for their role in thrombosis [4].

The $P2Y_1$ receptor, coupled to $G\alpha q$, triggers calcium mobilization from internal stores resulting in platelet shape change and weak and transient aggregation in response to ADP. Studies in $P2Y_1$-deficient mice or the use of selective $P2Y_1$ receptor antagonists have demonstrated the role of this receptor in various models of experimental thrombosis [5–7]. The $P2X_1$ receptor also plays a role in platelet shape change and in platelet activation by collagen. Its role in experimental thrombosis has also been reported [8].

However, to date, only the $P2Y_{12}$ receptor has been the target of antithrombotic drugs in clinical use. This receptor, previously named $P2T_{AC}$, $P2_{CYC}$ or $P2Y_{ADP}$, was cloned in 2001 [9,10]. Its tissue distribution is restricted to platelets and subregions of the brain, which makes it an attractive target for selective antiplatelet drugs. Much of our knowledge about this receptor accumulated long before its actual identification. Numerous studies, using ticlopidine and clopidogrel as well as the ATP analogues such as AR-C69931MX (cangrelor), established the role of this receptor in the amplification of platelet activation, the stabilization of platelet aggregation and thrombosis [11]. The $P2Y_{12}$ receptor is coupled to the $G\alpha_{i2}$ G protein subunit [12]. Downstream of $G\alpha_{i2}$, several signaling pathways are involved in the amplification mechanism. First, the inhibition of cyclic adenosine monophosphate (cAMP) production, although not sufficient to trigger platelet aggregation, has a facilitating effect on activation [13,14] by inhibition of the cAMP-dependent protein kinase (PKA)-mediated phosphorylation of the vasodilator-stimulated phosphoprotein (VASP). VASP is an actin regulatory protein and a negative modulator of the $\alpha IIb\beta 3$ integrin activation [15–17]. Thus, levels of VASP phosphorylation/ dephosphorylation reflect $P2Y_{12}$ inhibition/activation state, which constitutes a sensitive marker to identify the effects of $P2Y_{12}$ antagonists [18,19]. Secondly, $P2Y_{12}$ has been shown to stimulate phosphatidyl inositol-3 kinase (PI-3K) activity, which is important to sustain aggregation [20,21]. In addition, $P2Y_{12}$ is known to activate the small GTPase Rap1b through a PI-3K dependent mechanism

[22–25]. These multiple pathways triggered by P2Y$_{12}$ explain why this receptor is required for completion of aggregation in response to ADP [26] and for the ADP-dependent amplification of platelet aggregation induced by agents such as the Gαq-coupled serotonin receptor 5HT$_{2A}$ [27] or the Gαq and G$_{12/13}$-coupled TXA$_2$ and PAR-1 receptors [28,29]. Similarly, the P2Y$_{12}$ receptor is an important cofactor of platelet aggregation and secretion induced by cross-linking FcγRIIa receptor with specific antibodies or by serum from patients with heparin-induced thrombocytopenia [30–34], or when platelets are activated by collagen through the GPVI/tyrosine kinase/PLCγ2 pathway [35]. The P2Y$_{12}$ receptor is also involved in potentiation of platelet secretion [36,37]. Finally, the P2Y$_{12}$ receptor is involved in the procoagulant activity of platelets through phosphatidyl serine exposure at the surface of platelets [38–41]. Thus, overall, the P2Y$_{12}$ receptor appears to be a key mediator or platelet function by serving as the target of ADP in amplification of platelet activation induced by low concentrations of agonists such as TXA$_2$, thrombin, collagen, chemokines or immune complexes.

Patients with congenital selective defect of ADP-induced platelet aggregation were shown to display a mild to severe bleeding diathesis comparable to a "clopidogrel-like" syndrome and mutated P2Y$_{12}$ receptor genes resulting in absence of protein expression or expression of a dysfunctional receptor [9,37,42–45].

The central role of the P2Y$_{12}$ receptor in experimental thrombosis has been established in a number of studies using the thienopyridine compounds or ATP analogues of the ARC or, more recently, taking advantage of the generation of P2Y$_{12}$ knock out mice. Consistent across models and species, blocking the P2Y$_{12}$ receptor results in inhibition of experimental thrombosis, which underlines its prominent role and its relevance as a key target for efficient antithrombotic therapy [46,47].

P2Y$_{12}$ receptor blockade acts early in the cascade of events leading to the formation of the platelet thrombus and effectively inhibits platelet aggregation. In fact, platelet P2Y$_{12}$ blockade prevents platelet degranulation and the release reaction, thereby inhibiting elaboration of prothrombotic and inflammatory mediators from the platelet, and also inhibits the transformation of the GP IIb/IIIa receptor to the form that binds fibrinogen and links platelets (Figure 5.1).

Thienopyridines: A heterogeneous class

Mode of action of ticlopidine and clopidogrel

The active metabolites of orally administered thienopyridines, ticlopidine, clopidogrel and prasugrel, irreversibly antagonize the platelet P2Y$_{12}$ adenosine diphosphate (ADP) receptor and inhibit selectively and irreversibly ADP-induced platelet activation and aggregation [48]. Thienopyridines are inactive

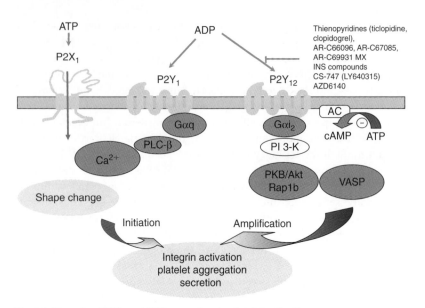

Fig. 5.1 The role of P2Y$_1$ and P2Y$_{12}$ receptors in platelet activation.

prodrugs and the active moiety of their active metabolites is a reactive thiol derivative that targets P2Y$_{12}$ on platelets (Figure 5.2). Although ticlopidine was discovered more than 30 years ago, it was only recently that the mechanism of action of ADP-receptor antagonists was characterized in detail. Ticlopidine was largely replaced by clopidogrel because the additional methoxycarbonyl

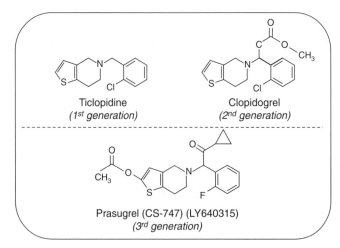

Fig. 5.2 Thienopyridine structures.

group on the benzylic position of the clopidogrel molecule provided increased pharmacological activity and a better safety and tolerability profile as compared with ticlopidine.

The prodrug clopidogrel requires oxidation by the hepatic cytochrome P450 (CYP) system to generate active metabolites. However, more than 85% of the prodrug is hydrolyzed by esterases in the blood to an inactive carboxylic acid derivative, and only <15% of the prodrug is metabolized by the cytochrome P 450 (CYP) system in the liver to generate an active metabolite. In particular, the thiophene ring of clopidogrel is oxidized to form an intermediate metabolite (2-oxo-clopidogrel), which is further oxidized, resulting in the opening of the thiophene ring and the formation of a carboxyl and thiol group (Figure 5.3). The reactive thiol group of the active metabolite of clopidogrel forms a disulfide bridge between one or more cysteine residues of the P2Y$_{12}$ receptor. This interaction is irreversible, accounting for the observation that platelets are inhibited, even if no active metabolite is detectable in plasma. This results in inhibition of the binding of the P2Y$_{12}$ agonist 2-methylthio-ADP and the ADP-induced downregulation of adenylyl cyclase. Platelet aggregation is affected not only when triggered by ADP but also by other substances requiring released ADP as an amplifier.

Clinical utility

Two major clinical trials have established the superiority of ticlopidine over aspirin in patients with TIA/stroke [49,50] but also over placebo in patients

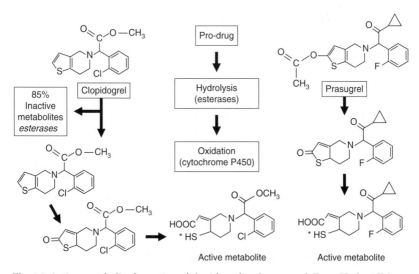

Fig. 5.3 Active metabolite formation of clopidogrel and prasugrel. From Herbert JM *et al. Sem Vasc Med* 2003; **3**: 113–122.

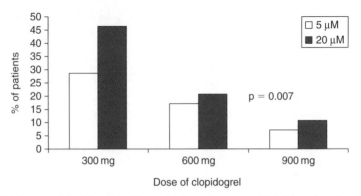

Fig. 5.4 Impact of clopidogrel loading on biological response. Definition of a suboptimal responder was IPA <10% at 6 hours. From Montalescot G *et al. J Am Coll Cardiol* 2006; **48**: 931–938 [56].

with recent history of major ischemic cerebral event related to atherosclerosis [49] and in patients with Peripheral Artery Disease (PAD). The CAPRIE mega trial has established the superiority of clopidogrel over aspirin in patients with symptomatic atherothrombosis. Dual oral antiplatelet therapy has become a standard of care for patients with acute coronary syndromes (ACS) and for patients undergoing percutaneous coronary intervention (PCI) with stenting. In these particular setting, clopidogrel has largely replaced ticlopidine due to its proven better tolerability profiles [51] and is currently the antiplatelet treatment of choice in combination with aspirin for prevention of stent thrombosis [52]. The long-term clinical benefit associated with dual antiplatelet therapy has been observed overall in patients with ACS, independent of clinical presentation and use or mode of coronary revascularization [53,54]. However, recurrent cardiovascular events remain with dual oral antiplatelet therapy. One concern in this regard has been the variable antiplatelet response to clopidogrel with some subjects having a limited response, especially in the setting of PCI for unstable coronary artery disease (CAD) [55] (Chapter 6). The delayed onset of platelet inhibition after receiving a thienopyridine has also been identified as a clinical limitation. Enhancing loading with clopidogrel has been shown to reduce the rate of suboptimal responders (Figure 5.4) and to further decrease the release of troponin prior to PCI [56]. Another way to overcome the persistence of enhanced platelet reactivity despite the use of higher loading dose of clopidogrel is to use novel $P2Y_{12}$ inhibitors, including prasugrel and non-thienopyridine agents.

The third generation thienopyridine: Prasugrel

Prasugrel (2-acetoxy-5-(•-cyclopropylcarbonyl-2-fluorobenzyl)-4,5,6,7-tetrahydrothieno [3,2-c]pyridine) is a member of the thienopyridine class of oral platelet aggregation inhibitors. The antiplatelet action of prasugrel, like ticlopidine and clopidogrel, is due to irreversible and selective blockade of platelet P2Y$_{12}$ ADP receptors by its active metabolite R-138727.

A single oral administration of prasugrel produced a dose-related inhibition of platelet aggregation in rats that is approximately 10- and 100-fold more potent than that of clopidogrel and ticlopidine, respectively [57]. The antiaggregatory effect of this agent was evident at 30 minutes and lasted until 72 hours after dosing, indicating fast onset and long duration of action. Prasugrel showed more potent antithrombotic activity compared with clopidogrel and ticlopidine with the same rank order as the antiaggregatory potencies. Combined administration of prasugrel with aspirin to rats produced substantially greater inhibition of both platelet aggregation and thrombus formation compared with each agent alone.

In phase I studies, a single oral dose of prasugrel produced >50% inhibition of ADP-induced platelet aggregation, with rapid onset (1 hour) and long duration (>48 hours) of action. In healthy volunteers, once-daily administration of 10 mg of prasugrel for 10 days showed significant cumulative inhibition of platelet aggregation from 2 days after the first dose until at least 2 days after the final dose. A double-blind, placebo-controlled trial was designed to evaluate the pharmacodynamics, pharmacokinetics, safety and tolerability of prasugrel, versus clopidogrel during multiple oral dosing in healthy subjects. Inhibition of ADP-induced platelet aggregation reached steady state by day 3 following prasugrel 10 and 20 mg compared with 5 days for clopidogrel 75 mg or prasugrel 5 mg. Compared with clopidogrel 75 mg, prasugrel 10 mg and 20 mg daily for 10 days resulted in more rapid, more consistent and higher levels of platelet inhibition [58]. In stable aspirin-treated patients with CAD, prasugrel (40–60 mg loading dose and 10–15 mg maintenance dose) has been shown to achieve greater inhibition of platelet aggregation (IPA) and a lower proportion of pharmacodynamic non-responders compared with the approved clopidogrel dosing (Figure 5.5) [59].

The greater *in vivo* antiplatelet potency of prasugrel compared to clopidogrel has been shown to reflect more efficient *in vivo* generation of its active metabolite (Figure 5.6). Indeed, both active metabolites of prasugrel and of clopidogrel display similar *in vitro* activity (Figure 5.6). These later findings further suggest that the limiting step for maximal effect of thienopyridine in general and clopidogrel in particular is not bioavailability but biotransformation [60].

Studies conducted to date indicate that prasugrel is a highly effective antiplatelet and antithrombotic agent [61]. In the Joint Utilization of Medications to Block Platelets Optimally-Thrombolysis In Myocardial Infarction 26 (JUMBO-TIMI 26), a phase 2, randomized, dose-ranging, double-blind safety trial of different prasugrel regimens versus standard dosing with clopidogrel in 904 patients undergoing elective or urgent percutaneous coronary intervention, have shown no significant difference in the primary safety endpoint (TIMI

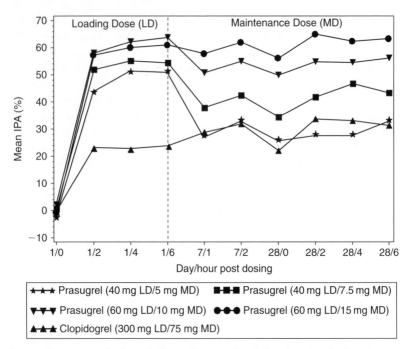

Fig. 5.5 Comparative biological effects of prasugrel and clopidogrel in CAD patients treated with aspirin – inhibition of platelet aggregation induced by 20 mM ADP. From Jernberg T *et al. Eur Heart J* 2006; **27**: 1166–1173.

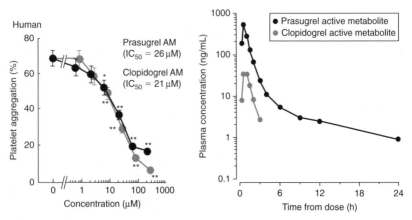

PRP = Platelet-Rich Plasma.

Fig. 5.6 Comparative biological efficacy of active metabolites of prasugrel and clopidogrel – *in vitro* antiplatelet effects of active metabolites in platelet-rich plasma. *$P < 0.05$; **$p < 0.01$ vs. control. From Ogawa T *et al.* Presented at ESC 2005.

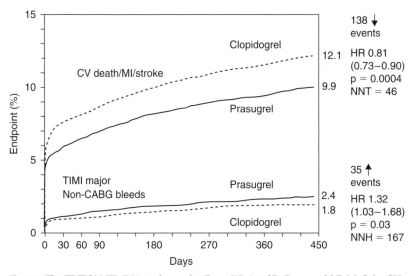

Fig. 5.7 The TRITON-TIMI 38 study results. From Wiviott SD, Braunwald E, McCabe CH *et al. New Eng J Med* 2007 [63].

major plus minor non-CABG-related bleeding events) [62]. In addition, in prasugrel-treated patients, there were numerically lower incidences of the primary efficacy composite end point (30-day major adverse cardiac events) and of the secondary end points, myocardial infarction, recurrent ischemia and clinical target vessel thrombosis. This trial served as a foundation for the large phase 3 clinical trial designed to assess both efficacy and safety, the Trial to Assess Improvement in Therapeutic Outcomes by Optimizing Platelet Inhibition with Prasugrel–Thrombolysis in Myocardial Infarction (TRITON–TIMI) 38 study (Figure 5.7).

The TRITON–TIMI 38 study included patients across the spectrum of ACS including (UA/NSTEMI and STEMI) with planned PCI; 13,608 patients were enrolled and randomized to receive a loading dose of prasugrel 60 mg followed by 10 mg daily or 300 mg of clopidogrel followed by 75 mg daily for 6 to 15 months. The primary efficacy endpoint was cardiovascular death, non-fatal myocardial infarction and non-fatal stroke. Patients randomized to prasugrel had a 19% lower rate of the composite endpoint than those receiving clopidogrel (9.9% vs. 12.1%, HR 0.81, P = 0.0004, Figure 5.7) [63]. Prasugrel also reduced stent thrombosis by more than 50%, a finding that was robust regardless of stent type used [64]. However, the beneficial effects seen as a reduction of ischemic events was accompanied by an increase in the key safety endpoint of TIMI major bleeding not related to coronary artery bypass surgery with prasugrel compared to clopidogrel (1.8 vs. 2.4%, HR 1.32, P = 0.03, Figure 5.7). In addition to establishing the efficacy and safety relationship between prasugrel and clopidogrel, the TRITON–TIMI 38 study served as a key proof of concept study that more rapid, consistent and greater inhibition of the $P2Y_{12}$ receptor resulted in a reduction of ischemic events.

Oral reversible $P2Y_{12}$ receptor antagonists

The oral, reversible $P2Y_{12}$ receptor antagonist AZD6140 is the first of a new chemical class of antiplatelet agents, the cyclopentyltriazolopyrimidines (Figure 5.8). Like the thienopyridines, AZD6140 blocks the platelet $P2Y_{12}$ receptor to inhibit ADP's prothrombotic effects. However, unlike the thienopyridines, this effect is reversible. This agent allows for a nearly complete inhibition of ADP-induced platelet aggregation *ex vivo* and as a direct-acting compound does not require any metabolic activation. AZD6140 has one known active metabolite, namely the AR-C126910 that is present in blood at about one-third the concentration of the parent in studies in healthy volunteers. This metabolite is approximately as potent as AZD6140 at blocking the $P2Y_{12}$ receptor *in vitro* and is thought to contribute to antiplatelet effects after oral dosing with AZD6140. When given orally as single oral doses of 100–400 mg, AZD6140 display a linear pharmacokinetics profile and provide a rapid onset of action (within 2 hours) and a more rapid offset of effect with a lessening of inhibition over the 24-hour post-dose period [65].

A randomized, double blind, parallel-group study has been conducted to assess the pharmacodynamics, pharmacokinetics, safety and tolerability of AZD6140 with aspirin relative to those of clopidogrel with aspirin in patients with atherosclerotic disease. A range of AZD6140 doses was assessed with the aim of identifying doses for further investigation in larger clinical studies (50–400 mg) [66]. AZD6140 100 mg b.i.d., 200 mg b.i.d. and 400 mg q.d. rapidly and nearly completely inhibited $P2Y_{12}$-mediated platelet aggregation as measured by optical aggregometry after initial dosing and at steady state. These

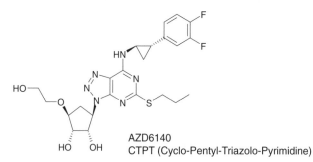

AZD6140
CTPT (Cyclo-Pentyl-Triazolo-Pyrimidine)

Fig. 5.8 Chemical structure of AZD 6140.

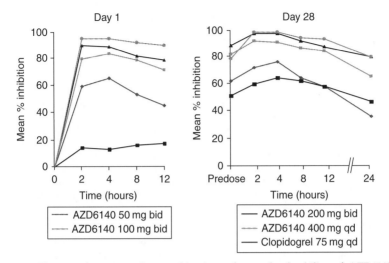

Fig. 5.9 Pharmacodynamics, pharmacokinetics, safety and tolerability of AZD6140. DISPERSE final extent of inhibition of platelet aggregation (IPA) on day 1 and day 28. From Husted S *et al. Eur Heart J* 2006; **27**: 1038–1047.

three doses of AZD6140 were also associated with greater steady-state IPA than AZD6140 50 mg b.i.d. or clopidogrel 75 mg q.d. (Figure 5.9). Of importance, no loading doses of AZD6140 and clopidogrel were administered in this study. AZD6140 was generally well tolerated with only a single major bleeding event in a patient receiving 400 mg q.d. Other reported side effects include dyspnea and, rarely, bradycardia or cardiac pauses.

In the randomized DISPERSE-2 trial, patients with unstable coronary artery disease were assigned to receive AZD6140 90 mg and 300 mg after a loading dose of 270 mg. This was compared to a standard regimen of clopidogrel including 300 mg loading and 75 mg maintenance dose (Figure 5.10). Both AZD6140 dose regimens provided a significant better inhibition of platelet aggregation both at 4 hours post-loading and at steady state, with a similar tolerance profile as compared to clopidogrel.

Figure 5.11 shows the pattern of IPA according to different type of dosing for both AZD6140 and prasugrel as compared to clopidogrel.

In the ongoing PLATO randomized trial, AZD6140 a dose regimen of 180 mg followed by 90 b.i.d. do is being compared to the standard regimen of clopidogrel 300/75 in moderate to high-risk ACS patients (Figure 5.12).

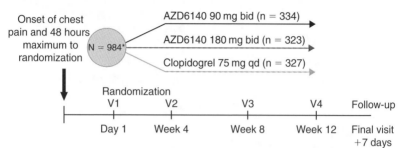

- All patients received aspirin (≤325 mg first dose, then 75–100 mg qd) and heparin/LMWH and/or GP IIb//IIIa inhibition
  - 50% of AZD6140 patients in each arm received a 270 mg loading dose
  - In the clopidogrel group, thienopyridine-naïve patients received a 300 mg loading dose

Fig. 5.10 Comparison of different dose regimens of prasugrel loading and maintenance dose DISPERSE 2 study design with standard regimen of clopidogrel. *Randomized patients who received ≥1 dose of the study drug. GP = glycoprotein; LMWH = low molecular weight heparin. From Cannon CP *et al. J Am Coll Cardiol* 2006; **47** (Suppl. A): 119A (abstract 974-242).

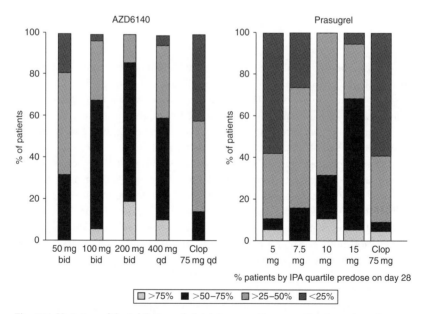

Fig. 5.11 Variation of the inhibition of platelet aggregation according to various dose regimens of AZD6140 as compared to a standard regimen of clopidogrel. Adapted from Husted S *et al. Eur Heart J* 2006; **27**: 1038–1047 and Jernberg T *et al. Eur Heart J* 2006; **27**: 1166–1173.

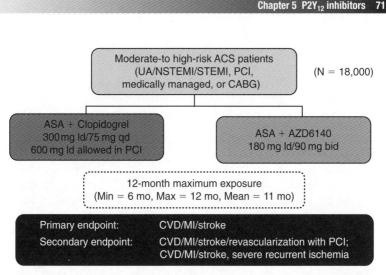

Fig. 5.12 PLATO study design. ASA = acetylsalicylic acid; bid = twice daily; CVD = cardiovascular disease; ld = loading dose; MI = myocardial infarction; NSTEMI = non-ST-segment elevation MI; qd = once daily; STEMI = ST-segment elevation MI; UA = unstable angina. Clinical Trials.gov Identifier: NCT00391872.

Conclusions and future directions

The P2Y$_{12}$ receptor has proven to be a key target in the prevention of complications associated with atherosclerotic vascular disease. Three generations of thienopyridines – ticlopidine, clopidogrel and prasugrel – have proven efficacy in the prevention of ischemic vascular events but with increased bleeding. Ongoing study of non-thienopyridine P2Y$_{12}$ antagonists will help to determine whether these benefits are limited to one class of agents or generalizable to antagonists of this receptor. Future rational use of these agents will require attention to disease and patient features to strike the optimal balance of benefit to risk.

References

1 Born GV. Adenosine diphosphate as a mediator of platelet aggregation in vivo: an editorial view. *Circulation* 1985; **72**: 741–746.
2 Maffrand JP, Bernat A, Delebassée D, Defreyn G, Cazenave JP, Gordon JL. ADP plays a key role in thrombogenesis in rats. *Thromb Haemost* 1988; **59**: 225–230.
3 Gachet C. Regulation of platelet functions by P2 receptors. *Annu Rev Pharmacol Toxicol* 2006; **46**: 277–300.
4 Gachet C, Hechler B. The platelet P2 receptors in thrombosis. *Semin Thromb Haemost* 2005; **31**: 162–167.
5 Hechler B, Nonne C, Roh EJ, Cattaneo M, Cazenave JP, Lanza F, Jacobson KA, Gachet C. MRS2500 [2-iodo-N6-methyl-(N)-methanocarba-2′-deoxyadenosine-3′,5′-bisphosphate],

a potent, selective, and stable antagonist of the platelet P2Y1 receptor with strong antithrombotic activity in mice. *J Pharmacol Exp Ther* 2006; **316**: 556–563.

6 Leon C, Freund M, Ravanat C, Baurand A, Cazenave JP, Gachet C. Key role of the P2Y(1) receptor in tissue factor-induced thrombin-dependent acute thromboembolism: studies in P2Y(1)-knockout mice and mice treated with a P2Y(1) antagonist. *Circulation* 2001; **103**: 718–723.

7 Léon C, Hechler B, Freund M, Eckly A, Vial C, Ohlmann P, Dierich A, LeMeur M, Cazenave JP, Gachet C. Defective platelet aggregation and increased resistance to thrombosis in purinergic P2Y(1) receptor-null mice. *J Clin Invest* 1999; **104**: 1731–1737.

8 Hechler B, Lenain N, Marchese P, Vial C, Heim V, Freund M, Cazenave JP, Cattaneo M, Ruggeri ZM, Evans R, Gachet C. A role of the fast ATP-gated P2X1 cation channel in thrombosis of small arteries in vivo. *J Exp Med* 2003; **198**: 661–667.

9 Hollopeter G, Jantzen HM, Vincent D, Li G, England L, Ramakrishnan V, Yang RB, Nurden P, Nurden A, Julius D, Conley PB. Identification of the platelet ADP receptor targeted by antithrombotic drugs. *Nature* 2001; **409**: 202–207.

10 Zhang FL, Luo L, Gustafson E, Lachowicz J, Smith M, Qiao X, Liu YH, Chen G, Pramanik B, Laz TM, Palmer K, Bayne M, Monsma FJ, Jr. ADP is the cognate ligand for the orphan G protein-coupled receptor SP1999. *J Biol Chem* 2001; **276**: 8608–8615.

11 Gachet C. ADP receptors of platelets and their inhibition. *Thromb Haemost* 2001; **86**: 222–232.

12 Ohlmann P, Laugwitz KL, Nurnberg B, Spicher K, Schultz G, Cazenave JP, Gachet C. The human platelet ADP receptor activates Gi2 proteins. *Biochem J* 1995; **312**: 775–779.

13 Haslam RJ. Interactions of the pharmacological receptors of blood platelets with adenylate cyclase. *Ser Haematol* 1973; **6**: 333–350.

14 Savi P, Pflieger AM, Herbert JM. cAMP is not an important messenger for ADP-induced platelet aggregation. *Blood Coagul Fibrinolysis* 1996; **7**: 249–252.

15 Horstrup K, Jablonka B, Honig-Liedl P, Just M, Kochsiek K, Walter U. Phosphorylation of focal adhesion vasodilator-stimulated phosphoprotein at Ser157 in intact human platelets correlates with fibrinogen receptor inhibition. *Eur J Biochem* 1994; **225**: 21–27.

16 Hauser W, Knobeloch KP, Eigenthaler M, Gambaryan S, Krenn V, Geiger J, Glazova M, Rohde E, Horak I, Walter U, Zimmer M. Megakaryocyte hyperplasia and enhanced agonist-induced platelet activation in vasodilator-stimulated phosphoprotein knockout mice. *Proc Natl Acad Sci USA* 1999; **96**: 8120–8125.

17 Waldmann R, Nieberding M, Walter U. Vasodilator-stimulated protein phosphorylation in platelets is mediated by cAMP- and cGMP-dependent protein kinases. *Eur J Biochem* 1987; **167**: 441–448.

18 Schwarz UR, Geiger J, Walter U, Eigenthaler M. Flow cytometry analysis of intracellular VASP phosphorylation for the assessment of activating and inhibitory signal transduction pathways in human platelets–definition and detection of ticlopidine/clopidogrel effects. *Thromb Haemost* 1999; **82**: 1145–1152.

19 Leil B, Ravanat C, Cazenave JP, Rochoux G, Heitz A, Gachet C. Flow cytometric analysis of intraplatelet VASP phosphorylation for the detection of clopidogrel resistance in patients with ischemic cardiovascular diseases. *J Thromb Haemost* 2005; **3**: 85–92.

20 Trumel C, Payrastre B, Plantavid M, Hechler B, Viala C, Presek P, Martinson EA, Cazenave JP, Chap H, Gachet C. A key role of adenosine diphosphate in the

irreversible platelet aggregation induced by the PAR1-activating peptide through the late activation of phosphoinositide 3-kinase. *Blood* 1999; **94**: 4156–4165.

21 Kauffenstein G, Bergmeier W, Eckly A, Ohlmann P, Léon C, Cazenave JP, Nieswandt B, Gachet C. The P2Y(12) receptor induces platelet aggregation through weak activation of the alpha(IIb)beta(3) integrin–a phosphoinositide 3- kinase-dependent mechanism. *FEBS Lett* 2001; **505**: 281–290.

22 Lova P, Paganini S, Sinigaglia F, Balduini C, Torti M. A Gi-dependent pathway is required for activation of the small GTPase Rap1B in human platelets. *J Biol Chem* 2002; **277**: 12009–12015.

23 Lova P, Paganini S, Hirsch E, Barberis L, Wymann M, Sinigaglia F, Balduini C, Torti M. A selective role for phosphatidylinositol 3,4,5-trisphosphate in the Gi-dependent activation of platelet Rap1B. *J Biol Chem* 2003; **278**: 131–138.

24 Woulfe D, Jiang H, Mortensen R, Yang J, Brass LF. Activation of Rap1B by G(i) family members in platelets. *J Biol Chem* 2002; **277**: 23382–23390.

25 Larson MK, Chen H, Kahn ML, Taylor AM, Fabre JE, Mortensen RM, Conley PB, Parise LV. Identification of P2Y$_{12}$-dependent and -independent mechanisms of glycoprotein VI-mediated Rap1 activation in platelets. *Blood* 2003; **101**: 1409–1415.

26 Hechler B, Eckly A, Ohlmann P, Cazenave JP, Gachet C. The P2Y1 receptor, necessary but not sufficient to support full ADP-induced platelet aggregation, is not the target of the drug clopidogrel. *Br J Haematol* 1998; **103**: 858–866.

27 Savi P, Beauverger P, Labouret C, Delfaud M, Salel V, Kaghad M, Herbert JM. Role of P2Y1 purinoceptor in ADP-induced platelet activation. *FEBS Lett* 1998; **422**: 291–295.

28 Nieswandt B, Schulte V, Zywietz A, Gratacap MP, Offermanns S. Costimulation of Gi- and G12/G13-mediated signaling pathways induces integrin alpha IIbbeta 3 activation in platelets. *J Biol Chem* 2002; **277**: 39493–39498.

29 Dorsam RT, Kim S, Jin J, Kunapuli SP. Coordinated signaling through both G12/13 and G(i) pathways is sufficient to activate GPIIb/IIIa in human platelets. *J Biol Chem* 2002; **277**: 47588–47595.

30 Polgar J, Eichler P, Greinacher A, Clemetson KJ. Adenosine diphosphate (ADP) and ADP receptor play a major role in platelet activation/aggregation induced by sera from heparin-induced thrombocytopenia patients. *Blood* 1998; **91**: 549–554.

31 Gratacap MP, Herault JP, Viala C, Ragab A, Savi P, Herbert JM, Chap H, Plantavid M, Payrastre B. FcgammaRIIA requires a Gi-dependent pathway for an efficient stimulation of phosphoinositide 3-kinase, calcium mobilization, and platelet aggregation. *Blood* 2000; **96**: 3439–3446.

32 Saci A, Pain S, Rendu F, Bachelot-Loza C. Fc receptor-mediated platelet activation is dependent on phosphatidylinositol 3-kinase activation and involves p120(Cbl). *J Biol Chem* 1999; **274**: 1898–1904.

33 Gratacap MP, Payrastre B, Viala C, Mauco G, Plantavid M, Chap H. Phosphatidylinositol 3,4,5-trisphosphate-dependent stimulation of phospholipase C-gamma2 is an early key event in FcgammaRIIA-mediated activation of human platelets. *J Biol Chem* 1998; **273**: 24314–24321.

34 Chacko GW, Brandt JT, Coggeshall KM, Anderson CL. Phosphoinositide 3-kinase and p72syk noncovalently associate with the low affinity Fc gamma receptor on human platelets through an immunoreceptor tyrosine-based activation motif. Reconstitution with synthetic phosphopeptides. *J Biol Chem* 1996; **271**: 10775–10781.

35 Nieswandt B, Bergmeier W, Eckly A, Schulte V, Ohlmann P, Cazenave JP, Zirngibl H, Offermanns S, Gachet C. Evidence for cross-talk between glycoprotein VI and Gi-coupled receptors during collagen-induced platelet aggregation. *Blood* 2001; **97**: 3829–3835.

36 Cattaneo M, Lombardi R, Zighetti ML, Gachet C, Ohlmann P, Cazenave JP, Mannucci PM. Deficiency of (33P)2MeS-ADP binding sites on platelets with secretion defect, normal granule stores and normal thromboxane A2 production. Evidence that ADP potentiates platelet secretion independently of the formation of large platelet aggregates and thromboxane A2 production. *Thromb Haemost* 1997; **77**: 986–990.

37 Cattaneo M, Lecchi A, Lombardi R, Gachet C, Zighetti ML. Platelets from a patient heterozygous for the defect of P2CYC receptors for ADP have a secretion defect despite normal thromboxane A2 production and normal granule stores: further evidence that some cases of platelet 'primary secretion defect' are heterozygous for a defect of P2CYC receptors. *Arterioscler Thromb Vasc Biol* 2000; **20**: E101–106.

38 Léon C, Freund M, Ravanat C, Baurand A, Cazenave JP, Gachet C. Key role of the P2Y(1) receptor in tissue factor-induced thrombin- dependent acute thromboembolism: studies in P2Y(1)-knockout mice and mice treated with a P2Y(1) antagonist. *Circulation* 2001; **103**: 718–723.

39 Léon C, Ravanat C, Freund M, Cazenave JP, Gachet C. Differential involvement of the $P2Y_1$ and $P2Y_{12}$ receptors in platelet procoagulant activity. *Arterioscler Thromb Vasc Biol* 2003; **23**: 1941–1947.

40 Dorsam RT, Tuluc M, Kunapuli SP. Role of protease-activated and ADP receptor subtypes in thrombin generation on human platelets. *J Thromb Haemost* 2004; **2**: 804–812.

41 Storey RF, Sanderson HM, White AE, May JA, Cameron KE, Heptinstall S. The central role of the P(2T) receptor in amplification of human platelet activation, aggregation, secretion and procoagulant activity. *Br J Haematol* 2000; **110**: 925–934.

42 Cattaneo M, Lecchi A, Randi AM, McGregor JL, Mannucci PM. Identification of a new congenital defect of platelet function characterized by severe impairment of platelet responses to adenosine diphosphate. *Blood* 1992; **80**: 2787–2796.

43 Cattaneo M, Gachet C. ADP receptors and clinical bleeding disorders. *Arterioscler Thromb Vasc Biol* 1999; **19**: 2281–2285.

44 Cattaneo M, Zighetti ML, Lombardi R, Martinez C, Lecchi A, Conley PB, Ware J, Ruggeri ZM. Molecular bases of defective signal transduction in the platelet $P2Y_{12}$ receptor of a patient with congenital bleeding. *Proc Natl Acad Sci USA* 2003; **100**: 1978–1983.

45 Cattaneo M. The P2 receptors and congenital platelet function defects. *Semin Thromb Haemost* 2005; **31**: 168–173.

46 Andre P, Delaney SM, LaRocca T, Vincent D, DeGuzman F, Jurek M, Koller B, Phillips DR, Conley PB. $P2Y_{12}$ regulates platelet adhesion/activation, thrombus growth, and thrombus stability in injured arteries. *J Clin Invest* 2003; **112**: 398–406.

47 Andre P, LaRocca T, Delaney SM, Lin PH, Vincent D, Sinha U, Conley PB, Phillips DR. Anticoagulants (thrombin inhibitors) and aspirin synergize with $P2Y_{12}$ receptor antagonism in thrombosis. *Circulation* 2003; **108**: 2697–2703.

48 Savi P, Herbert JM. Clopidogrel and ticlopidine: $P2Y_{12}$ adenosine diphosphate-receptor antagonists for the prevention of atherothrombosis. *Semin Thromb Hemost* 2005; **31**: 174–183.

49 Gent M, Blakely JA, Easton JD, Ellis DJ, Hachinski VC, Harbison JW, Panak E, Roberts RS, Sicurella J, Turpie AG. The Canadian American Ticlopidine Study (CATS) in thromboembolic stroke. *Lancet* 1989; **1**: 1215–1220.

50 Hass WK, Easton JD, Adams HP, Pryse-Phillips W, Molony BA, Anderson S, Kamm B. A randomized trial comparing ticlopidine hydrochloride with aspirin for the prevention of stroke in high-risk patients. Ticlopidine Aspirin Stroke Study Group. *New Engl J Med* 1990; **322**: 404–405.

51 Bertrand ME, Rupprecht HJ, Urban P, Gershlick AH, CLASSICS Investigators. Double-blind study of the safety of clopidogrel with and without a loading dose in combination with aspirin compared with ticlopidine in combination with aspirin after coronary stenting: the clopidogrel aspirin stent international cooperative study (CLASSICS). *Circulation* 2000; **102**: 624–629.

52 Smith SC Jr, Allen J, Blair SN, Bonow RO, Brass LM, Fonarow GC, Grundy SM, Hiratzka L, Jones D, Krumholz HM, Mosca L, Pasternak RC, Pearson T, Pfeffer MA, Taubert KA. AHA/ACC guidelines for secondary prevention for patients with coronary and other atherosclerotic vascular disease: 2006 update: endorsed by the National Heart, Lung, and Blood Institute. *Circulation* 2006; **113**: 2363–2372.

53 Steinhubl SR, Berger S, Mann JT, Fry ETA, DeLago A, Wilmer C, Topol EJ, for the Credo Investigators. Early and sustained dual oral antiplatelet therapy following percutaneous coronary intervention. *JAMA* 2002; **288**: 2411.

54 CURE Investigators. Effects of clopidogrel in addition to aspirin in patients with acute coronary syndromes without ST-segment elevation. *N Eng J Med* 2001; **345**: 494–502.

55 Snoep SD, Hovens MMC, Eikenboom JCJ, van der Bom JG, Jukema JW, Huisman MV. Clopidogrel nonresponsiveness in patients undergoing percutaneous coronary intervention with stenting: A systematic review and meta-analysis. *Am Heart J* 2007; **154**: 220–231.

56 Montalescot G, Sideris G, Meuleman C, Bal-dit-Sollier C, Lellouche N, Steg PG, Slama M, Milleron O, Collet JP, Henry P, Beygui F, Drouet L. A randomized comparison of high clopidogrel loading doses in patients with non-ST-segment elevation acute coronary syndromes: the ALBION (Assessment of the Best Loading Dose of Clopidogrel to Blunt Platelet Activation, Inflammation and Ongoing Necrosis) trial. *J Am Coll Cardiol* 2006; **48**: 931–938.

57 Niitsu Y, Jakubowski JA, Sugidachi A, Asai F. Pharmacology of CS-747 (prasugrel, LY640315), a novel, potent antiplatelet agent with in vivo P2Y₁₂ receptor antagonist activity. *Semin Thromb Hemost* 2005; **31**: 184–194.

58 Jakubowski JA, Matsushima N, Asai F, Naganuma H, Brandt JT, Hirota T, Freestone S, Winters KJ. A multiple dose study of prasugrel (CS-747), a novel thienopyridine P2Y₁₂ inhibitor, compared with clopidogrel in healthy humans. *Br J Clin Pharmacol* 2007; **63**: 421–430.

59 ernberg T, Payne CD, Winters KJ, Darstein C, Brandt JT, Jakubowski JA, Naganuma H, Siegbahn A, Wallentin L. Prasugrel achieves greater inhibition of platelet aggregation and a lower rate of non-responders compared with clopidogrel in aspirin-treated patients with stable coronary artery disease. *Eur Heart J* 2006; **27**: 1166–1173.

60 Sugidachi A, Ogawa T, Kurihara A, Hagihara K, Jakubowski JA, Hashimoto M, Niitsu Y, Asai F. The greater in vivo antiplatelet effects of prasugrel compared to

clopidogrel reflect more efficient generation of its active metabolite with similar antiplatelet activity to clopidogrel's active metabolite. *J Thromb Haemost* 2007; **19**: 1545–1551.

61 Wiviott SD, Trenk D, Frelinger AL, O'Donoghue M, Neumann FJ, Michelson AD, Angiolillo DJ, Hod H, Montalescot G, Miller DL, Jakubowski JA, Cairns R, Murphy SA, McCabe CH, Antman EM, Braunwald E, for The PRINCIPLE-TIMI 44 Investigators. Prasugrel compared to high loading and maintenance dose clopidogrel in patients with planned percutaneous coronary intervention: the PRINCIPLE-TIMI 44 trial. *Circulation* 2007; **116**: 2923–2932.

62 Wiviott SD, Antman EM, Winters KJ, Weerakkody G, Murphy SA, Behounek BD, Carney RJ, Lazzam C, McKay RG, McCabe CH, Braunwald E, JUMBO-TIMI 26 Investigators. Randomized comparison of prasugrel (CS-747, LY640315), a novel thienopyridine P2Y$_{12}$ antagonist, with clopidogrel in percutaneous coronary intervention: results of the Joint Utilization of Medications to Block Platelets Optimally (JUMBO)-TIMI 26 trial. *Circulation* 2005; **111**: 3366–3373.

63 Wiviott SD, Braunwald E, McCabe CH, Montalescot G, Ruzyllo W, Gottlieb S, Neumann FJ, Ardissino D, De Servi S, Murphy SA, Riesmeyer J, Weerakkody G, Gibson CM, EM; A, the TRITON-TIMI 38 Investigators. Prasugrel versus clopidogrel in patients with acute coronary syndromes. *New Engl J Med* 2007; **357**: 2001–2015.

64 Wiviott SD, Braunwald E, McCabe CH, Horvath I, Keltai M, Herrman JP, Van de Werf F, Downey WE, Scirica BM, Murphy SA, Antman EM, TRITON-TIMI 38 Investigators. Intensive oral antiplatelet therapy for reduction of ischaemic events including stent thrombosis in patients with acute coronary syndromes treated with percutaneous coronary intervention and stenting in the TRITON-TIMI 38 trial: a sub-analysis of a randomised trial. *Lancet* 2008; **371**: 1353–1363.

65 Peters G, Robbie G. Single-dose pharmacokinetics and pharmacodynamics of AZD6140-an oral reversible ADP receptor antagonist (abstract). *Haematologica* 2004; **989** (Suppl. 7): 14.

66 Husted S, Emanuelsson H, Heptinstall S, Sandset PM, Wickens M, Peters G. Pharmacodynamics, pharmacokinetics, and safety of the oral reversible P2Y$_{12}$ antagonist AZD6140 with aspirin in patients with atherosclerosis: a double-blind comparison to clopidogrel with aspirin. *Eur Heart J* 2006; **27**: 1038–1047.

Chapter 6

Thienopyridine response variability and resistance

Udaya S. Tantry, Thomas A. Suarez and Paul A. Gurbel

Introduction

Platelet activation and aggregation are central to the development of athero-thrombotic complications of cardiovascular disease. Adenosine diphosphate (ADP) and thromboxane (TX) A2 are the major secondary agonists released by platelets [1]. These agonists play important roles in the amplification of platelet activation and aggregation and the generation of a stable thrombus at the site of plaque rupture (Figure 6.1). Dual antiplatelet therapy with a thienopyridine and aspirin has been demonstrated to be an effective strategy to prevent atherothrombotic complications in major clinical trials of acute coronary syndromes and coronary stenting [2] (Chapter 5). Despite significant benefits and wide-spread use of dual antiplatelet treatment, the continued occurrence of adverse ischemic events remains a serious clinical problem [3]. The current recommended dose of clopidogrel is based primarily on clinical trial results and not an assessment of the individual patient's response (a one size fits all principle) [2]. However, pharmacodynamic studies, based on the *ex vivo* measurement of ADP-induced platelet aggregation have revealed various limitations of clopidogrel therapy: (i) a delayed pharmacodynamic response; (ii) an overall modest degree of platelet inhibition (~30 to 50%); (iii) distinct response variability with a substantial percentage of patients exhibiting non-responsiveness or resistance; (iv) a potential influence of drug–drug interactions; and (v) the recent demonstration of an association between clinical adverse events including stent thrombosis and clopidogrel non-responsiveness [4].

Antiplatelet Therapy in Ischemic Heart Disease, 1st edition. Edited by Stephen D. Wiviott
© 2009 American Heart Association, ISBN: 9-781-4051-7626-2

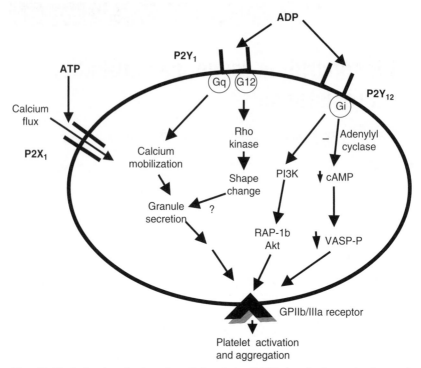

Fig. 6.1 Central role of adenosine diphosphate (ADP) in platelet activation and aggregation. There are 3 purinergic receptors in the platelet membrane; Binding of ADP to $P2Y_1$ results in shape change and intracellular calcium mobilization through Gq/G_{12} coupled intracellular signaling pathways. Binding of ADP to P2Y12 receptor leads to sustained platelet activation and aggregation through Gi coupled pathways. Binding of ATP to P2X1 affects calcium flux.
PI3K = phosphoionisitide-3-kinase , VASP-P = vasodilator stimulated phosphoprotein - phosphorylated
cAMP = cyclic adenosine monophophate

Mechanism of action

Clopidogrel is a prodrug that requires hepatic conversion to an active metabolite in order to block the $P2Y_{12}$ receptor. Clopidogrel is rapidly absorbed from the intestine. Approximately 85% of the drug is hydrolyzed to an inactive carboxylic acid metabolite (SR26334) by esterases. The remaining 15% of clopidogrel is first converted to 2-oxo-clopidogrel and subsequently to an active thiol metabolite, R-130964, by hepatic cytochrome P450 isoenzymes CYP3A4 and 3A5 and to a smaller extent by CYP2B6, 1A2, 2C9 and 2C19 [5,6]. The short-lived active metabolite permanently binds to the $P2Y_{12}$ receptor via a disulfide bridge between the reactive thiol group and two cysteine residues (Cys17 and Cys270) present in the extracellular domains of the $P2Y_{12}$ receptor [7]. The half-life of the platelet-bound clopidogrel metabolite was found to be 11 days as demonstrated by radioligand studies. Clopidogrel specifically inhibits ADP-induced platelet activation and aggregation and also less effectively inhibits collagen-, and thrombin-induced aggregation [8]. The effect of clopidogrel in the inhibition of platelet aggregation induced by latter agonists can be overcome by increased concentrations of the respective agonists. The latter evidence indicates the ability of clopidogrel to inhibit ADP-mediated amplification of the platelet response to multiple agonists. Clopidogrel does not have any effect on ADP binding to the $P2Y_1$ receptor or the platelet response to $P2Y_1$ activation that induces shape change and intracellular Ca^{+2} mobilization [9]. Clopidogrel has also been reported to attenuate platelet–leukocyte aggregate formation, and levels of C-reactive protein, P-selectin and CD-40L, as well as the rate of thrombin formation [8].

Clopidogrel resistance – definition

Platelet activation and aggregation involve multiple receptor signaling pathways. Therefore, it is unlikely that a single treatment strategy directed against a specific receptor will be able to overcome all thrombotic events. Thus, treatment failure should not be considered synonymous with drug resistance. The resistance or non-responsiveness to an antiplatelet agent can be defined as the failure of the antiplatelet agent to inhibit the target of its action. Clopidogrel resistance has been demonstrated by evidence of residual post-treatment $P2Y_{12}$ activity by measuring ADP-induced platelet aggregation [4]. Other assays detecting residual activity of $P2Y_{12}$ are shown in Table 6.1.

Laboratory evaluation of clopidogrel responsiveness

A standardized laboratory method, as well as definition for clopidogrel resistance, is still lacking. Since clopidogrel specifically inhibits one of two ADP receptors, ex vivo measurement of ADP-induced maximum platelet aggregation by light transmittance aggregometry (LTA) has been the most commonly used method [10]. However, the assessment of clopidogrel responsiveness by LTA may be affected by the anticoagulant (citrate or D-Phenylalanyl-L-prolyl-L-arginine chloromethyl ketone (PPACK)), the measurement of maximum or final aggregation, the occurrence of ex vivo platelet activation during preparation, the mandatory measurement of pre- and post-treatment platelet function, the use of a specific and standardized agonist and agonist concentration (e.g. 5 and 20 µM ADP). Although PPACK/hirudin and measurement of late aggregation were suggested to be better indicators of clopidogrel responsiveness in a small study, a subsequent study indicated that there were no significant differences in the assessment of clopidogrel non-responsiveness between studies conducted with citrate or PPACK. Moreover, the prevalence of

Table 6.1 Definition of clopidogrel nonresponsiveness and laboratory methods to study clopidogrel metabolism and responsiveness

No single pathway mediates all thrombotic events – there are multiple pathways of platelet activation

Antiplatelet drug non-responsivenes/resistance = failure to inhibit target

Antiplatelet drug non-responsivenes/resistance ≠ clinical failure

Clopidogrel non-responsiveness = ⩽10% absolute change in platelet aggregation
(baseline aggregation–post-treatment aggregation)

Laboratory methods to study clopidogrel metabolism [1,2] and responsiveness [3,4]

1. Plasma unchanged clopidogrel, active and inactive metabolites liquid chromatography/mass-spectroscopy

2. Hepatic CYP3A4 activity erythromycin breath test

3. Adenosine diphosphate-induced platelet aggregation light transmittance aggregation with platelet rich plasma

4. Adenosine diphosphate-induced P-selectin, active glycoprotein (GP) IIb/IIIa expression, and $P2Y_{12}$ receptor reactivity (phosphorylated vasodilator stimulated phosphoprotein levels) flow cytometry

5. Point-of-care assays thrombelastography (Platelet Mapping Assay); VerifyNow $P2Y_{12}$ assay with ADP as agonist

non-responsiveness was the same whether measured by maximum or late aggregation [11,12]. Flow cytometric measurements of the expression of the active GP IIb/IIIa receptor and P-selectin expression after ADP stimulation have also demonstrated wide response variability to clopidogrel [10].

In addition, measurements of ADP-induced platelet–fibrin clot strength by whole blood thrombelastography and the VerifyNow $P2Y_{12}$ receptor assay using ADP as the agonist have also been used to measure clopidogrel responsiveness as point-of-care assays and have been correlated with LTA [13,14]. However, the cutoff values for non-responsiveness and their relation to adverse clinical events have not been standardized in large studies. The PFA-100 method using collagen-ADP based cartridges and whole blood aggregometry are associated with inconsistent estimates of platelet reactivity to ADP [4].

The phosphorylation state of vasodilator-stimulated phosphoprotein is a specific intracellular marker of residual $P2Y_{12}$ receptor reactivity in patients treated with clopidogrel and can be measured by flow cytometry. This technique is perhaps the most specific indicator of residual $P2Y_{12}$ activity in patients treated with a $P2Y_{12}$ inhibitor. However, the methodology is labor intensive; requiring permeation of the platelet membrane and the use of monoclonal antibodies specific for phosporylated vasodilator-stimulated phosphoprotein [15].

Effect of time of treatment and dose on platelet responsiveness to clopidogrel

Response variability to clopidogrel treatment has been demonstrated mostly in patients undergoing coronary stenting [10,16–24] (Table 6.2). It has been demonstrated that the prevalence of clopidogrel non-responsiveness or resistance, defined as a ≤10% absolute change in *ex vivo* ADP-induced platelet aggregation by LTA from pre- to post-treatment, is dependent upon the loading dose and time when platelet function is assessed after treatment [10]. In the initial study demonstrating response variability to clopidogrel, patients undergoing stenting were treated with a 300-mg loading dose at the time of the procedure followed by a 75-mg/day maintenance dose; 53–63% of patients were resistant to clopidogrel treatment at 2 hours post-stenting; 31–35% were resistant at day 1 and day 5 post-stenting; 13–21% were resistant at day 30 post-stenting; and the response profile followed a normal distribution (Figure 6.2a and b). In a subsequent pharmacodynamic study, treatment with a 600-mg loading dose during elective stenting, reduced clopidogrel non-responsiveness to 8% compared to 28–32% after a 300-mg loading dose (Figure 6.3) [16]. Similar superior responsiveness to high dose clopidogrel treatment was demonstrated in other studies [22–24]. Finally, a 150-mg maintenance dose therapy was associated with increased platelet inhibition compared to the 75-mg maintenance dose [25].

Mechanism of clopidogrel resistance

The mechanisms responsible for clopidogrel response variability and resistance are incompletely defined. Clopidogrel treatment is associated with overall submaximal inhibition (30–50%) of ADP-induced platelet aggregation following either a clopidogrel maintenance dose or a loading dose. Recent studies have indicated incomplete active metabolite generation as the primary cause for response variability rather than receptor-related causes [4].

Functional and genetic variability in the hepatic cytochrome CYP3A has been reported as a cause of clopidogrel response variability [26]. Pharmacologic stimulation of CYP3A4 activity by rifampin enhances the inhibitory effect of clopidogrel, whereas agents that compete with clopidogrel for CYP 3A4 (e.g. erythromycin) attenuate the antiplatelet effect of clopidogrel [26]. In addition, cigarette smoking, possibly by the effect of nicotine as an inducer of CYP1A2 activity and St Johns Wort, an inducer of CYP3A4, have also been associated with enhanced clopidogrel responsiveness [27,28]. However, co-administration of lipophilic statins (that compete with clopidogrel for CYP3A4) such as atorvastatin or simvastatin have been shown to attenuate the platelet inhibitory effect of clopidogrel in pharmacodynamic studies [29]. Although, the lipophilic statin–clopidogrel interaction has not been definitively demonstrated in retrospective analyses of large scale clinical trials,

Table 6.2 Clopidogrel resistance studies

Investigators	n	Patients	Clopidogrel dose (mg, load/q.d.)	Definition of clopidogrel resistance	Time	Incidences
Gurbel et al. [10]	92	PCI	300/75	5 and 20 µM ADP-induced aggregation ≤10% absolute change	24 h	31–35%
Jaremo et al. [17]	18	PCI	300/75	ADP-induced fibrinogen binding <40% of baseline	24 h	28%
Muller et al. [18]	119	PCI	600/75	5 and 50 µM ADP-induced aggregation <10% relative change	4 h	5–11%
Mobely et al. [19]	50	PCI	300/75	1 µM ADP-induced aggregation, TEG and Ichor PW; <10% absolute inhibition	Pre and post	30%
Lepantalo et al. [20]	50	PCI	300/75	2 or 5 µM ADP- induced aggregation and PFA-100; 10% inhibition and 170s	2.5 h	40%
Matetzky et al. [38]	60	STEMI	300/75	5 µM ADP-induced aggregation and CPA <10% inhibition	Daily for 5 days	25%
Lev El et al. [21]	150	PCI	300	5 µM ADP-induced aggregation ≤10% absolute change	20–24 h	24%
Gurbel et al. [16]	190	PCI	300 or 600/75	5 and 20 µM ADP-induced aggregation <10% absolute change	24 h	28–32% with 300 mg 8% with 600 mg

PCI = percutaneous coronary interventions; ADP = adenosine diphosphate; CAD = coronary artery disease; TEG = thrombelastography; PW = Plateletworks; PFA-100 = Platelet function analyzer; CPA = Cone and platelet analyzer; STEMI = ST-segment elevation myocardial infarction.

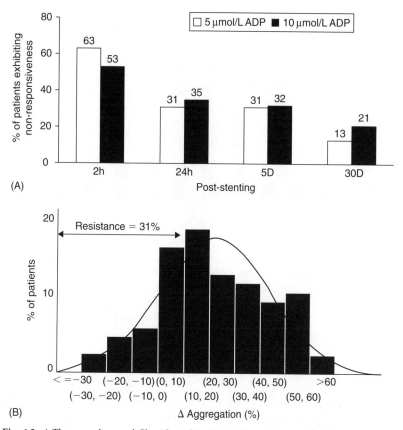

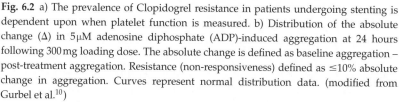

Fig. 6.2 a) The prevalence of Clopidogrel resistance in patients undergoing stenting is dependent upon when platelet function is measured. b) Distribution of the absolute change (Δ) in 5μM adenosine diphosphate (ADP)-induced aggregation at 24 hours following 300mg loading dose. The absolute change is defined as baseline aggregation – post-treatment aggregation. Resistance (non-responsiveness) defined as $\leq$10% absolute change in aggregation. Curves represent normal distribution data. (modified from Gurbel et al.[10])

a trend towards a better clinical outcome in patients co-administered clopidogrel and non-CYP3A4 metabolized statins compared to lipophilic statins has been reported [30].

Prasugrel is a thienopyridine that also requires conversion to an active metabolite by hepatic cytochromes (see below). In a small study involving human volunteers the effects of the CYP3A4 inhibitor, ketoconazole, on the pharmacokinetics and *ex vivo* platelet inhibitory effects of prasugrel and clopidogrel were investigated. In this study, ketoconazole co-administration did

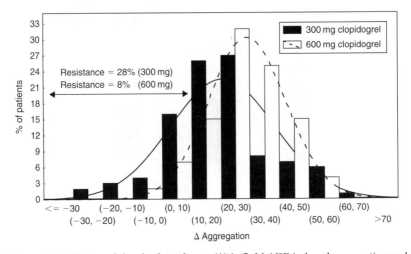

Fig. 6.3 Distribution of the absolute change (Δ) in 5μM ADP-induced aggregation and prevalence of clopidogrel resistance measured at 24 hours following 300 mg and 600 mg clopidogrel loading dose. All of the patients under double- headed arrow meet the definition of clopidogrel resistance. The distribution is shifted rightward and a narrower in the 600 mg group indicating greater inhibition (responsiveness to clopidogrel) and lower incidence of resistance.
(Adapted from Gurbel et al.[16]).

not affect prasugrel active metabolite generation or prasugrel-induced platelet inhibition, whereas clopidogrel-induced platelet inhibition following a loading dose and maintenance dose was associated with less active metabolite generation [6]. Similarly, in another study, prasugrel treatment was associated with superior active metabolite generation and platelet inhibition together with a lower incidence of non-responsiveness compared to clopidogrel treatment [31]. Furthermore, the demonstration of an approximately similar IC_{50} (inhibitory constant) for the active metabolites of prasugrel and clopidogrel in inhibiting *in vitro* ADP-induced platelet aggregation is strong evidence that suboptimal inhibition of platelet aggregation associated with clopidogrel treatment is due to insufficient active metabolite generation [32].

Recent pharmacokinetic studies measuring free drug and active metabolite levels after different doses of clopidogrel have suggested that individual differences in drug absorption may also be an important factor in the occurrence of response variability [25,33]. In support of the latter concept, the intestinal efflux transporter P-glycoprotein has been proposed to be a limiting factor in the absorption of clopidogrel. In addition, MDR1 genotype-related differences in functional P-glycoprotein expression may be, in part, responsible for clopidogrel response variability [34].

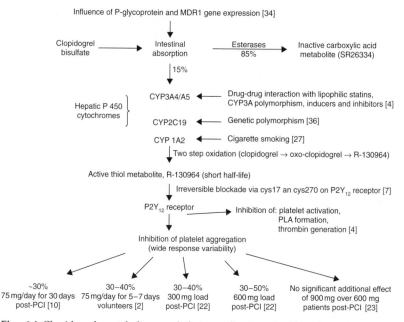

Fig. 6.4 Clopidogrel metabolism and factors affecting clopidogrel responsiveness. MDR1 = P-gycoprotein gene
CYP = hepatic cytochrome P450, PCI = percutaneous coronary intervention
PLA = platelet-leukocyte aggregate.

Polymorphisms of the CYP3A5 gene have also been shown to affect clopidogrel responsiveness in healthy volunteers and moreover, worse outcomes were seen in patients undergoing stent implantation with the CYP3A5 non-expressor genotype following treatment with clopidogrel [35]. Similarly, the influence of the CYP2C19 genotype and polymorphism of the CYP3A4 gene on clopidogrel response variability have also been demonstrated in small studies [36]. Genetic polymorphisms of platelet GP IIb/IIIa, and P2Y$_{12}$ receptors have been reported to affect platelet function, but their influence on clopidogrel responsiveness is not clearly defined [4]. Heightened platelet reactivity in diabetic patients undergoing stenting has been reported despite a 600-mg clopidogrel loading dose [37]. Finally, the effect of pre-existing variability in platelet function on clopidogrel responsiveness has also been suggested [10].

Thus, several lines of evidences indicate that clopidogrel response variability and non-responsiveness are a pharmacokinetic problem associated with insufficient active metabolite generation. The latter is influenced by effect of P-glycoprotein on intestinal absorption, and functional and genetic variability in the cytochrome P450 isoenzymes (Figure 6.4).

Relation of clopidogrel non-responsiveness and high post-treatment platelet reactivity to adverse clinical events

Poor responsiveness to clopidogrel and high post-treatment platelet reactivity to ADP have been associated with ischemic risk following PCI. In a study of patients with ST-elevation myocardial infarction, those with poor responsiveness to clopidogrel (first quartile according to the percentage reduction in pre-treatment ADP-induced aggregation) had a 40% probability for a recurrent cardiovascular event within 6 months [38]. It has subsequently been suggested that post-treatment platelet reactivity to ADP might be a better indicator of adverse clinical events in patients receiving clopidogrel treatment than the measurement of clopidogrel non-responsiveness [39]. To support this hypo-thesis, recent studies have demonstrated the link between high-post-treatment platelet reactivity to adverse clinical events [13,22,42–51]. In the initial study demonstrating this relation, patients suffering a recurrent ischemic event within 6 months of elective stenting had significantly higher post-stent plate-let reactivity to ADP compared to patients without ischemic events despite dual antiplatelet therapy [40]. Similarly, an increased risk of post-stenting myonecrosis and inflammation markers release were associated with high post-treatment platelet reactivity [22,41–46]. Finally, a significantly greater incidence of ischemic events occurring within 1 year of PCI was observed in patients with high pre-procedure ADP-induced platelet aggregation who were on chronic clopidogrel therapy prior to undergoing elective coronary stenting [13] (Table 6.3).

Table 6.3 Clinical relevance of clopidogrel non-responsiveness

Study	n	Results	Clinical relevance
1. Matetzky *et al.* [38]	60	↓ inhibition of ADP-induced platelet aggregation (1st quartile)	Recurrent cardiac events (6 months)
2. Gurbel *et al.* [40] (PREPARE Post-Stenting Study)	192	↑ Periprocedural platelet aggregation	Post-PCI ischemic events (6 months)
3. Gurbel *et al.* [22,46] (CLEAR PLATELETS and CLEAR PLATELETS Ib)	120	↑ Periprocedural platelet aggregation	Myonecrosis and inflammation marker release
4. Bliden *et al.* [13]	100	↑ Preprocedural platelet aggregation inpatients who were on chronic clopidogrel.	Post-PCI ischemic events (6 months)

(Continued)

Table 6.3 (Continued)

Study	n	Results	Clinical relevance
5. Cuisset et al. [41]	106	↑ Platelet aggregation	30 day post-PCI recurrent events
6. Lev et al. [21]	120	Clopidogrel/aspirin resistant patients	Post-PCI myonecrosis
7. Geisler et al. [42]	485	↑ Post-treatment platelet aggregation in diabetic patients with ACS	Acute coronary events
8. Hochholzer et al. [43]	802	↑ Post-treatment platelet aggregation	30 day MACE
9. Bonello et al. [44]	144	↑ $P2Y_{12}$ reactivity ratio (VASP-levels)	6 months MACE
10. Bonello et al. [45]	162	↑ $P2Y_{12}$ reactivity ratio (VASP-levels)	1 month MACE Additional clopidogrel load decreased MACE
11. Barragen et al. [47]	36	↑ $P2Y_{12}$ reactivity ratio (VASP-levels)	Stent thrombosis
12. Gurbel et al. [48] (CREST Study)	120	↑ $P2Y_{12}$ reactivity ratio ↑ platelet aggregation ↑ stimulated GPIIb/IIIa expression	Stent thrombosis
13. Ajzenberg et al. [49]	49	↑ Shear-induced platelet aggregation	Stent thrombosis
14. Buonamici et al. [50]	804	↑ Post-treatment platelet aggregation	Stent thrombosis
15. Price et al. [51]	280	↑ Post-treatment platelet Reactivity by VerifyNow P2Y12 assay	Stent thrombosis

ADP = Adenosine diphosphate; CLEAR PLATELETS Study = Clopidogrel loading with eptifibatide to arrest the reactivity of platelets: results of the Clopidogrel Loading With Eptifibatide to Arrest the Reactivity of Platelets study; CREST Study = Clopidogrel effect on platelet reactivity in patients with stent thrombosis; GP = Glycoprotein; MACE = major adverse clinical events, PCI = Percutaneous coronary intervention; PREPARE POST-Stenting Study = Platelet reactivity in patients and recurrent events post-stenting study; VASP = Vasodilator-stimulated phosphoprotein.

High post-treatment platelet reactivity has been associated with the occurrence of stent thrombosis based on the analysis of flow cytometric measurements of intracellular VASP phosphorylation levels [47,48]. In the CREST study, higher ADP-induced platelet aggregation; greater ADP-stimulated expression of active GP IIb/IIIa expression; and a higher $P2Y_{12}$ reactivity ratio measured by VASP phosphorylation were observed in patients with stent thrombosis compared to patients without stent thrombosis [48]. Other investigators have reported that high *ex vivo* shear-induced platelet aggregation despite dual antiplatelet therapy [49]. Subsequent investigations have supported these initial findings [50,51] (Table 6.3).

Management of clopidogrel resistance

Higher doses

In clinical studies of patients undergoing stenting, a 600-mg clopidogrel loading dose was associated with a greater platelet inhibition, lower mean post-treatment reactivity to ADP, and a lower incidence of non-responsiveness when compared to a 300-mg dose [16,22–24]. In the CLEAR PLATELETS studies, a 600-mg clopidogrel loading dose was associated with superior early platelet inhibition compared to a 300-mg loading dose and accompanied by a decrease in release of myocardial necrosis and inflammation markers [22]. In the ISAR-CHOICE study there was a ceiling effect in unchanged clopidogrel, clopidogrel metabolite levels and platelet inhibition after a 600-mg loading dose. No significant additional effect was seen with a 900-mg loading dose. Similar increased platelet inhibition was observed in patients receiving 150-mg maintenance dose compared to patients receiving a 75-mg dose [23]. Thus, higher loading doses may be considered for selected patients exhibiting high platelet reactivity to ADP during treatment with standard clopidogrel doses.

However, the superiority of a high-dose regimen in reducing ischemic events and the associated risk profile compared to standard dosing has yet to be established in large-scale clinical trials. Despite these limitations, the current ACC/AHA guidelines for PCI provide a Class IIa recommendation that "a regimen of greater than 300 mg is reasonable to achieve higher levels of antiplatelet activity more rapidly". Finally, the ACC/AHA Guidelines provide a Class IIb recommendation that "in patients in whom subacute thrombosis may be catastrophic or lethal… platelet aggregation studies may be considered and the dose of clopidogrel increased to 150 mg per day if less than 50% inhibition of platelet aggregation is demonstrated" [52]. The latter guidelines, however, do not specify the methodology that should be used to assess inhibition. Moreover, there are very limited clinical data to support a cut-point of 50% inhibition [22,45,48]. In the CLEAR PLATELETS Study periprocedural myocardial infarction was observed only in those patients with 5μM ADP-induced aggregation >50% [22]. In the CREST Study the cutpoint for stent thrombosis was 20μM ADP-induced aggregation >40% [48].

New P2Y$_{12}$ receptor antagonists

Prasugrel, a third generation thienopyridine

Prasugrel is an irreversible P2Y$_{12}$ inhibitor with a more rapid, predictable and potent antiplatelet effect than clopidogrel [53,54]. Superior active metabolite generation associated with prasugrel is due to: (i) an effective one-step conversion instead of a multistep conversion associated with clopidogrel; (ii) conversion by various CYP isoenzymes: CYP3A4 and CYP2B6 mainly with minor contribution from CYP2C9, CYP2C19 and CYP2D6 [6,53]; and (iii) lack of vulnerability to esterase inactivation as compared to clopidogrel. Preliminary evidence from a phase II trial suggests a similar safety profile compared to clopidogrel treatment with less response variability and non-responsiveness [53]. The superior pharmacokinetic characteristics make prasugrel a potential alternative to clopidogrel therapy in the treatment of high-risk patients with acute coronary syndromes and patients undergoing stenting [54].

AZD 6140 and cangrelor are reversible, direct and potent inhibitors of the P2Y$_{12}$ receptor. AZD 6140 is an oral inhibitor whereas cangrelor is administered parentally. Both agents exhibit more consistent and greater platelet inhibition compared to clopidogrel. The short onset and offset of action make these agents appealing adjunctive antiplatelet agents during PCI when maximum and rapid platelet inhibition of ADP-induced aggregation is desired [55–57]. The reversibility of these agents reduces the concerns for excessive bleeding following surgery observed with the irreversible inhibitor, clopidogrel [58].

Conclusion

The use of the second generation thienopyridine, clopidogrel has increased following its effectiveness with aspirin therapy in reducing adverse events in large-scale clinical trials. At the same time, based on the laboratory evaluation of the platelet response, wide response variability and non-responsiveness in selected patients are also present. In recent studies, heightened post-treatment platelet reactivity in patients treated with clopidogrel has been associated with the occurrence of adverse ischemic events, including stent thrombosis. The primary cause of clopidogrel response variability is attributed to suboptimal generation of active metabolite secondary to limitation in intestinal absorption, and variability in the activities of hepatic cytochrome P450 isoenzymes. The use of higher loading or maintenance doses of clopidogrel and more potent, new P2Y$_{12}$ receptor blockers are future alternative strategies under investigation.

References

1 Jackson SP. The growing complexity of platelet aggregation. *Blood* 2007; **109**: 5087–5095.

2 Patrono C, Coller B, FitzGerald GA, et al. Platelet-active drugs: the relationships among dose, effectiveness, and side effects: the Seventh ACCP Conference on Antithrombotic and Thrombolytic Therapy. *Chest* 2004; **126** (3 Suppl.): 234S–264S.

3 Gurbel PA, Tantry US. The relationship of platelet reactivity to the occurrence of post-stenting ischemic events: emergence of a new cardiovascular risk factor. *Rev Cardiovasc Med* 2006; **7** (Suppl. 4): S20–28.

4 Gurbel PA, Tantry US. Clopidogrel resistance? *Thromb Res* 2007; **120**: 311–321.

5 Savi P, Combalbert J, Gaich C, et al. The antiaggregating activity of clopidogrel is due to a metabolic activation by the hepatic cytochrome P450-1A. *Thromb Haemost* 1994; **72**: 313–317.

6 Farid NA, Payne CD, Small DS, et al. Cytochrome P450 3A inhibition by ketoconazole affects prasugrel and clopidogrel pharmacokinetics and pharmacodynamics differently. *Clin Pharmacol Ther* 2007; **81**: 735–741.

7 Ding Z, Kim S, Dorsam RT, Jin J, Kunapuli SP. Inactivation of the human $P2Y_{12}$ receptor by thiol reagents requires interaction with both extracellular cysteine residues, Cys17 and Cys270. *Blood* 2003; **101**: 3908–3914.

8 Tantry US, Bliden KP, Gurbel PA. Resistance to antiplatelet drugs: current status and future research. *Expert Opin Pharmacother* 2005; **6**: 2027–2045.

9 Foster CJ, Prosser DM, Agans JM, et al. Molecular identification and characterization of the platelet ADP receptor targeted by thienopyridine antithrombotic drugs. *J Clin Invest* 2001; **107**: 1591–1598.

10 Gurbel PA, Bliden KP, Hiatt BL, et al. Clopidogrel for coronary stenting: response variability, drug resistance, and the effect of pretreatment platelet reactivity. *Circulation* 2003; **107**: 2908–2913.

11 Labarthe B, Theroux P, Angioi M, Ghitescu M. Matching the evaluation of the clinical efficacy of clopidogrel to platelet function tests relevant to the biological properties of the drug. *J Am Coll Cardiol* 2005; **46**: 638–645.

12 Gurbel PA, Bliden KP, Etherington A, Tantry US. Assessment of clopidogrel responsiveness: measurements of maximum platelet aggregation, final platelet aggregation and their correlation with vasodilator-stimulated phosphoprotein in resistant patients. *Thromb Res* 2007; **121**: 107–115.

13 Bliden KP, DiChiara J, Tantry US, et al. Increased risk in patients with high platelet aggregation receiving chronic clopidogrel therapy undergoing percutaneous coronary intervention: is the current antiplatelet therapy adequate? *J Am Coll Cardiol* 2007; **49**: 657–666.

14 van Werkum JW, van der Stelt CA, Seesing TH, et al. A head-to-head comparison between the VerifyNow $P2Y_{12}$ assay and light transmittance aggregometry for monitoring the individual platelet response to clopidogrel in patients undergoing elective percutaneous coronary intervention. *J Thromb Haemost* 2006; **4**: 2516–2518.

15 Aleil B, Ravanat C, Cazenave JP, et al. Flow cytometric analysis of intraplatelet VASP phosphorylation for the detection of clopidogrel resistance in patients with ischemic cardiovascular diseases. *J Thromb Haemost* 2005; **3**: 85–92.

16 Gurbel PA, Bliden KP, Hayes KM, et al. The relation of dosing to clopidogrel responsiveness and the incidence of high post-treatment platelet aggregation in patients undergoing coronary stenting. *J Am Coll Cardiol* 2005; **45**: 1392–1396.

17 Jaremo P, Lindahl TL, Fransson SG, Richter A. Individual variations of platelet inhibition after loading doses of clopidogrel. *J Intern Med* 2002; **252**: 233–238.

18 Muller I, Besta F, Schulz C, et al. Prevalence of clopidogrel non-responders among patients with stable angina pectoris scheduled for elective coronary stent placement. *Thromb Haemost* 2003; **89**: 783–787.

19 Mobley JE, Bresee SJ, Wortham DC, et al. Frequency of nonresponse antiplatelet activity of clopidogrel during pretreatment for cardiac catheterization. *Am J Cardiol* 2004; **93**: 456–458.

20 Lepantalo A, Virtanen KS, Heikkila J, et al. Limited early antiplatelet effect of 300 mg clopidogrel in patients with aspirin therapy undergoing percutaneous coronary interventions. *Eur Heart J* 2004; **25**: 476–483.

21 Lev EI, Patel RT, Maresh KJ, et al. Aspirin and clopidogrel drug response in patients undergoing percutaneous coronary intervention: the role of dual drug resistance. *J Am Coll Cardiol* 2006; **47**: 27–33.

22 Gurbel PA, Bliden KP, Zaman KA, et al. Clopidogrel loading with eptifibatide to arrest the reactivity of platelets: results of the Clopidogrel Loading With Eptifibatide to Arrest the Reactivity of Platelets (CLEAR PLATELETS) study. *Circulation* 2005; **111**: 1153–1159.

23 von Beckerath N, Taubert D, Pogatsa-Murray G, et al. A. Absorption, metabolization, and antiplatelet effects of 300-, 600-, and 900-mg loading doses of clopidogrel: results of the ISAR-CHOICE (Intracoronary Stenting and Antithrombotic Regimen: Choose Between 3 High Oral Doses for Immediate Clopidogrel Effect) Trial. *Circulation* 2005; **112**: 2946–2950.

24 Muller I, Seyfarth M, Rudiger S, et al. Effect of a high loading dose of clopidogrel on platelet function in patients undergoing coronary stent placement. *Heart* 2001; **85**: 92–93.

25 von Beckerath N, Kastrati A, Wieczorek A, Pogatsa-Murray G, Sibbing D, Graf I, Schömig A. A double-blind, randomized study on platelet aggregation in patients treated with a daily dose of 150 or 75 mg of clopidogrel for 30 days. *Eur Heart J* 2007; **28**: 1814–1819.

26 Lau WC, Gurbel PA, Watkins PB, et al. Contribution of hepatic cytochrome P450 3A4 metabolic activity to the phenomenon of clopidogrel resistance. *Circulation* 2004; **109**: 166–171.

27 Bliden KP, Dichiara J, Lawal L, Singla A, Antonino MJ, Baker BA, Bailey WL, Tantry US, Gurbel PA. The association of cigarette smoking with enhanced platelet inhibition by clopidogrel. *J Am Coll Cardiol* 2008; **52**: 531–533.

28 Lau WC, Gurbel PA, Carville DG, et al. Saint Johns wort enhances clopidogrel responsiveness in clopidogrel resistant volunteers and patients by induction of CYP3A4 isoenzyme. *J Am Coll Cardiol* 2007; **49**: 343A.

29 Lau WC, Waskell LA, Watkins PB, Neer CJ, Horowitz K, Hopp AS, Tait AR, Carville DG, Guyer KE, Bates ER. Atorvastatin reduces the ability of clopidogrel to inhibit platelet aggregation: a new drug-drug interaction. *Circulation* 2003; **107**: 32–37.

30 Neubauer H, Mugge A. Thienopyridines and statins: assessing a potential drug–drug interaction. *Curr Pharm Des* 2006; **12**: 1271–1280.

31 Jernberg T, Payne CD, Winters KJ, et al. Prasugrel achieves greater inhibition of platelet aggregation and a lower rate of non-responders compared with clopidogrel in aspirin-treated patients with stable coronary artery disease. *Eur Heart J* 2006; **27**: 1166–1173.

32 Sugidachi A, Ogawa T, Kurihara A, Hagihara K, Jakubowski JA, Hashimoto M, Niitsu Y, Asai F. The greater in vivo antiplatelet effects of prasugrel as compared

to clopidogrel reflect more efficient generation of its active metabolite with similar antiplatelet activity to that of clopidogrel's active metabolite. *J Thromb Haemost* 2007; **5**: 1545–1551.

33 Taubert D, Kastrati A, Harlfinger S, *et al.* Pharmacokinetics of clopidogrel after administration of a high loading dose. *Thromb Haemost* 2004; **92**: 311–316.

34 Taubert D, von Beckerath N, Grimberg G, *et al.* Impact of P-glycoprotein on clopidogrel absorption. *Clin Pharmacol Ther* 2006; **80**: 486–501.

35 Suh JW, Koo BK, Zhang SY, *et al.* Increased risk of atherothrombotic events associated with cytochrome P450 3A5 polymorphism in patients taking clopidogrel. *Can Med Assoc J* 2006; **174**: 1715–1722.

36 Hulot JS, Bura A, Villard E, Azizi M, Remones V, Goyenvalle C, Aiach M, Lechat P, Gaussem P. Cytochrome P450 2C19 loss-of-function polymorphism is a major determinant of clopidogrel responsiveness in healthy subjects. *Blood* 2006; **108**: 2244–2247.

37 Geisler T, Anders N, Paterok M, Langer H, Stellos K, Lindemann S, Herdeg C, May AE, Gawaz M. Platelet response to clopidogrel is attenuated in diabetic patients undergoing coronary stent implantation. *Diabetes Care* 2007; **30**: 372–374.

38 Matetzky S, Shenkman B, Guetta V, *et al.* Clopidogrel resistance is associated with increased risk of recurrent atherothrombotic events in patients with acute myocardial infarction. *Circulation* 2004; **109**: 3171–3175.

39 Samara WM, Bliden KP, Tantry US, Gurbel PA. The difference between clopidogrel responsiveness and posttreatment platelet reactivity. *Thromb Res* 2005; **115**: 89–94.

40 Gurbel PA, Bliden KP, Guyer K, *et al.* Platelet reactivity in patients and recurrent events post-stenting: results of the PREPARE POST-STENTING Study. *J Am Coll Cardiol* 2005; **46**: 1820–1826.

41 Cuisset T, Frere C, Quilici J, Barbou F, *et al.* High post-treatment platelet reactivity identified low-responders to dual antiplatelet therapy at increased risk of recurrent cardiovascular events after stenting for acute coronary syndrome. *J Thromb Haemost* 2006; **4**: 542–549.

42 Geisler T, Langer H, Wydymus M, *et al.* Low response to clopidogrel is associated with cardiovascular outcome after coronary stent implantation. *Eur Heart J* 2006; **27**: 2420–2425.

43 Hochholzer W, Trenk D, Bestehorn HP, *et al.* Impact of the degree of peri-interventional platelet inhibition after loading with clopidogrel on early clinical outcome of elective coronary stent placement. *J Am Coll Cardiol* 2006; **48**: 1742–1750.

44 Bonello L, Paganelli F, Arpin-Bornet M, *et al.* Vasodilator-stimulated phosphoprotein phosphorylation analysis prior to percutaneous coronary intervention for exclusion of postprocedural major adverse cardiovascular events. *J Thromb Haemost* 2007; **5**: 1630–1636.

45 Bonello L, Camoin-Jau L, Arques S, *et al.* Adjusted clopidogrel loading doses according to vasodilator-stimulated phosphoprotein phosphorylation index decrease rate of major adverse cardiovascular events in patients with clopidogrel resistance: a multicenter randomized prospective study.*J Am Coll Cardiol* 2008; **51**: 1404–1411.

46 Gurbel PA, Bliden KP, Tantry US. The effect of clopidogrel with and without eptifibatide on tumor necrosis factor-alpha and C-reactive protein release after elective stenting: Results of the CLEAR PLATELETS-Ib study. *J Am Coll Cardiol* 2006; **48**: 2186–2191.

47 Barragan P, Bouvier JL, Roquebert PO, *et al.* Resistance to thienopyridines: clinical detection of coronary stent thrombosis by monitoring of vasodilator-stimulated phosphoprotein phosphorylation. *Catheter Cardiovasc Interv* 2003; **59**: 295–302.

48 Gurbel PA, Bliden KP, Samara W, *et al*. Clopidogrel effect on platelet reactivity in patients with stent thrombosis: results of the CREST Study. *J Am Coll Cardiol* 2005; **46**: 1827–1832.

49 Ajzenberg N, Aubry P, Huisse MG, *et al*. Enhanced shear-induced platelet aggregation in patients who experience subacute stent thrombosis: a case-control study. *J Am Coll Cardiol* 2005; **45**: 1753–1756.

50 Buonamici P, marcucci R, Miglironi A, *et al*. Impact of platelet reactivity after clopidogrel administration on drug-eluting stent thrombosis. *J Am Coll Cardiol* 2007; **49**: 2312–2317.

51 Price JM, Wong GB, Valenica R, *et al*. Measurement of clopidogrel inhibition with a point-of-care assay identifies patients at risk for stent thrombosis after percutaneous coronary intervention. *Am J Cardiol* 2006; **98**: 204M [abstract].

52 Smith SC Jr, Feldman TE, Hirshfeld JW, Jr., *et al*. ACC/AHA/SCAI 2005 guideline update for percutaneous coronary intervention-summary article: a report of American Collage of Cardiology/ American Heart Association Task Force on Practice Guidelines (ACC/AHA/SCAI Writing Committee to update the 2001 Guidelines for Percutaneous Coronary Intervention). *Circulation* 2006; **113**: e166–286.

53 Tantry US, Bliden KP, Gurbel PA. Prasugrel. *Expert Opin Investig Drugs* 2006; **15**: 1627–1633.

54 Wiviott SD, Antman EM, Winters KJ, *et al*. E JUMBO-TIMI 26 Investigators. Randomized comparison of prasugrel (CS-747, LY640315), a novel thienopyridine P2Y$_{12}$ antagonist, with clopidogrel in percutaneous coronary intervention: results of the Joint Utilization of Medications to Block Platelets Optimally (JUMBO)-TIMI 26 trial. *Circulation* 2005 28; **111**: 3366–3373.

55 Tantry US, Etherington A, Bliden KP, Gurbel PA. Antiplatelet therapy: current strategies and future trends. *Future Cardiol* 2006; **2**: 343–366.

56 Husted S, Emanuelsson H, Heptinstall S, *et al*. Pharmacodynamics, pharmacokinetics, and safety of the oral reversible P2Y$_{12}$ antagonist AZD6140 with aspirin in patients with atherosclerosis: a double-blind comparison to clopidogrel with aspirin. *Eur Heart J* 2006; **27**: 1038–1047.

57 Greenbaum AB, Ohman EM, Gibson CM, Borzak S, Stebbins AL, Lu M, Le May MR, Stankowski JE, Emanuelsson H, Weaver WD. Preliminary experience with intravenous P2Y$_{12}$ platelet receptor inhibition as an adjunct to reduced-dose alteplase during acute myocardial infarction: results of the Safety, Tolerability and Effect on Patency in Acute Myocardial Infarction (STEP-AMI) angiographic trial. *Am Heart J* 2007; **154**: 702–709.

58 Kapetanakis EI, Medlam DA, Boyce SW, *et al*. Clopidogrel administration prior to coronary artery bypass grafting surgery: the cardiologist's panacea or the surgeon's headache? *Eur Heart J* 2005; **26**: 576–583.

PART III

Pharmacology of Intravenous Antiplatelet Agents

Chapter 7

Pharmacology of intravenous glycoprotein IIb/IIIa antagonists

James C. Blankenship and Peter B. Berger

Glycoprotein IIb/IIIa receptors and platelet physiology

Platelets play a key role in atherosclerosis and thrombosis. Inhibition of platelet function was first proved valuable with aspirin, decades after its use became widespread. In 1981, the platelet membrane IIb/IIIa receptor was first identified. Because of its key role in platelet aggregation, it was a logical target of efforts to control the platelet response to vascular injury.

The IIb/IIIa receptor plays only a minor role in platelet adhesion, the first step in the process of hemostasis [1]. Damage to vascular endothelium exposes the subendothelial matrix, including adhesive proteins. Platelets adhere to the subendothelium when platelet membrane glycoproteins bind to its adhesive proteins. Many of the platelet membrane glycoproteins are integrins, a term used to describe heterodimeric molecules composed of a series of alpha and beta subunits. At least five integrins and two other glycoproteins are involved in platelet adhesion. One of these integrins is the IIb/IIIa receptor, which thereby plays a minor role in platelet adhesion.

Platelet activation follows platelet adhesion and is initiated by various mechanical and biochemical processes. Platelet activation stimulates metabolic pathways, induces conformational changes in platelet structure, activates the IIb/IIIa receptor and stimulates the clotting cascade. Activated platelets release adenosine diphosphate (ADP), serotonin, thromboxane A2 and other signaling molecules; these trigger the recruitment and activation of other platelets. A layer of platelets spreads over the injured endothelial surface.

Antiplatelet Therapy in Ischemic Heart Disease, 1st edition. Edited by Stephen D. Wiviott.
© 2009 American Heart Association, ISBN: 9-781-4051-7626-2

After platelet adhesion occurs, platelet aggregation produces a platelet plug. Over 100 agonists of aggregation have been identified, but there are only three major stimuli of platelet aggregation: thromboxane A2 via cyclooxygenase, ADP and thrombin. All agonists and aggregation pathways ultimately mediate platelet aggregation via the IIb/IIIa receptor.

The IIb/IIIa receptor is found only in cells of megakaryocyte lineage. In platelets, the IIb/IIIa receptor is the most numerous integrin on the surface membrane. Each platelet has 50,000 to 90,000 IIb/IIIa receptors in the resting state [2]. The IIb/IIIa receptor consists of a large extracellular region and a small intracellular region. The extracellular portion facilitates ligand binding. The intracellular portion mediates signal transduction within the cell. In the resting state, platelet IIb/IIIa receptors have a low affinity for fibrinogen binding. When a platelet is activated, changes in the intracellular cytoskeleton induce changes in the structure of the receptor such that it has high affinity for fibrinogen binding. This is termed "inside-to-outside" signaling [3].

Any molecule that binds to the IIb/IIIa receptor induces conformational changes in the ligand–receptor complex, thereby inducing "outside-to-inside" changes in the platelet (platelet membrane fluidity, cystoskeletal activity) and in the receptor (receptor epitopes or ligand-induced binding sites). These changes in turn induce platelet granule secretion and P-selectin expression. Different molecules bind to different sites in the IIb/IIIa receptor and, depending on which site is bound, different "outside-to-inside" changes occur. Thus, different synthetic molecules that bind to the IIb/IIIa receptor may have a similar inhibitory effect on platelet aggregation (via receptor occupancy) but may have very different effects on platelet secretion or platelet procoagulant activity.

The binding of fibrinogen to IIb/IIIa receptors is the most important mechanism responsible for platelet aggregation. Other ligands also bind to IIb/IIIa receptors, including von Willebrand factor (vWf), vitronection and fibronectin. These other ligands play a more important role in platelet adhesion to subendothelial structures.

Binding of ligands to the IIb/IIIa receptor depends on two peptide sequences. The more important is the Lys-Gln-Ala-Gly-Asp-Val sequence unique to the fibrinogen molecule. In contrast, the Arg-Gly-Asp (RGD) sequence is found in vWF, vitronection and fibronectin, as well as in the IIb/IIIa receptor. Binding sites for these two peptide sequences may overlap on the IIb/IIIa receptor, and these sequences can bind at several sites within the IIb/IIIa receptor. The number and conformation of these peptide sequences in IIb/IIIa receptor ligands contributes to their affinity for the IIb/IIIa receptor [4].

Development of glycoprotein IIb/IIIa receptor antagonists

Any compound that occupies IIb/IIIa receptors and prevents them from binding to fibrinogen will inhibit platelet aggregation. The first IIb/IIIa receptor antagonists were murine monoclonal antibodies against the IIb/IIIa receptor that blocked fibrinogen binding, thus inhibiting platelet aggregation. One such murine antibody, 7E3, was modified to minimize immunogenicity, and its Fab fragments were bonded to human immunoglobulin to form abciximab. This became the first Food and Drug Administration (FDA) approved IIb/IIIa receptor antagonist.

Natural products have been examined for IIb/IIIa receptor inhibitory properties. Venom of the viper *Trimeresurus gramineus* was found to contain peptides that inhibit fibrinogen binding to IIb/IIIa receptors, and subsequently venoms from several other snakes have been discovered to have similar properties [5]. These inhibitory peptides are labeled disintegrins for their anti-integrin properties. Their inhibitory effects are due to RGD peptide sequences. Due to their immunogenicity, they have been most useful as models for the design of synthetic IIb/IIIa receptor antagonists.

Eptafibitide is based on a 73-amino acid peptide called barbourin, a constituent of the venom of the pigmy rattlesnake *Sistrurus m. barbouri*. Unlike most disintegrins, eptifibitide is very selective for the IIb/IIIa receptor. Eptifibitide contains a Lys-Gly-Asp sequence (KGD) that is a more effective inhibitor than the RGD sequence.

Tirofiban, another FDA-approved IIb/IIIa receptor antagonist, is a non-peptide compound. It is termed peptidomimetic because it mimics a peptide with the RGD sequence. After the IIb/IIIa receptor was characterized in the 1980s and the importance of the RGD sequence was realized, several RGD peptides and proteins were identified and tested for ability to inhibit the IIb/IIIa receptor. Because these contained molecular structures in addition to the RGD complex required for IIb/IIIa binding, chemists synthesized a low molecular weight compound, tirofiban, containing little more than the RGD sequence [6].

Pharmacokinetics and pharmacodynamics of glycoprotein IIb/IIIa receptor antagonists

Abciximab

The binding site of abciximab is located on the beta chain of the IIb/IIIa receptor [1], a different site than that which binds eptifibitide or tirofiban. The abciximab is large (molecular weight 50 kD) and sterically hinders other ligands from binding to sites on the IIb/IIIa molecule. A standard bolus of abciximab 0.25 mg/kg produces >80% blockade of receptors and reduces platelet aggregation to <20% of baseline values, using citrated collection tubes and ADP as an agonist. This degree of inhibition persists for the duration of the infusion (0.125 μg/kg/min up to 10 μg/min). After bolus injection, 50% of abciximab molecules are bound to platelets within 10 minutes. The half-life of dissociation of abciximab from platelets is 4 hours, due to its high affinity for the IIb/IIIa receptors. In contrast, abciximab is rapidly cleared from the plasma with a half-life of 5 minutes. Because abciximab binds with very high affinity to IIb/IIIa receptors and dissociates very slowly, it occupies 13% of IIb/IIIa receptors even 15 days after administration [7], and is detectable on circulating platelets for at least 21 days.

The ability of abciximab to dissociate from platelets explains the efficacy of platelet transfusions in halting abciximab-induced bleeding. After transfusion, abciximab molecules will redistribute to the new platelets. When the percent of IIb/IIIa receptor occupancy drops below a threshold level, aggregation can occur [8].

Abciximab is non-specific and will bind to vitronectin receptors on endothelial cells and MAC-1 receptor on leukocytes. The clinical significance of these effects remains unclear.

Eptifibitide

The pharmacokinetics of eptifibitide are linear for boluses and infusion rates throughout the therapeutic doses that have been used in clinical trials. Plasma elimination half-life is 2.5 hours. Renal clearance accounts for 50% of total body clearance, with most of it excreted as the unchanged drug in the urine. Clinical studies recruited patients with creatinine up to 2 mg/dL, and dosing recommendations state that dosing adjustment is unnecessary for patients with creatinine <2 mg/dL. Reliable data on patients with higher creatinine is not available. It has a very rapid association ("on-rate") and dissociation ("off-rate") with the IIb/IIIa receptor. Its small size is responsible for its lack of immunogenicity.

Estimates of *in vivo* platelet inhibition are based primarily on *ex vivo* platelet aggregation testing. *Ex vivo* platelet aggregation is affected by two factors: the type of anticoagulant used for blood collection and the agonist used for platelet activation [9].

Blood samples used in *ex vivo* aggregation studies are often anticoagulated with citrate. Citrate prevents clotting by reducing the calcium concentration in the sample from physiologic levels 25-fold (from 1 mM to 0.04 mM). However, this has the unintended consequence of reducing the amount of calcium bound to IIb/IIIa receptors, thereby enhancing binding of eptifibitide to the IIb/IIIa receptor, making eptifibitide appear to be a more potent antagonist of the IIb/IIIa receptor. Furthermore, in citrated samples, binding of *fibrinogen* to the IIb/IIIa receptor is less effective due to the lower calcium concentrations. Thus, using citrate as an anticoagulant in blood sample tubes leads to overestimates of the potency of eptifibitide as a IIb/IIIa receptor antagonist.

In contrast, when the direct thrombin inhibitor PPACK (D-phenylalanyl-L-propyl-L-arginyl-chloromethyl ketone) is used as anticoagulant, calcium concentrations remain physiologic. Calcium remains normally bound to the IIb/IIIa receptor. The eptifibitide concentration required for platelet aggregation is four times higher than that estimated to be necessary from citrate-collected blood.

When assessing inhibition of platelet aggregation, platelets in the blood sample must be activated. More potent agonists produce activated platelets whose aggregation can only be inhibited by very high doses of IIb/IIIa receptor antagonist. ADP and thrombin receptor agonist peptide (TRAP) are two substances used as agonists. While both activate the IIb/IIIa receptors on the platelet surface, TRAP also induces *de novo* expression of IIb/IIIa receptors from the intracellular pool of alpha granules to the platelet surface. This makes it a more potent agonist than ADP. If TRAP is used to activate platelets, the concentration of eptifibitide needed for inhibition will be higher. ADP is thought to be the more physiologic agonist, with activity close to that found in the circulation, so it is predominantly used in assays of platelet inhibition.

Phase I studies of eptifibitide pharmacokinetics used citrated tubes, and thus tended to overestimate the inhibitory power of eptifibitide. This led to doses of eptifibitide in clinical trials that were at the lower end of the therapeutic range. For the first large study of eptifibitide, Integrilin to Minimize Platelet Aggregation and Coronary Thrombosis Trial II (IMPACT II), bolus and infusion doses of 135μg/kg and 0.5 or 0.75μg/kg/min were used [10]. The results of IMPACT II showed marginal benefit from eptifibitide, and subsequent pharmacokinetic studies estimated that *in vivo* platelet inhibition achieved in IMPACT II was only 50–60% [11]. A subsequent study, Enhanced Suppression of the Platelet IIb/IIIa Receptor with Integrilin (ESPRIT), used a double bolus of 180μg/kg and infusion of 2μg/kg/min, and achieved dramatically better clinical results [12]. This is the dose currently used in patients undergoing PCI. An ongoing trial, Early Glycoprotein IIb/IIIa Inhibition in Non ST segment Elevation Acute Coronary Syndrome (EARLY ACS), is comparing the upstream administration of Eptifibatide versus the more selective in-lab use of Eptifibatide in only those patients who undergo PCI; the double bolus dose is being used in both arms of the trial.

Tirofiban

Tirofiban is a non-peptide. The pharmacokinetics of tirofiban are similar to those of eptifibitide. Tirofiban is a reversible antagonist of IIb/IIIa receptors with an affinity intermediate between abciximab and eptifibitide [13]. Its inhibitory effect is dose and concentration-dependent. Plasma elimination half-life is 2 hours. After discontinuation of infusion, *ex vivo* platelet aggregation returns to near baseline in 90% of patients in 4–8 hours. Renal clearance accounts for 65% of total body clearance, with most of it excreted as the drug in the urine. Renal clearance is decreased in patients with creatinine clearance <30mL/min, and recommended doses are decreased in these patients. Tirofiban's affinity for IIb/IIIa receptors is much stronger than Eptifibatide's and more closely resembles that of abciximab; the significance of this is unknown.

In the Tirofiban And ReoPro Give similar Efficacy outcomes Trial (TARGET) trial, tirofiban yielded ischemic outcomes inferior to those of abciximab [14]. One explanation centered around the adequacy of tirofiban dosing (10μg/kg bolus and 0.15μg/kg/min infusion). Pharmacokinetic studies on which dosing was based used citrate as an anticoagulant and low doses of the agonist

ADP (5 μM). Both choices probably contributed to underestimation of the dose of tirofiban needed to inhibit platelet aggregation under physiologic conditions [15]. Several clinical studies [16–18] have been conducted with "high dose" tirofiban using a two and a half times greater bolus dose with the same infusion dose (25 μg/kg and 0.15 μg/kg/min). Results have been promising in five small, randomized trials in which a total of 1392 patients were enrolled, but have not yet been confirmed by large studies [19].

Measurement of efficacy of IIb/IIIa receptor antagonists

In contrast to most drugs, monitoring of IIb/IIIa receptor antagonists tends to focus on their effect on their target organ, the platelet [20]. Several methods have been used to measure the efficacy of IIb/IIIa receptor antagonists. None are completely satisfactory, and none has come into common clinical use.

Bleeding times in the pre- IIb/IIIa era failed to correlate with clinical bleeding events, and early studies with abciximab showed bleeding time did not predict bleeding complications [21].

The most commonly used technique is light transmission aggregometry. Platelet-rich plasma is prepared from anticoagulated blood, and a platelet agonist is added to the stirring suspension of platelets [22]. The results of aggregometry vary depending on the agonist used and on the choice of anti-coagulant. As noted above, use of non-physiologic agents has led to under-dosing of small-molecule IIb/IIIa receptor antagonists in major clinical trials. In addition, aggregometry is time consuming and difficult to use for large numbers of samples. These factors make it a poor candidate for routine clinical monitoring of patients receiving IIb/IIIa receptor antagonists [23].

A promising alternative is the Rapid Platelet Function Assay (RPFA), which relies on an interaction between IIb/IIIa receptors and fibrinogen-coated beads to agglutinate the beads [24]. IIb/IIIa receptor antagonists block this agglutination. The degree of receptor inhibition is proportional to the reduction in agglutination, which is closely related to platelet aggregation. Blood samples can be anticoagulated with either citrate or PPACK. A modified form of TRAP, lyophilized iso-TRAP, is used as an agonist.

The AU-Assessing Ultegra (GOLD) study used RPFA to assess platelet function after usual doses of IIb/IIIa receptor antagonists: abciximab (0.25 mg/kg bolus and 0.125 μg/kg/min), tirofiban (10 μg/kg bolus and 0.15 μg/kg/min), and eptifibitide (180 μg/kg and 2 μg/kg/min) [25]. Citrate was used as anticoagulant for eptifibitide and abciximab, and PPACK was used for eptifibitide. At 10 minutes post bolus, all three drugs achieved >90% platelet inhibition. All three drugs achieved 1 hour inhibition of at least 89% and 8 hour inhibition >93%. At 1 hour post bolus, the mean level of platelet inhibition was 96%. The incidence of major adverse events in the lowest quartile of inhibition (i.e. <95% inhibition) was 14% compared to 6% (p = 0.006) in patients with >95% platelet inhibition.

Although the study was quite small, the relationship between agglutination and clinical outcome was assessed at many different time points, and different cut-points were retrospectively identified at each time point, the study does suggest that there does indeed exist a relationship between the degree of inhibition of aggregation and clinical outcome with IIb/IIIa inhibitors.

Beneficial clinical effects of IIb/IIIa receptor antagonists

In the ESPRIT [12] trial and the IMPACT II trial [10], eptifibitide significantly decreased the incidence of myocardial infarction as measured by CK-MB enzyme elevation in patients with angiographically uncomplicated procedures [26,27]. In these studies, eptifibitide decreased or tended to decrease both the incidence of angiographic complications and the incidence of creatine-kinase-MB (CK-MB) enzyme elevation when angiographic complications did occur.

In contrast, in Evaluation of Platelet IIb/IIIa Inhibition in Stenting Trial (EPISTENT) [28], abciximab did decrease the incidence of angiographic complications compared to placebo (17% versus 24%, p = 0.001) as well as the incidence of CK-MB rises in patients without angiographic complications (6.5% versus 10.7%, p = 0.007) [29].

Thus, the major beneficial effects of IIb/IIIa receptors in PCI are not only to prevent angiographic complications, but rather to reduce the incidence of CK-MB elevation, which most often occurs in patients with uncomplicated procedures. Presumably this is due to prevention of angiographically inapparent distal embolization. The IIb/IIIa antagonists decrease the overall Major Adverse Cardiac Event (MACE) rate, principally through a 30 to 50% reduction in CK-MB enzyme rises (non-ST-elevation MI). Some studies have demonstrated survival benefits to receiving IIb/IIIa antagonists during PCI [28,30].

While these drugs are frequently used as adjunctive therapy ("bail out") in the setting of difficult or complicated PCI procedures, they have not been shown to decrease post-PCI vessel occlusion or be beneficial in this setting. It may be that embolization and resultant infarction has already occurred by the time that angiographic evidence of a complication becomes apparent.

Clinical use of GP IIb/IIIa antagonists are discussed in detail elsewhere in this book.

Detrimental clinical effects of glycoprotein IIb/IIIa receptor antagonists

Bleeding

There is a fundamental tension between the need to prevent coronary thrombosis in patients with acute coronary syndromes or coronary intervention and the need for therapeutic hemostasis at sites of vascular injury or disruption. The most important complication of IIb/IIIa receptor antagonists is bleeding.

The first large study of IIb/IIIa receptor antagonists, Evaluation of 7E3 for the Prevention of Ischemic Complications (EPIC), demonstrated a 50% increase in major bleeding attributable to abciximab [31]. Subsequent studies demonstrated a lesser increase in bleeding complications [32] as various strategies to prevent bleeding were implemented [33]. These strategies included weight-adjusted heparin dosing, early vascular sheath removal, the use of smaller sheaths, and avoiding femoral sheath placement during PCI. These practices, innovative in the late 1990s, have since become common practice. An additional strategy to minimize bleeding is the use of radial access, which reduces hemorrhagic and other vascular site complications. Vascular closure devices have become commonplace but have not decreased bleeding and other complications.

Thrombocytopenia

All three FDA-approved IIb/IIIa antagonists have been associated with thrombocytopenia [34,35]. However, abciximab causes thrombocytopenia much more frequently and to a more severe degree (often to <20,000) compared to the small molecule IIb/IIIa antagonists. In a pooled analysis of eight trials, abciximab (but not tirofiban or eptifibitide) significantly increased the incidence of thrombocytopenia compared to placebo (4.2% versus 2.0%, $p < 0.001$, odds ratio 2.1) [36].

Abciximab-induced thrombocytopenia (AIT) has been extensively studied. AIT typically occurs within 24 hours of first exposure to the drug. This raises the possibility that it is non-immune, but non-immune mechanisms have not been identified. AIT is more likely due to antibodies induced by prior exposure to murine sequences that are part of the chimeric abciximab molecule. AIT may be delayed (3–7 days). Delayed thrombocytopenia is likely caused by antibodies induced by exposure to the drug that destroy platelets still carrying the drug several days after first exposure [37].

AIT must be distinguished from heparin-induced thrombocytopenia (HIT). HIT is identified by antibodies reactive to heparin–platelet factor 4 complexes [38]. Furthermore, the time course over which the thrombocytopenia develops usually allows one to distinguish between the two entities. Clopidogrel only rarely causes thrombocytopenia. Pseudothrombocytopenia is an *in vitro* artifact that can lead to an incorrect diagnosis of thrombocytopenia; it is important to distinguish this from true thrombocytopenia [39]. Pseudothrombocytopenia accounts for about one-third of what appears to be thrombocytopenia after abciximab. It is caused by platelet clumping in blood samples collected with ethylene diaminetetra acetic acid (EDTA) as the anticoagulant. Cell counters count each clump as a single platelet, so the number of platelets *in vivo* is under-reported. This can easily be distinguished from true thrombocytopenia by collecting a blood sample in a tube with citrate as the anticoagulant, or by microscopic detection of platelet clumps in the original sample. Pseudothrombocytopenia has been observed with abciximab but not with the small molecule antagonists.

Thrombocytopenia associated with the small molecule IIb/IIIa antagonists is likely due to "drug-dependent antibodies". These are naturally-occurring antibodies that react with platelets only in the presence of a drug such as eptifibitide or tirofiban. [40]. The mechanism of action may be through these antibodies binding to ligand-induced binding sites that are exposed when the IIb/IIIa antagonist binds to the IIb/IIIa receptor, inducing conformational changes in the receptor [41].

Bleeding associated with IIb/IIIa antagonist-induced thrombocytopenia is rare [36] but can occur. Generally, thrombocytopenia reverses within several days. Platelet or blood transfusions are usually discouraged unless there is active bleeding or a drop in platelet count below 10,000.

Pulmonary alveolar hemorrhage

Individual cases of pulmonary hemorrhage associated with abciximab have been reported. Iskandar *et al.* retrospectively reviewed 5458 patients undergoing PCI and found an increased incidence of alveolar hemorrhage in patients treated with IIb/IIIa antagonists compared to placebo. The incidence of pulmonary hemorrhage was 0.33% in patients treated with eptifibitide and 0.14% in patients treated with abciximab [42].

Re-administration

Re-administration of abciximab produced severe thrombocytopenia more frequently than in first-time users [43]. A 500 patient registry [44] of patients receiving abciximab twice demonstrated a 4.6% incidence of thrombocytopenia with the second administration. There were no cases of hypersensitivity or anaphylaxis. The authors noted that human antichimeric antibodies (HACA) were present in 5% of patients after first administration and in 24% after second administration. HACA did not correlate with clinical events or interfere with the antagonist effect of the IIb/IIIa receptor antagonist. The authors recommend checking platelet counts 4 hours and 24 hours after each administration of abciximab and with any bleeding.

Cross-administration of IIb/IIIa antagonists

There does not appear to be cross-sensitivity among the IIb/IIIa receptor antagonists. For patients requiring a IIb/IIIa antagonist after prior treatment with abciximab, eptifibitide or tirofiban may be preferable over repeat abciximab, particularly if it is within 2 months. [45,46]

Contraindications

Contraindications to IIb/IIIa receptor antagonists are principally related to risk of bleeding. These include major surgery, trauma or internal bleeding in the past 30 days; intracranial pathology that would predispose to bleeding including recent bleeding, aneurysm, stroke or vascular malformations; systolic/diastolic blood pressure above 180/110, acute pericarditis, possible aortic dissection, concomitant coumadin use, and hemmorrhagic retinopathy. In patients with thrombocytopenia, history of IIb/IIIa antagonist-induced thrombocytopenia or IIb/IIIa receptor antagonist therapy in the past 48 hours, the benefits of the drug should be weighed against the risks of severe thrombocytopenia. Allergy to any component of a IIb/IIIa formulation is also a contraindication. Small molecule IIb/IIIa antagonists should be used cautiously in patients with renal failure. Eptifibitide should be avoided if the creatinine is above 4 mg/dL or the creatinine clearance is markedly reduced.

Alternative dosing strategies

Bolus only IIb/IIIa antagonists

The EPIC trial included a bolus-only arm, but it provided less protection against ischemic events than did the bolus–infusion arm. Consequently, the bolus-only strategy was abandoned. It should be remembered, however, that EPIC was a balloon angioplasty trial, with multiple prolonged inflations, elastic recoil, deep injury to the vessel wall and a significant risk of abrupt closure, all of which are reduced by stent placement. The applicability of the results of EPIC to the modern era and the need for a prolonged infusion have been called into question. A recent analysis of the EPIC data noted that the rates of thrombocytopenia and bleeding were significantly less in the bolus-only arm (compared to the bolus-infusion arm) [47]. Also the ischemic complication rate was lower in the abciximab bolus-only arm than for placebo. The authors concluded that in the current era of early discharges and concerns over bleeding, a bolus-only strategy might have some merit.

Marmur *et al.* performed an observational analysis of patients treated with abciximab using only a bolus and eptfibitide using only a bolus during PCI [48] and found that ischemic complications were infrequent, bleeding was rare and both ischemic and bleeding complications with bolus-only strategies compared favorably to historic controls.

Bertrand *et al.* examined bolus-only abciximab as part of a strategy of early, same-day discharge after PCI [49]. The early discharge group received only a bolus of abciximab, while the overnight group received a bolus and 12-hour infusion. There were no significant differences in ischemic outcomes, and there was only a non-significant trend towards more bleeding in the bolus and infusion group.

Intracoronary administration

Kakkar *et al.* compared ischemic outcomes during PCI with intravenous (14%) versus intracoronary (6%, $p = 0.04$) abciximab [50]. Wohrle *et al.* confirmed this finding [51]. The mechanism by which local administration of IIb/IIIa antagonists acts to confer a benefit over intravenous administration is unknown.

References

1 Lefkovits J, Plow EF, Topol EJ. Platelet glycoprotein IIb–IIIa receptors in cardiovascular medicine. *N Eng J Med* 1995; **332**: 1553–1559.

2 Wagner CL, Mascelli MA, Neblock DS, Weisman HF, Coller BS, Jordan RE. Analysis of GP IIb–IIIa receptor number by quantification of 7E3 binding to human platelets. *Blood* 1996; **88**: 907–914.

3 Chew DP, Moliterno DJ. A critical appraisal of platelet glycoprotein IIb–IIIa inhibition. *J Am Coll Cardiol* 2000; **36**: 2028–2035.

4 Schror K, Weber A-A. Comparative pharmacology of GP IIb–IIIa antagonists. *J Thrombosis Thrombolysis* 2003; **15**: 71–80.

5 Phillips DR, Scarborough RM. Clinical pharmacology of eptifibitide. *Am J Cardiol* 1997; **80**: 11B–20B.

6 Kondo K, Umemura K. Clinical pharmacokinetics of tirofiban, a nonpeptide glycoprotein IIb–IIIa receptor antagonist. *Clin Pharmacokinet* 202; **41**: 187–195.

7 Casserly IP, Topol EJ. Glycoprotein IIb–IIIa antagonists – from bench to bedside practice. *Cell Mol Life Sci* 2002; **59**: 1–23.

8 Kleiman NS. Pharmacology of the intravenous platelet receptor glycoprotein IIb–IIIa antagonists. *Cor Art Dis* 1998; **9**: 603–616.

9 Phillips DR, Teng W, Arfsten A, Nannizzi-Alaimo L, White MM, Longhurst C, Shattil SJ, Randolph A, Jakubowski JA, Jennings LK, Scarborough RM. Effect of Ca^{2+} on GP IIb–IIIa interactions with integrilin; enhanced GP IIb–IIIa binding and inhibition of platelet aggregation by reductions in the concentration of ionized calcium in plasma anti-coagulated with citrate. *Circulation* 1997; **96**: 1488–1494.

10 The IMPACT-II Investigators. Randomised placebo-controlled trial of effect of eptifibatide on complications of percutaneous coronary intervention: IMPACT-II. *Lancet* 1997; **349**: 1422–1428.

11 Schneider DJ, Aggarwal A. Development of glycoprotein IIb–IIIa antagonists: translation of pharmacodynamic effects into clinical benefit. *Expert Rev Cardiovasc Ther* 2004; **2**: 903–913.

12 The ESPRIT Investigators. A randomised, placebo-controlled trial of a novel dosing regimen of eptifibatide in planned coronary stent implantation. *Lancet* 2000; **356**: 2037–2044.

13 Gowda RM, Khan IA, Vasavada BC, Sacchi TJ. Therapeutics of platelet glycoprotein IIb–IIIa receptor antagonism. *Am J Therapeutics* 2004; **11**: 302–307.

14 Topol EJ, Moliterno DJ, Herrmann HC, Powers ER, Grines CL, Cohen DJ, Cohen EA, Bertrand M, Neumann F-J, Stone GW, DiBattiste PM, Yakubov SJ, DeLucca PT, Demopoulos L. Comparison of two platelet glycoprotein IIb–IIIa antagonists, tirofiban and abciximab, for the prevention of ischemic events with percutaneous coronary revascularization. *New Engl J Med* 2001; **344**: 1888–1894.

15 Moliterno DJ, Topol EJ. The TARGET trial: hit or miss? *Eur Heart J* 2002; **23**: 835–837.

16 Gunasekara AP, Walters DL, Aroney CN. Comparison of abciximab with "high-dose" tirofiban in patients undergoing percutaneous coronary intervention. *Int J Cardiol* 2006; **109**: 16–20.

17 Valgimigli M, Percoco G, Barbieri D, Ferrari F, Guardigli G, Parrinello G, Soukhomovskaia O, Ferrari R. The additive value of tirofiban administered with the high-dose bolus in the prevention of ischemic complications during high-risk coronary angioplasty: the ADVANCE trial. *J Am Coll Cardiol* 2004; **44**: 14–19.

18 Valgimigli M, Percoco GF, Cicchitelli G, Ferrari F, Barbieri D, Ansani L, Guardigli G, Parrinello G, Malagutti P, Soukhomovskaia O, Bettini A, Campo G, Ferrari R. High dose boluS TiRofibAn and sirolimus eluting sTEnt versus abciximab and bare metal stent in acute mYocardial infarction (STRATEGY) study-protocol design and demography of the first 100 patients. *Cardiovasc Drugs Ther* 2004; **18**: 225–230.

19 Dawson CB, Valgimigli M, Charnigo R, Walters DL, Danzi GB, Bolognese L, Moliterno DJ, Topol EJ. Meta-analysis of high-dose single-bolus tirofiban versus abciximab in patients undergoing percutaneous coronary interventions. *Circulation* 2006; **114**: II–647.

20 Coller BS. Monitoring platelet GP IIa/IIIb antagonist therapy. *Circulation* 1998; **97**: 5–9.

21 Bernardi MM, Califf RM, Kleiman N, Ellis SG, Topol EJ. Lack of usefulness of prolonged bleeding times in predicting hemorrhagic events in patients receiving the 7E3 glycoprotein IIb–IIIa platelet antibody. *Am J Cardiol* 1993; **72**: 1121–1125.

22 Jennings LK, Jacoski MV, White MM. The pharmacodynamics of parenteral glycoprotein IIb–IIIa antagonists. *J Interv Cardiol* 2002; **15**: 45–60.

23 Matzdorff A. Platelet function tests and flow cytometry to monitor antiplatelet therapy. *Sem Thrombosis Hemostasis* 2005; **31**: 393–399.

24 Kereiakes DJ, Broderick TM, Roth EM, Whang D, Mueller M, Lacock P, Anderson LC, Howard W, Blanck C, Schneider J, Abbottsmith CA. Time course, magnitude, and consistency of platelet inhibition by abciximab, tirofiban, or eptifibitide in patients with unstable angina pectoris undergoing percutaneous coronary intervention. *Am J Cardiol* 1999; **84**: 226–233.

25 Steinhubl SR, Talley JD, Braden GA, Tcheng JE, Casterella PJ, Moliterno DJ, Navetta FI, Berger PB, Popma JJ, Dangas G, Gallo R, Sane DC, Saucedo J, Jia G, Lincoff AM, Theroux P, Holmes DR, Teirstein PS, Kereiakes DJ. Point-of-care measured platelet inhibition correlates with a reduced risk of an adverse cardiac event after percutaneous coronary intervention: results of the GOLD (AU-assessing Ultegra) Multicenter Study. *Circulation*. 2001; **103**: 2572–2578.

26 Blankenship JC, Tasissa G, O'Shea JC, Iliadis EA, Bachour FA, Cohen DJ, Lui HK, Mann T, Cohen E, Tcheng JE. Effect of glycoprotein IIb–IIIa receptor inhibition on angiographic complications during percutaneous coronary intervention in the ESPRIT trial. *J Am Coll Cardiol* 2001; **38**: 653–658.

27 Blankenship JC, Sigmon KN, Pieper KS, O'Shea CO, Tardiff BE, Tcheng JE. Effect of eptifibatide on angiographic complications during percutaneous coronary intervention in the IMPACT (Integrilin to Minimize Platelet Aggregation and Coronary Thrombosis) II Trial. *Am J Cardiol* 2001; **88**: 969–973.

28 The EPISTENT Investigators. Randomised placebo-controlled and balloon angioplasty-controlled trial to assess safety of coronary stenting with use of platelet glycoprotein-IIb–IIIa blockade. *Lancet* 1998; **352**: 87–92.

29 Islam MA, Blankenship JC, Balog C, Iliadis EA, Lincoff AM, Tcheng JE, Califf RM, Topol EJ. Effect of abciximab on angiographic complications during percutaneous

coronary stenting in the Evaluation of Platelet IIb–IIIa Inhibition in Stenting Trial (EPISTENT). *Am J Cardiol* 2002; **90**: 916–921.

30 Mukherjee D, Reginelli JP, Moliterno DJ, Yadav JS, Schneider JP, Raymond R, Whitlow PL, Franco I, Topol EJ, Ellis SG. Unexpected mortality reduction with abciximab for in-stent restenosis. *J Invasive Cardiol* 2000; **12**: 540–544.

31 Blankenship JC, Hellkamp AS, Aguirre FV, Demko SL, Topol EJ, Califf RM. Vascular access site complications after percutaneous coronary interventions with abciximab in the Evaluation of c7E3 for the Prevention of Ischemic Complications (EPIC) trial. *Am J Cardiol* 1998; **81**: 36–40.

32 Blankenship JC, Balog C, Sapp SK, Califf RM, Lincoff AM, Tcheng JE, Topol EJ. Reduction in vascular access site bleeding in sequential abciximab coronary intervention trials. *Catheter Cardio Inte* 2002; **57**: 476–483.

33 Blankenship JC. Bleeding complications of glycoprotein IIb–IIIa receptor antagonists. *Am Heart J* 1999; **138**: S287–S296.

34 Mulot A, Moulin F, Fohlen-Walter A, Angioi M, Sghaier M, Carteaux JP, Lecompte T, de Maistre E. Practical approach to the diagnosis and management of thrombocytopenia associated with tirofiban treatment. *Am J Hemat* 2004; **77**: 67–71.

35 Khaykin Y, Paradiso-Hardy FL, Madan M. Acute thrombocytopenia associated with eptifibatide therapy. *Canadian J Cardiol* 2003; **19**: 797–801.

36 Dasgupta H, Blankenship JC, Demko SL, Menapace FJ. Thrombocytopenia complicating treatment with intravenous glycoprotein IIb–IIIa receptor antagonists: a pooled analysis. *Am Heart J* 2000; **140**: 206–211.

37 Curtis BR, Divgi A, Garritty M, Aster RH. Delayed thrombocytopenia after treatment with abciximab: a distinct clinical entity associated with immune response to the drug. *J Thromb Haemost* 2004; **2**: 985–992.

38 Astor RH. Warkentin TE, Laboratory testing for heparin-induced thrombocytopenia. *J Thromb Thrombolysis* 2000; **10** (Suppl. 1): 35–45.

39 Sane DC, Damaraju LV, Topol EJ, Cabot CF, Mascelli MA, Harrington RA, Simoons ML, Califf RM. Occurrence and clinical significance of pseudothrombocytopenia during abciximab therapy. *J Am Coll Cardiol* 2000; **36**: 75–83.

40 Astor RH, Curtis BR, Bougie DW. Thrombocytopenia resulting from sensitivity to GPII-IIIa antagonists. *Sem Thrombosis and Hemostasis* 2004; **30**: 569–577.

41 Bougie DW, Wilker PR, Wuitschick ED, Curtis BR, Malik M, Levine S, Lind RN, Pereira J, Aster RH. Acute thrombocytopenia after treatment with tirofiban or eptifibatide is associated with antibodies specific for ligand-occupied GPIIb–IIIa. Citation is *Blood* 2002; **100**: 2071–2076.

42 Iskandar SB, Kasasbeh ES, Mechleb BK, Garcia I, Jackson A, Fahrig S, Albalbissi K, Henry PD. Alveolar hemorrhage: an underdiagnosed complication of treatment with glycoprotein IIb–IIIa antagonists. *J Intervent Cardiol* 2006; **19**: 356–363.

43 Madan M, Kereiakes DJ, Hermiller JB, Rund MM, Tudor G, Anderson L, McDonald MB, Berkowitz SD, Sketch MH Jr, Phillips HR 3rd, Tcheng JE. Efficacy of abciximab readministration in coronary intervention. *Am J Cardiol* 2000; **85**: 435–440.

44 Tcheng JE, Kereiakes DJ, Lincoff AM, George BS, Kleiman NS, Sane DC, Cines DB, Jordan RE, Mascelli MA, Langrall MA, Damaraju L, Schantz A, Effron MB, Braden GA. Abciximab readministration: results of the ReoPro Readministration Registry. *Circulation* 2001; **104**: 870–875.

45 Lev EI, Osende JI, Richard MF, Robbins JA, Delfin JA, Rodroguez O, Sharma SK, Jayasundera T, Badimon JJ, Marmur JD. Administration of abciximab to patients receiving tirofiban or eptifibitide: effect on platelet function. *J Am Coll Cardiol* 2001; **37**: 847–855.

46 Rao J, Mascarenhas DA. Successful use of eptifibatide as an adjunct to coronary stenting in a patient with abciximab-associated acute profound thrombocytopenia. *J Invasive Cardiol* 2001; **13**: 471–473.

47 Marmur JD, Mitre CA, Barnathan E, Cavusoglu. Benefit of bolus-only platelet glycoprotein IIb–IIIa inhibition during percutaneous coronary intervention: insights from the very early outcomes in the Evaluation of 7E3 for the Prevention of Ischemic Complications (EPIC) trial. *Am Heart J* 2006; **152**: 876–881.

48 Marmur JD, Poludasu S, Agarwal A, Vladutiu P, Lapin R, Cavusoglu E. Bolus-only platelet glycoprotein IIb–IIIa inhibition during percutaneous coronary intervention. *J Inv Cardiol* 2006; **18**: 521–526.

49 Bertrand OF, De Larochelliere R, Rodes-Cabau J, Proulx G, Gleeton O, Nguyen CM, Dery JP, Barbeau G, Noel B, Larose E, Poirier P, Roy L. Early Discharge After Transradial Stenting of Coronary Arteries Study Investigators. A randomized study comparing same-day home discharge and abciximab bolus only to overnight hospitalization and abciximab bolus and infusion after transradial coronary stent implantation. *Circulation* 2006; **114**: 2636–2643.

50 Kakkar AK, Moustapha A, Hanley HG, Weiss M, Caldito G, Misra P, Reddy PC, Tandon N. Comparison of intracoronary vs. intravenous administration of abciximab in coronary stenting. *Catheter Cardio Diag* 2004; **61**: 31–34.

51 Wohrle J, Grebe OC, Nusser T, Al-Khayer E, Schaible S, Kochs M, Hombach V, Hoher M. Reduction of major adverse cardiac events with intracoronary compared to intravenous bolus application of abciximab in patients with acute myocardial infarction or unstable angina undergoing coronary angioplasty. *Circulation* 2003; **107**: 1840–1843.

Chapter 8

Intravenous P2Y$_{12}$ inhibitors

Steven P. Dunn and Steven R. Steinhubl

Introduction

Therapeutic modalities that inhibit platelet aggregation, such as the thienopy-ridine P2Y$_{12}$ inhibitors (Chapter 5), aspirin (Chapter 3) and glycoprotein IIb/IIIa inhibitors (Chapter 7), are critically important in the treatment and prevention of intra-arterial thrombosis, whether spontaneous or related to mechanical injury such as during a percutaneous coronary intervention (PCI). Thienopyridines, while initially discovered by chance with the target of inhibition being unknown for several decades after the initiation of clinical use, are now known to inhibit the effects of the platelet agonist adenosine diphosphate (ADP) via irreversible inhibition of one of two platelet ADP receptors – the P2Y$_{12}$ receptor. The impact of P2Y$_{12}$ inhibition on platelet function is demonstrated *ex vivo* through its effects on platelet aggregation and activation, but most importantly and convincingly through an impressive array of clinical evidence in the setting of a PCI, non-ST-segment elevation acute coronary syndrome (ACS) and acute myocardial infarction [1–4].

Clopidogrel and ticlopidine are approved for human use, with several other compounds in development [5]. Clopidogrel is generally preferred over ticlopidine due to its superior safety profile [6] and its ability to achieve a more rapid onset of antiplatelet effect by administration of a loading dose. Beyond this, however, the two share several similarities and limitations. Both drugs are only approved in oral dosage formulations and they are also both irreversible inhibitors of the P2Y$_{12}$ receptor [7]. Both are also prodrugs [8,9], which require metabolism by the liver in order to achieve biologic effect. These limitations

Antiplatelet Therapy in Ischemic Heart Disease, 1st edition. Edited by Stephen D. Wiviott.
© 2009 American Heart Association, ISBN: 9-781-4051-7626-2

translate into several therapeutic challenges with the use of these agents. First, even with larger loading doses of clopidogrel (up to 900 mg), onset of antiplatelet effect is relatively slow, requiring at least 2 hours after ingestion to reach maximal ADP inhibition [10].

Second, since both drugs are irreversible inhibitors of the $P2Y_{12}$ receptor, offset of antiplatelet effect equates to the lifespan of the platelet [10–12]. This limits the early use of thienopyridines in some clinical settings in which the patient's risk for requiring a surgical procedure and the increased risk of bleeding associated with it must be weighed against the potential for a thrombotic complication [2,13,14]. This concern prompted recommendations from the American College of Cardiology and the American Heart Association for at least 5 days between discontinuation of thienopyridines and surgical procedures (Chapters 15, 16) [15], which may cause delays in surgical revascularization in patients who receive clopidogrel but also presenting barriers to pretreatment until coronary artery anatomy is known. This highlights the need for a rapid acting, intravenous, *reversible* $P2Y_{12}$ receptor inhibitor. Such a treatment modality would allow for the near-instantaneous onset of full $P2Y_{12}$ inhibition, and minimized bleeding concerns when rapidly reversed by termination of the infusion. By offering greater control of antiplatelet therapy, agents with these characteristics could potentially improve outcomes and concurrently decrease the risk for bleeding events.

There are several intravenous, reversible inhibitors of the $P2Y_{12}$ ADP receptor in development. Cangrelor (AR-C69931MX, The Medicines Company; Parsippany, NJ), INS50589 (Inspire Pharmaceuticals; Durham, NC), PRT060128 (Portola Pharmaceuticals; South San Francisco, CA), and BX667 (Berlex Biosciencies; Richmond, CA) are four such compounds that have shown promise in Phase I and II trials. Cangrelor is the first agent to be evaluated in Phase III trials in patients with ACS and those undergoing PCI. Development on INS50589 has since been halted following an excess of bleeding events in a Phase II trial investigating the impact of $P2Y_{12}$ inhibitors on graft patency in patients undergoing coronary artery bypass grafting (CABG) surgery [16]. PRT060128 and BX667 are being investigated for both oral and parenteral use and are undergoing early investigational trials in humans and animals.

Pharmacology of intravenous $P2Y_{12}$ antagonists

Upon vascular injury and endothelial dysfunction, a cascade of events is unleashed in order to promote clot formation at the site of injury, including platelet activation. Platelets are initially activated at the site of injury by subendothelial proteins such as vWF and collagen, in addition to many other agonists. These initial interactions and activations cause the release of ADP from platelet dense granules. ADP further interacts with the platelet via the purinergic $P2Y_1$ and $P2Y_{12}$ (formerly $P2_T$) receptors (Figure 8.1) [17,18]. Stimulation

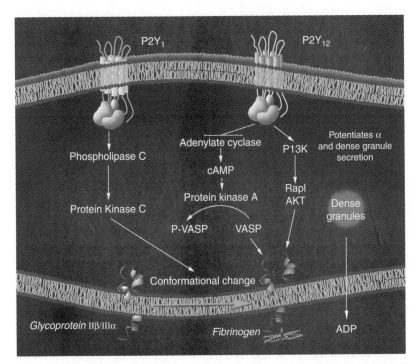

Fig. 8.1 Representation of the G-protein coupled platelet surface receptors for ADP and some of their intracellular mechanisms of action. Activation of the P2Y1 receptor results in transient platelet aggregation through its effect on phospholipase C and protein kinase C, leading to increased calcium mobilization. Activation of the P2Y$_{12}$ receptor sustains platelet aggregation through two mechanisms. First, by dephophorylating vasodilator-stimulated phosphoprotein (VASP), a substrate of cyclic AMP (cAMP) dependant protein kinases, and second, by stimulation of the GTPase RapI through phosphatidylinositol-3 kinase (PI3K).

of the P2Y$_1$ receptor is largely responsible for conformational changes in plate-let shape via activation of protein kinase C, leading to increased intracellular calcium levels as well as transient platelet aggregation. However, the P2Y$_{12}$ receptor has been shown TO govern more sustained platelet aggregation by its inhibitory effects on adenylate cyclase via G$_i$, leading to a decrease in cyclic AMP (cAMP), and resulting in platelet aggregation. Antagonism of the P2Y$_{12}$ receptor with clopidogrel, a relatively weak antagonist *ex vivo*, inhibits approximately 50–70% of aggregatory activity induced by ADP, expanding further to an effect on global *ex vivo* platelet aggregation induced by thrombin and TRAP. However, significant interindividual variability in the antagonism of ADP induced platelet aggregation with clopidogrel (sometimes referred to as clopidogrel resistance or non-responsiveness) has been demonstrated (see Chapter 6) [19–21], although the clinical implications of these findings are as yet unclear. Platelet inhibition with $P2Y_{12}$ antagonists has also been shown to have an effect on platelet–leukocyte interactions via P-selectin, thereby contributing a potentially critical anti-inflammatory component of these agents in the treatment of vascular thrombosis.

The intravenous $P2Y_{12}$ inhibitors in development, similar to the theinopyridines, antagonize the purinerigic $P2Y_{12}$ receptor on the platelet surface. However, they have a distinctly different molecular chemistry. Cangrelor and INS50589 were synthesized as structural analogs of the competitive $P2Y_{12}$ antagonist adenosine triphosphate (ATP). ATP itself is a relatively weak $P2Y_{12}$ antagonist, but an ATP analog would allow the analogous compound to be reversible; a stark contrast to the irreversible theinopyridines. ATP is also a highly polar molecule, which aids in the formulation of an intravenous solution. Chemical manipulations of the molecule could also improve the poor affinity for the $P2Y_{12}$ receptor. The first ATP analogs suitable for clinical investigation were developed by AstraZeneca R&D Charnwood [22] and cangrelor was later developed and initially referred to in publications by its chemical name AR-C69931MX [23]. Initial experiments with ATP analogs revealed compounds with short half-lives and very rapid onset/offset receptor properties in animal models. AR-C69931MX showed significant promise as a therapeutic agent by exhibiting dose-dependent, 100% inhibition of ADP induced *ex vivo* platelet aggregation in canines, as well as significantly decreased bleeding time when compared to the glycoprotein IIb/IIIa inhibitor lamifiban at equivalent levels of ADP inhibition [23]. These findings paved the way for further investigation of cangrelor in humans. PRT060128 and BX667 also selectively inhibit the $P2Y_{12}$ receptor, but unlike cangrelor and INS50589, they are not structural analogs of ATP (Figure 8.2).

Little information is available about the clinical pharmacology of the intravenous $P2Y_{12}$ antagonists, including the method of elimination (and ramifications for those patients with altered drug clearance) or significant drug–drug interactions. BX667 is known to produce an active metabolite, however. Unlike clopidogrel, the intravenous $P2Y_{12}$ inhibitors do not require metabolism by the liver to achieve clinical effect and are active *in vitro*, indicating a significant role for these agents as research tools to further explore the role of ADP in thrombosis. Research is underway with cangrelor to expanded knowledge about the interactions of ADP with P2 receptors on the platelet surface and throughout the body. While specific data on the terminal half-life of these compounds is not available, initial research suggests this is on the order of several minutes for most intravenous $P2Y_{12}$ inhibitors [24–26].

While detailed information on drug–drug interactions with the intravenous $P2Y_{12}$ inhibitors are not known, there is evidence for a competitive pharmacodynamic interaction between cangrelor and clopidogrel. Effects of this were

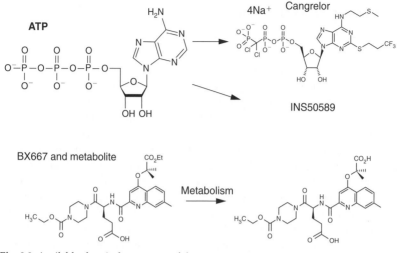

Fig. 8.2 Available chemical structures of the intravenous P2Y$_{12}$ inhibitors that have undergone or are undergoing clinical testing. Adenosine triphosphate (ATP), which served as a base from which cangrelor and INS50589 were synthesized and BX667 (and its active metabolite), which is not an analog of ATP.

demonstrated in a randomized, open-label study in 20 healthy volunteers [27]. Group 1 (n = 10) received cangrelor (30 μg/kg IV bolus followed by 4 μg/kg/min infusion for 1 hour) followed by 600 mg of clopidogrel immediately *after* termination of the infusion. Group 2 (n = 10) received clopidogrel 600 mg (group 2A) and then were readmitted after a 2-week washout period and given 600 mg of clopidogrel *simultaneously* with cangrelor (same dose as above) (group 2B). Subjects in group 1 achieved maximal ADP inhibition with cangrelor and although normalization of platelet function occurred after discontinuation of cangrelor, platelet aggregation began to decline by 1 hour and was completely inhibited by 3 hours after the receipt of clopidogrel. However, in group 2, the effect of clopidogrel when given simultaneously with cangrelor was completely attenuated at 6 hours after ingestion. This effect was demonstrated with ADP-induced aggregation (5 mmol/L and 20 mmol/L) measured by flow cytometry, whole-blood electrical impedance, light-transmittance aggregometry, and, additionally, P-selectin expression. This data indicates that patients on baseline thienopyridine therapy who receive cangrelor will likely require administration of a loading dose of clopidogrel after discontinuation of the infusion in order to prevent a potentially critical gap in antiplatelet therapy, particularly after PCI with stent placement.

Effects on platelet aggregation

The most robust data available on the pharmacodynamic effects of the intravenous $P2Y_{12}$ inhibitors in humans is from substudies of the two main Phase II clinical trials with cangrelor. The first investigated the use of cangrelor in patients with acute coronary syndromes [28]. Cangrelor demonstrated nearly 100% inhibition of platelet aggregation induced by up to 10 mmol/L of ADP only 30 minutes after an infusion (with no bolus) of $2\mu g/kg/min$ (n = 8) or $4\mu g/kg/min$ (n = 5). This effect was not measurably greater at 21 hours or 69 hours after the onset of infusion. The *in vitro* pharmacodynamic effect of cangrelor was also compared in this study to the *ex vivo* effect of a group receiving clopidogrel (n = 11) for elective PCI after 4–7 days. Cangrelor showed statistically greater effect on ADP (2 mmol/L) induced platelet aggregation and also a larger effect on TRAP (20 mmol/L) induced aggregation when compared with the clopidogrel group. Effects on platelet aggregation were again examined with cangrelor in a substudy of a 2-part, Phase II, multicenter, randomized, placebo- and active-controlled trial [25]. Cangrelor again demonstrated near 100% inhibition of *ex vivo* platelet aggregation induced by 3 mmol/L of ADP beginning 15 minutes after initiation of infusion when compared with placebo. In part 2 of the study, $4\mu g/kg/min$ of cangrelor demonstrated equivalent (100%) inhibition to 3 mmol/L of ADP when compared to abciximab after 15 minutes. However, the effects of cangrelor on platelet aggregation began to dissipate 15 minutes after termination, whereas abciximab still demonstrated nearly 100% inhibition 24 hours after termination. This is consistent with the known near-irreversible inhibition of platelet aggregation with abciximab.

Several smaller trials have also investigated the pharmacological effects of cangrelor on platelet aggregation in humans in comparison with other antiplatelet agents. It was first compared to aspirin in healthy volunteers [29], demonstrating significantly greater inhibitory effect on platelet function induced by ADP, TRAP, PAF and collagen, illustrating the importance of the $P2Y_{12}$ receptor in sustaining platelet aggregation. A subsequent study also showed the superior *in vitro* antiplatelet effect of 100 nmol/L of cangrelor in comparison to aspirin and dipyridamole on platelet aggregation induced by ADP and PAF [30]. Cangrelor by itself appeared superior to either drug alone and to the combination of aspirin and dipyridamole, but the most effective inhibition occurred when all three drugs were used together. This again is consistent with the central, but not all-inclusive, role of ADP in platelet activation and aggregation.

P-selectin is expressed on the platelet surface upon activation and appears to play a major role in the recruitment of leukocytes into thrombus formation and the subsequent inflammatory response. The effects of intravenous $P2Y_{12}$ inhibitors on this interaction were examined in a substudy of a Phase II trial in patients with acute coronary syndromes receiving cangrelor [31]. Samples were also obtained from healthy volunteers and cangrelor induced P-selectin expression and platelet–leukocyte conjugate formation was evaluated *in vitro* in addition to the *ex vivo* results from the Phase II study. This data was examined alongside the *ex vivo* effects of clopidogrel, aspirin, and clopidogrel plus aspirin in 12 healthy volunteers after 10 days of treatment. The results of this study demonstrated that ADP inhibition with either cangrelor or clopidogrel, but not aspirin, resulted in significant reductions in P-selectin expression and, consequently, platelet–monocyte and platelet–neutrophil conjugation. However, *in vitro* cangrelor (100mmol/L) added significantly to the effects of clopidogrel, causing further decrease in P-selectin expression and platelet–monocyte conjugation, likely due to its superior inhibition of ADP-induced platelet aggregation. Additionally, no significant difference was noted between 2µg/kg/min and 4µg/kg/min infusions of cangrelor.

The pharmacokinetics and pharmacodynamics of cangrelor as a bolus followed by an infusion have also been evaluated. Twenty-two healthy volunteers were recruited and randomized to receive either a 15µg/kg bolus followed by a 2µg/kg/min infusion or a 30µg/kg bolus followed by a 4µg/kg/min infusion [24]. Maximal platelet inhibition was achieved only 2 minutes after bolus administration with complete recovery of platelet function 60 minutes after termination of the infusion. This indicates that near-instantaneous onset of antiplatelet effect can be achieved with this method of administration.

Less information is known about the pharmacology of INS50589, PRT060128 and BX667. Results from a Phase I trial with INS50589 in 36 healthy volunteers has been presented [32]. This study evaluated the safety and tolerability of 4-hour IV infusions of INS50589 at doses of 0.1mg/kg/h, 0.3mg/kg/h, 1mg/kg/h, and 3mg/kg/h versus placebo. The drug exhibited dose-dependant, linear pharmacokinetics as well as dose-dependant, near-100% inhibition of ADP-induced *ex vivo* platelet aggregation in addition to the rapid onset/offset properties that characterize the ATP analog P2Y$_{12}$ inhibitor. These data paved the way for a larger Phase II trial in CABG patients, a novel market for intravenous antiplatelet agents. Similar "first in human" trials exist describing the pharmacologic profile of PRT060128 [33], which also exhibits dose-dependent, 100% inhibition of ADP-induced platelet aggregation.

Animal studies

To date, two studies evaluating cangrelor in animal models of thrombosis have been published. The first study examined the efficacy of cangrelor (4µg/kg/min for 6 hours) in a canine model for the prevention of occlusive thrombus formation after electrolytically induced deep vessel wall injury [34]. Incidence of thrombus formation was 16.7% in the drug-treated group (n = 6), versus 100% in the group receiving infusions of normal saline (n = 5, p < 0.05). A second study, again in a canine coronary electrolytic injury thrombosis model, used cangrelor ($4\mu g/kg/min$ for 2 hours beginning 10 minutes prior to administration of t-PA) in conjunction with thrombolytic therapy versus placebo [35]. No significant difference between groups was found with regards to reperfusion rate (100% for both groups), or time to reflow (24.7 ± 7.9 in the cangrelor group versus 20.9 ± 9.1 minutes in the placebo group). However, cangrelor did demonstrate statistically improved reflow duration time (75.0 ± 39.9 vs. 120 ± 0 minutes, $p < 0.05$) cyclic flow variation (50% vs. 0%, $p < 0.05$), and reocclusion rate (60% vs. 0%, $p < 0.05$). In addition, myocardial infarct size was statistically lower with the cangrelor group when assessed via the *ex vivo* dual-perfusion histochemical method.

BX667 has been evaluated intravenously in a rat arterial–venous (AV) shunt model of thrombosis [36]. A bolus injection of $3\,mg/kg$ inhibited ~80% of thrombus formation, but this was not further improved with a higher dose of $10\,mg/kg$. BX667 also appeared to cause significantly less dose-dependant bleeding in this study when compared to clopidogrel, with threefold increases in clopidogrel concentration resulting in a nearly tenfold increase in bleeding time versus a 4.4-fold increases in the concentration of BX667 only causing a twofold increase in bleeding time ($p < 0.05$ at ED_{50}). This may indicate that selective inhibition of the $P2Y_{12}$ receptor could result in a wider therapeutic index with concurrently improved efficacy and safety.

Clinical studies in humans

The safety and tolerability of cangrelor in humans has been evaluated in two Phase II studies. The first was an open-label, multicenter, dose-escalation study in 39 patients presenting with unstable angina or non-Q wave myocardial infarction [26]. Cangrelor was infused at stepped dose increments over 3 hours to a maximum of either $2\mu g/kg/min$ for 21 hours (Part 1; n = 12), $2\mu g/kg/min$ for 69 hours (Part 2; n = 13), or $4\mu g/kg/min$ for 69 hours (Part 3; n = 14). No bolus was given prior to initiation of the infusion. Blood samples were also obtained for pharmacodynamic studies, as discussed above. The drug appeared to be well tolerated, with no deaths, or major or minor bleeding events (using TIMI criteria) on 30-day follow-up.

A second Phase II program in elective or urgent PCI further confirmed the safety and tolerability of cangrelor [25]. Part 1 of this study randomized patients (n = 200) to receive 18 to 24 hours of 1, 2 or $4\mu g/kg/min$ infusions (with no bolus) of cangrelor versus placebo initiated immediately prior to PCI. In part 2, patients (n = 199) were further randomized to receive the highest dose of cangrelor ($4\mu g/kg/min$) or abciximab ($0.25\,mg/kg$ bolus, followed by $0.125\mu g/kg/min$ infusion up to $10\mu g/min$ for 12 hours) directly prior to PCI. The primary endpoint of the study was the composite endpoint of major and minor bleeding through 7 days. Blood samples were also obtained for platelet aggregometry studies, as discussed previously. Results revealed no significant difference in the primary endpoint between cangrelor (all doses) and placebo in part 1 (13% vs. 8%, p = NS) and no significant difference between cangrelor (4µg/kg/min) and abciximab 7.6% vs. 5.3%, p = NS) in part 2. However, a trend towards increased major bleeding was observed with the 4µg/kg/min dose versus placebo in part 1 (8% vs. 0%, p = 0.052; 95% CI 0.048, 0.277). This increase in major bleeding was not observed in part 2 when compared with abciximab (1% vs. 2%, p = NS). Statistically less frequent thrombocytopenia was also observed with cangrelor versus abciximab for part 2 (1% vs. 7%, p = 0.025). In addition, no significant difference in 30-day major adverse cardiac events (death, MI, unplanned repeat PCI) was noted between cangrelor and abciximab in part 2 (7.6% vs. 5.3%, respectively, p = NS).

More definitive clinical data on the safety and efficacy of intravenous P2Y$_{12}$ inhibitors will likely begin with the Phase III Cangrelor versus standard tHerapy to Achieve optimal Management of Platelet inhibitION (CHAMPION) trials designed to assess the use of cangrelor in the treatment of ACS and as adjunctive antiplatelet therapy during PCI. The CHAMPION-PLATFORM trial is a randomized, double-blind, placebo control trial set to enroll a total of 6400 patients with ACS and will compare cangrelor versus placebo plus standard therapy [37]. The primary endpoint of the trial will be a composite endpoint of all-cause mortality, myocardial infarction, and ischemia-driven revascularization (IDR). CHAMPION-PCI (Figure 8.3) will enroll 9000 ACS patients and will compare cangrelor to clopidogrel in the setting of higher-risk PCI [38]. The primary endpoint will be the same composite endpoint as above measured 48 hours after PCI. Enrollment is currently underway for both Phase III trials.

Summary/conclusion

The P2Y$_{12}$ receptor plays a vital role in sustaining platelet aggregation. Therapies that currently target inhibition of this receptor have disadvantages relating to their pharmacological profile, which makes the concept of a reversible, intravenous P2Y$_{12}$ inhibitor attractive. Such an agent will potentially decrease bleeding events by its rapid onset and offset, resulting in more limited and controlled exposure to high levels of drug-induced platelet dysfunction. It may also improve treatment in ACS by yielding faster onset of antiplatelet therapy, leading to decreased myocardial ischemia and improved coronary artery patency prior to PCI. Early administration of antiplatelet therapy in the acute setting appears to be critical and time-dependence has been shown with multiple agents, dating back to the International Study of Infarct Survival (ISIS)-2 trial with aspirin [39] and potentially continuing today with abciximab [40]. Early studies with reversible intravenous P2Y$_{12}$ inhibitors have been promising, demonstrating significant effects on platelet aggregation and appearing to be well tolerated, but further clinical data will be required

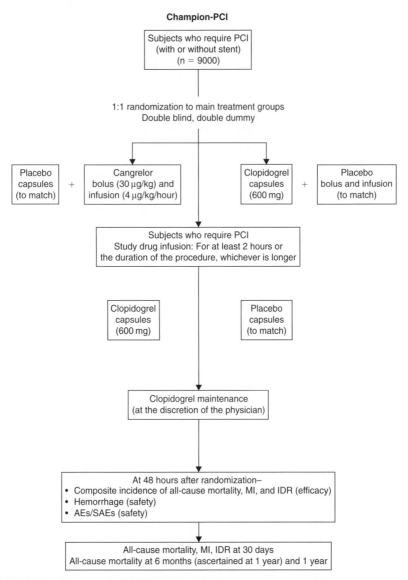

Fig. 8.3 Design of the CHAMPION-PCI trial.

to justify their use over existing thienopyridines and glycoprotein IIb/IIIa inhibitors.

Trials with intravenous $P2Y_{12}$ inhibitors, which have unique molecular chemistry in comparison to the thienopyridine class, may help to answer whether the effects of thienopyridines are limited to ADP inhibition. These trials, in combination with results from high-dose clopidogrel and novel thienopyridines studies, will help to definitively establish the role of ADP in platelet aggregation and thrombosis-related infarction. Additionally, these studies may serve to validate measures of ADP inhibition as a treatment benchmark in the acute and chronic setting.

As discussed previously, development on INS50589 has been halted due to excess bleeding events in a CABG population [16]. While bleeding risk with the higher levels of ADP inhibition is of concern, the results of this trial may simply reflect the extremely high bleeding risk of this population. The results of the ongoing CHAMPION trials with cangrelor and the Phase II and III trials with PRT060128 and BX667 will assess the safety and efficacy of rapid and reversible maximal inhibition of ADP in the pharmacotherapeutic treatment of acute coronary syndromes and PCI.

References

1 Steinhubl SR, Berger PB, Mann JT, 3rd, Fry ET, DeLago A, Wilmer C, *et al.* Early and sustained dual oral antiplatelet therapy following percutaneous coronary intervention: a randomized controlled trial. *JAMA* 2002; **288**: 2411–2420.

2 Yusuf S, Zhao F, Mehta SR, Chrolavicius S, Tognoni G, Fox KK. Effects of clopidogrel in addition to aspirin in patients with acute coronary syndromes without ST-segment elevation. *New Engl J Med* 2001; **345**: 494–502.

3 Sabatine MS, Cannon CP, Gibson CM, Lopez-Sendon JL, Montalescot G, Theroux P, *et al.* Addition of clopidogrel to aspirin and fibrinolytic therapy for myocardial infarction with ST-segment elevation. *New Engl J Med* 2005; **352**: 1179–1189.

4 Chen ZM, Jiang LX, Chen YP, Xie JX, Pan HC, Peto R, *et al.* Addition of clopidogrel to aspirin in 45,852 patients with acute myocardial infarction: randomised placebo-controlled trial. *Lancet* 2005; **366**: 1607–1621.

5 Cattaneo M. Platelet P2 receptors: old and new targets for antithrombotic drugs. *Expert Rev Cardiovasc Ther* 2007; **5**: 45–55.

6 Bertrand ME, Rupprecht HJ, Urban P, Gershlick AH. Double-blind study of the safety of clopidogrel with and without a loading dose in combination with aspirin compared with ticlopidine in combination with aspirin after coronary stenting: the clopidogrel aspirin stent international cooperative study (CLASSICS). *Circulation* 2000; **102**: 624–629.

7 Savi P, Herbert JM. Clopidogrel and ticlopidine: P2Y$_{12}$ adenosine diphosphate-receptor antagonists for the prevention of atherothrombosis. *Semin Thromb Hemost* 2005; **31**: 174–183.

8 Savi P, Combalbert J, Gaich C, Rouchon MC, Maffrand JP, Berger Y, *et al.* The antiaggregating activity of clopidogrel is due to a metabolic activation by the hepatic cytochrome P450-1A. *Thromb Haemost* 1994; **72**: 313–317.

9 Savi P, Herbert JM, Pflieger AM, Dol F, Delebassee D, Combalbert J, *et al.* Importance of hepatic metabolism in the antiaggregating activity of the thienopyridine clopidogrel. *Biochem Pharmacol* 1992; **44**: 527–532.

10 Price MJ, Coleman JL, Steinhubl SR, Wong GB, Cannon CP, Teirstein PS. Onset and offset of platelet inhibition after high-dose clopidogrel loading and standard daily

therapy measured by a point-of-care assay in healthy volunteers. *Am J Cardiol* 2006; **98**: 681–684.

11 Weber AA, Braun M, Hohlfeld T, Schwippert B, Tschope D, Schror K. Recovery of platelet function after discontinuation of clopidogrel treatment in healthy volunteers. *Br J Clin Pharmacol* 2001; **52**: 333–336.

12 Thebault JJ, Kieffer G, Lowe GD, Nimmo WS, Cariou R. Repeated-dose pharmaco-dynamics of clopidogrel in healthy subjects. *Semin Thromb Hemost* 1999; **25** (Suppl. 2): 9–14.

13 Chu MW, Wilson SR, Novick RJ, Stitt LW, Quantz MA. Does clopidogrel increase blood loss following coronary artery bypass surgery? *Ann Thorac Surg* 2004; **78**: 1536–1541.

14 Kapetanakis EI, Medlam DA, Boyce SW, Haile E, Hill PC, Dullum MK, *et al.* Clopidogrel administration prior to coronary artery bypass grafting surgery: the cardiologist's panacea or the surgeon's headache? *Eur Heart J* 2005; **26**: 576–583.

15 Braunwald E, Antman EM, Beasley JW, Califf RM, Cheitlin MD, Hochman JS, *et al.* ACC/AHA 2002 guideline update for the management of patients with unstable angina and non-ST-segment elevation myocardial infarction – summary article: a report of the American College of Cardiology/ American Heart Association task force on practice guidelines (Committee on the Management of Patients With Unstable Angina). *J Am Coll Cardiol* 2002; **40**: 1366–1374.

16 Inspire Pharmaceuticals. *Study of INS50589 Intravenous Infusion in Subjects Undergoing Coronary Artery Bypass Grafting (CABG) Involving Cardiopulmonary Bypass.* In: ClinicalTrials.gov [Internet]. Bethesda (MD): National Library of Medicine (US), 2000–2006. Available from: http://www.clinicaltrials.gov/ct/show/NCT00316212? order=1 NLM Identifier: NCT00316212.

17 Abbracchio MP, Burnstock G, Boeynaems JM, Barnard EA, Boyer JL, Kennedy C, *et al.* International Union of Pharmacology LVIII: update on the P2Y G protein-coupled nucleotide receptors: from molecular mechanisms and pathophysiology to therapy. *Pharmacol Rev* 2006; **58**: 281–341.

18 Nylander S, Mattsson C, Ramstrom S, Lindahl TL. The relative importance of the ADP receptors, $P2Y_{12}$ and $P2Y_1$, in thrombin-induced platelet activation. *Thromb Res* 2003; **111**: 65–73.

19 Barragan P, Bouvier JL, Roquebert PO, Macaluso G, Commeau P, Comet B, *et al.* Resistance to thienopyridines: clinical detection of coronary stent thrombosis by monitoring of vasodilator-stimulated phosphoprotein phosphorylation. *Catheter Cardiovasc Interv* 2003; **59**: 295–302.

20 Gurbel PA, Bliden KP, Samara W, Yoho JA, Hayes K, Fissha MZ, *et al.* Clopidogrel effect on platelet reactivity in patients with stent thrombosis: results of the CREST Study. *J Am Coll Cardiol* 2005; **46**: 1827–1832.

21 Matetzky S, Shenkman B, Guetta V, Shechter M, Bienart R, Goldenberg I, *et al.* Clopidogrel resistance is associated with increased risk of recurrent atherothrombotic events in patients with acute myocardial infarction. *Circulation* 2004; **109**: 3171–3175.

22 van Giezen JJ, Humphries RG. Preclinical and clinical studies with selective reversible direct $P2Y_{12}$ antagonists. *Semin Thromb Hemost* 2005; **31**: 195–204.

23 Ingall AH, Dixon J, Bailey A, Coombs ME, Cox D, McInally JI, *et al.* Antagonists of the platelet P2T receptor: a novel approach to antithrombotic therapy. *J Med Chem* 1999; **42**: 213–220.

24 Akers WS, Oh JJ, Oestreich JH, Ferraris S, Nessel CC, Schwabe KD, *et al.* The pharmacokinetics and pharmacodynamics of a bolus and infusion of cangrelor: a direct, parenteral P2Y$_{12}$ receptor antagonist. *In press*, 2007.

25 Greenbaum AB, Grines CL, Bittl JA, Becker RC, Kereiakes DJ, Gilchrist IC, *et al.* Initial experience with an intravenous P2Y$_{12}$ platelet receptor antagonist in patients undergoing percutaneous coronary intervention: results from a 2-part, phase II, multicenter, randomized, placebo- and active-controlled trial. *Am Heart J* 2006; **151**: 689 e1–689 e10.

26 Storey RF, Oldroyd KG, Wilcox RG. Open multicentre study of the P2T receptor antagonist AR-C69931MX assessing safety, tolerability and activity in patients with acute coronary syndromes. *Thromb Haemost* 2001; **85**: 401–407.

27 Steinhubl SR, Oh JJ, Oestreich JH, Ferraris S, Charnigo R, Akers WS. Transitioning patients from cangrelor to clopidogrel: pharmacodynamic evidence of a competitive effect. *Thromb Res* 2008; **121**(4): 527-34. Epub 2007 Jul 13.

28 Storey RF, Wilcox RG, Heptinstall S. Comparison of the pharmacodynamic effects of the platelet ADP receptor antagonists clopidogrel and AR-C69931MX in patients with ischaemic heart disease. *Platelets* 2002; **13**: 407–413.

29 Storey RF, Sanderson HM, White AE, May JA, Cameron KE, Heptinstall S. The central role of the P(2T) receptor in amplification of human platelet activation, aggregation, secretion and procoagulant activity. *Br J Haematol* 2000; **110**: 925–934.

30 Zhao L, Bath P, Heptinstall S. Effects of combining three different antiplatelet agents on platelets and leukocytes in whole blood in vitro. *Br J Pharmacol* 2001; **134**: 353–358.

31 Storey RF, Judge HM, Wilcox RG, Heptinstall S. Inhibition of ADP-induced P-selectin expression and platelet-leukocyte conjugate formation by clopidogrel and the P2Y$_{12}$ receptor antagonist AR-C69931MX but not aspirin. *Thromb Haemost* 2002; **88**: 488–494.

32 Johnson FL, Boyer JL, Leese PT, Durham T, Crean CS, Krishnamoorthy R, *et al.* Pharmacological evaluation of a novel, rapidly reversible intravenous platelet P2Y$_{12}$ ADP receptor antagonist, INS50589, in healthy volunteers. *J Am Coll Cardiol* 2006; **47**: 51B.

33 Lieu HD, Conley PB, Andre P, Leese PT, Romanko K, Phillips DR, Jurek M, Meloni A, Hutchaleelaha A, Gretler DD. INITIAL INTRAVENOUS EXPERIENCE WITH PRT060128 (PRT128), AN ORALLY-AVAILABLE, DIRECT-ACTING, AND REVERSIBLE P2Y$_{12}$ INHIBITOR. *J Thromb Haemost* 2007; **5** Supplement 2: P-T-292.

34 Huang J, Driscoll EM, Gonzales ML, Park AM, Lucchesi BR. Prevention of arterial thrombosis by intravenously administered platelet P2T receptor antagonist AR-C69931MX in a canine model. *J Pharmacol Exp Ther* 2000; **295**: 492–499.

35 Wang K, Zhou X, Zhou Z, Tarakji K, Carneiro M, Penn MS, *et al.* Blockade of the platelet P2Y$_{12}$ receptor by AR-C69931MX sustains coronary artery recanalization and improves the myocardial tissue perfusion in a canine thrombosis model. *Arterioscler Thromb Vasc Biol* 2003; **23**: 357–362.

36 Wang YX, Vincelette J, da Cunha V, Martin-McNulty B, Mallari C, Fitch RM, *et al.* A novel P2Y(12) adenosine diphosphate receptor antagonist that inhibits platelet aggregation and thrombus formation in rat and dog models. *Thromb Haemost* 2007; **97**: 847–855.

37 The Medicines Company. *Cangrelor versus standard therapy to achieve optimal management of platelet inhibition.* In: ClinicalTrials.gov [Internet]. Bethesda (MD): National

Library of Medicine (US), 2000–2006. Available from: http://www.clinicaltrials.gov/ct/show/NCT00385138?order=1 NLM Identifier: NCT00385138.

38 The Medicines Company. *A clinical trial to demonstrate the efficacy of cangrelor*. In: ClinicalTrials.gov [Internet]. Bethesda (MD): National Library of Medicine (US). 2000–2006. Available from: http://www.clinicaltrials.gov/ct/show/NCT00305162?order=2 NLM Identifier: NCT00305162.

39 ISIS-2 (Second International Study of Infarct Survival) Collaborative Group. Randomised trial of intravenous streptokinase, oral aspirin, both, or neither among 17,187 cases of suspected acute myocardial infarction. *Lancet* 1988; **2**: 349–360.

40 Maioli M, Bellandi F, Leoncini M, Toso A, Dabizzi RP. Randomized early versus late abciximab in acute myocardial infarction treated with primary coronary intervention (RELAx-AMI Trial). *J Am Coll Cardiol* 2007; **49**: 1517–1524.

Chapter 9

Antiplatelet effects of thrombin inhibitors and fibrinolytic agents

Nicolai Mejevoi, Anjum Tanwir and Marc Cohen

In physiologic conditions platelets participate in hemostasis by adhesion to the damaged vessel wall, activation and, finally, platelet aggregation. Platelet activation is marked by the release of vasoactive and thromboactive substances. The surfaces formed during activation and aggregation are crucial to the propagation of the coagulation cascade, resulting in the deposition of thrombus. Strategies for antiplatelet therapy focused on their activation pathways and surface receptors, resulting in three main groups of medications approved presently for patients with coronary artery disease: (1) cyclooxygenase inhibitors – aspirin; adenosine diphosphate (ADP); (2) $P2Y_{12}$ receptor inhibitors – ticlopidine, clopidogrel, prasugrel and newer agents currently being studied; and (3) glycoprotein (GP) IIb/IIIa receptor inhibitors – abciximab, eptifibatide and tirofiban (Figure 9.1).

Platelet activation and coagulation cascade

Concurrently, anticoagulants are widely used for the patients with acute coronary syndromes (ACS), including unstable angina (UA) and non-ST elevation myocardial infarction (NSTEMI), and fibrinolytic agents are often used during ST-elevation myocardial infarction (STEMI). These agents are used along with dual or even triple antiplatelet therapy (Table 9.1). The focus of this chapter is on the effects of fibrinolytic agents and antithrombins on platelets, and benefits of their use in patients with ACS already receiving recommended antiplatelet therapy.

Antiplatelet Therapy in Ischemic Heart Disease, 1st edition. Edited by Stephen D. Wiviott.
© 2009 American Heart Association, ISBN: 9-781-4051-7626-2

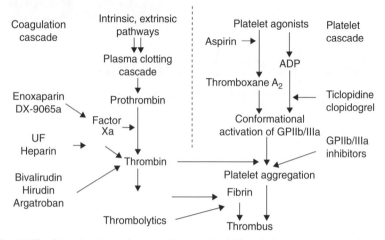

Fig. 9.1 Platelet activation and coagulation cascade. Although there are a variety of approaches to enhancing anticoagulant effects none are completely satisfactory when used as a single agent. Major categories of anticoagulant therapy include agents that target any one of three main components of the thrombotic process: thrombin, platelets or fibrin. Reproduced with permission from Selwyn AP. prothrombotic and antithrambotic pathways in acute coronary syndromes. *American Journal of Cardiology* 2003; **91**(12): 3–11.

Table 9. 1A Heparins and fibrinolytic agents in patients with ST-Elevation myocardial infarction (extract from ACC/AHA Guidelines).

Class I

- Anticoagulation with subcutaneous LMWH or intravenous UFH should be added to antiplatelet therapy with ASA and/or clopidogrel. (Level of Evidence: A)

- Patients undergoing percutaneous or surgical revascularization should receive UFH. *(Level of Evidence: C)*

- UFH should be given i.v. to patients undergoing reperfusion therapy with alteplase, reteplase, or tenecteplase with dosing as follows: bolus of 60 U/kg (maximum 4000 U) followed by an infusion of 12 U/kg/h (maximum 1000 U) initially adjusted to maintain activated partial thromboplastin time (aPTT) at 1.5 to 2.0 times control (approximately 50 to 70 seconds). *(Level of Evidence: C)*

- UFH should be given i.v. to patients treated with nonselective fibrinolytic agents (streptokinase, anistreplase, urokinase) who are at high risk for systemic emboli (large or anterior MI, atrial fibrillation (AF), previous embolus, or known LV thrombus). *(Level of Evidence: B)*

- Platelet counts should be monitored daily in patients taking UFH. *(Level of Evidence: C)*

(*Continued*)

Table 9.1A (Continued)

Class IIb

■ It may be reasonable to administer UFH intravenously to patients undergoing reperfusion therapy with streptokinase. *(Level of Evidence: B)*

Class III

■ Low-molecular-weight heparin should not be used as an alternative to UFH as ancillary therapy in patients aged more than 75 years who are receiving fibrinolytic therapy. *(Level of Evidence: B)*

■ Low-molecular-weight heparin should not be used as an alternative to UFH as ancillary therapy in patients less than 75 years who are receiving fibrinolytic therapy but have significant renal dysfunction (serum creatinine greater than 2.5 mg/dL in men or 2.0 mg/dL in women). *(Level of Evidence: B)*

Table 9.1B Heparins in patients with UA/NST-Elevation Myocardial Infarction (Extract from ACC/AHA Guidelines).

Class I

■ Anticoagulation with subcutaneous LMWH or intravenous unfractionated heparin (UFH) should be added to antiplatelet therapy with ASA and/or clopidogrel. *(Level of Evidence: A)*

Class IIa

■ Enoxaparin is preferable to UFH as an anticoagulant in patients with UA/NSTEMI, unless CABG is planned within 24 h. *(Level of Evidence: A)*

Table 9.1C Antithrombins in PCI (Extract from ACC/AHA/SCAI 2005 Guideline Update for Percutaneous Coronary Intervention).

Class I

■ Unfractionated heparin should be administered to patients undergoing PCI. *(Level of Evidence: C)*

■ For patients with heparin-induced thrombocytopenia, it is recommended that bivalirudin or argatroban be used to replace heparin. *(Level of Evidence: B)*

(Continued)

Table 9.1C (Continued)

Class IIa

- It is reasonable to use bivalirudin as an alternative to unfractionated heparin and glycoprotein IIb/IIIa antagonists in low-risk patients undergoing elective PCI. *(Level of Evidence: B)*

- Low-molecular-weight heparin is a reasonable alternative to unfractionated heparin in patients with UA/NSTEMI undergoing PCI. *(Level of Evidence: B)*

Class IIb

- Low-molecular-weight heparin may be considered as an alternative to unfractionated heparin in patients with STEMI undergoing PCI. *(Level of Evidence: B)*

Platelets and fibrinolysis

Fibrinolytic agents (Table 9.2), including streptokinase, urokinase and tissue plasminogen activator (t-PA), are established for acute treatment of patients with STEMI, resulting from a major coronary occlusion with fresh thrombus. First clinical evidence of survival benefits with aspirin and fibrinolytic agent came from the Second International Study of Infarct Survival (ISIS-2) [1]. Ever since, aspirin and fibrinolytics have become the standard of care for patients with STEMI, to which all newer strategies are compared. It is reasonable to expect benefit from the combined use of fibrinolytic and antiplatelet agents, considering that in the high velocity/high shear conditions of a 2–4 mm coronary artery formation of an occlusive, platelet-rich thrombus, loaded with fibrin is the final step in the pathophysiologic cascade of events leading to STEMI. While ostensibly fibrinolytics are selective for fibrin, they do have some impact on platelets. This interaction is complex and suggests both activation and inhibition, possibly with different time courses. However, both streptokinase and t-PA have been shown to activate platelets within minutes of administration, action which cannot be ascribed entirely to plasmin generation [2]. One of the proposed mechanisms of these interactions is related to the stimulation of platelets through urokinase type plasminogen activator (uPA) receptor, identified as CD87. Urokinase plasminogen activator receptor (uPAR, CD87) is a widely distributed 55-kD glycoprotein I-anchored surface receptor. This process involves formation of uPAR–uPA and plasminogen activator inhibitor-1 complex, delivering further activating or inhibitory signaling. It has been shown in animal studies that uPAR plays a critical role in platelet kinetics as well as in their activation and endothelium adhesion associated with inflammation [3]. Lenich *et al.* described a pathway of plasminogen activation by endogenous or exogenous u-PA, which is based on

Table 9.2 Comparative properties of fibrinolytic agents.

Feature	SK	t-PA Alteplace	r-PA Reteplase	Tenecteplace	UK
Fibrin-specific	–	++	+	++++	–
Brand Names	Kabikinase, Streptase	Activase, Cathflo Activase	Retavase	TNKase	Abbokinase
Half-life (minutes)	20	5	15	20	10–20
Direct plasminogen activator	Yes	Yes	Yes	Yes	No
Requires Concomitant heparin	+/–	Yes	Yes	Yes	Yes**
Weight adjusted dosing	No	Yes	Yes	Yes	Yes
Dose	1.5 ml units i.v. Over 30 to 60 min	15 mg i.v. bolus over 2 min, **then:** 0.75 mg/kg i.v./30 min (max 50 mg), **then:** 0.5 mg/kg i.v./60 minutes (max 35 mg)	10 U i.v. bolus Repeat bolus in 30 min	One time weight-based bolus: <60 kg = 30 mg, 60–69 kg = 35 mg 70–79 kg = 40 mg 80–89 kg = 45 mg >90 kg = 50 mg	240,000 U/h x 4 then 120,000 U/h
Bolus administration	No	No	Yes (double bolus)	Yes	Yes *
Cost ($ US)	$613	$3609	$3016	$2917	$5600

SK, streptokinase; t-PA, tissue plasminogen activator; r-PA, recombinant plasminogen activators; UK, urokinase; i.v. intravenous; U, units.
* Loading dose; **recommended following infusion.

its association with platelets, and which is specifically triggered by thrombin, is surface related, dependent on the formation of platelet-bound fibrin and involves a platelet lysosomal enzyme consistent with cathepsin C. This pathway targets u-PA to a platelet thrombus and may help explain the mechanism by which u-PA induces physiologic fibrinolysis [4].

Moser *et al.* found a decrease in platelet aggregation in patients with STEMI early after reteplase or streptokinase infusion, compared to alteplase [5]. Gurbel *et al.* studied platelet aggregation and activation in patients with STEMI before and up to 24 hours after infusion of fibrinolytic agents and demonstrated a gradual increase in platelet activity from 12 to 24 hours post-thrombolysis; more with reteplase compared to alteplase [6].

Regardless of the mechanism by which thrombolytic agents contribute to platelet activation and formation of new platelet-rich thrombi, concomitant antiplatelet therapy is warranted. Clarifying the mechanisms involved in the interaction between each individual fibrinolytic agent and platelets would allow for the development of more effective antiplatelet and fibrinolytic regimens for patients with STEMI and possibly ischemic stroke. As new antiplatelet strategies have been developed, their efficacy has been tested in patients with STEMI undergoing fibrinolysis. Addition of clopidogrel to aspirin, was studied in 3491 patients with STEMI treated with fibrinolytic agents in the Clopidogrel as Adjunctive Reperfusion Therapy (CLARITY)-TIMI 28 trial. Clopidogrel dramatically reduced the rate of the primary efficacy endpoint (composite of an occluded infarct-related artery on angiography, death or recurrent myocardial infarction) by 36%. By 30 days, clopidogrel therapy reduced the odds of the composite end-point of death from cardiovascular causes, recurrent myocardial infarction or recurrent ischemia leading to urgent revascularization by 20% [7].

Addition of clopidogrel to aspirin in 45,852 patients with acute myocardial infarction was studied in Clopidogrel and Metoprolol in Myocardial Infarction Trial – Second Chinese Cardiac Study (COMMIT-CCS 2) trial. In this study, 93% of patients presented with STEMI, half of whom received fibrinolytic agent prior to randomization. Overall, allocation to therapy with clopidogrel (without a loading dose) produced a highly significant 9% relative reduction in composite of death, reinfarction or stroke. This effect was independent from the use of fibrinolytic agent [8].

Based on evidence of the role of platelet-rich thrombi in coronary occlusion and preclinical studies of GP IIb/IIIa inhibitors (GPIs) efficacy for platelet disaggregation and clot dissolution, GPIs were proposed as a solitary agent for coronary reperfusion. Pilot angiographic studies showed lower rates of infarct-related artery patency with GPIs, compared to those shown with fibrinolytics. Combination of full-dose fibrinolytics and GPIs provided a modestly improved rate of reperfusion in patients with STEMI, which came with an increased rate of major bleeding, including intracranial bleed. These safety concerns led to the search for new regimens of reduced-dose fibrinolytic agent, combined with GPIs, to achieve better clinical outcome without increased bleeding complications.

Data from the Thrombolysis in Myocardial Infarction (TIMI) 14 trial showed that STEMI patients receiving abciximab, in combination with half-dose alteplase, experienced a significantly higher rate of TIMI 3 flow than those receiving full-dose alteplase at both 60 minutes (72% vs. 43%) and 90 minutes (77% vs. 62%). The increase in the rate and extent of thrombolysis resulted in markedly improved reperfusion without raising the risk of major hemorrhage [9].

GUSTO-V was a randomized, open-label trial to compare the effect of standard-dose reteplase alone with half-dose reteplase plus abciximab in 16,588 patients with STEMI. The primary end-point was 30-day mortality, and secondary end-points included complications of myocardial infarction. There was no significant change in mortality rate at 30 days (5.6% in combination group vs. 5.9% with reteplase alone). Combination therapy led to a consistent reduction in key secondary complications of myocardial infarction including reinfarction, major non-fatal ischemic complications and the need for urgent revascularization; however, these advantages were partly counterbalanced by an increase in non-intracranial severe bleeding complications [10].

Another large-scale clinical trial, Assessment of the Safety and Efficacy of a New Thrombolytic Regimen (ASSENT)-3, included 6095 patients with STEMI within 6 hours, and compared three different strategies: (1) full-dose tenecteplase and enoxaparin for a maximum of 7 days (enoxaparin group); (2) half-dose tenecteplase with weight-adjusted low-dose unfractionated heparin and a 12-hour infusion of abciximab (abciximab group); or (3) full-dose tenecteplase with weight-adjusted unfractionated heparin (UFH) for 48 hours (unfractionated heparin group). There were significantly fewer primary end-points (composites of 30-day mortality, in-hospital reinfarction or in-hospital refractory ischemia) in the enoxaparin and abciximab groups than in the UFH group (11.4%, 11.1% vs. 15.4%, respectively), the same was true when primary end-points were combined to prespecified safety end-points of in-hospital intracranial hemorrhage or in-hospital major bleeding complications (13.7%, enoxaparin group; 14,2%,abciximab group vs. 17% in UFH group) [11].

The suggested advantage of combined use of fibrinolytic agent and dual or triple antiplatelet therapy is likely related to primary reperfusion with fibrinolysis followed by prevention of coronary re-occlusion by antiplatelet therapy. Each combination strategy needs to be individually tested for efficacy and safety, as no assumptions can be made regarding a class effect. Fibrinolytics remain class IA indication for the patients presenting with STEMI within 12 hours of onset, when primary PCI is not an available option within 90 minutes from the first medical contact [12]. However, in the era when primary percutaneous coronary intervention (PCI) provides a better rate of infarct-related artery patency without increased risk of bleeding, resulting in improving clinical outcomes, action is shifted towards a more invasive approach in the management of patients with STEMI.

Interaction between platelets and heparins

Mechanisms of thrombogenesis are closely linked, with activation of both the coagulation and platelet aggregation pathways being responsible for thrombus formation. Thrombin, a key clotting enzyme generated by blood coagulation, is a very potent platelet activator. At the same time, activated platelets provide a platform for the coagulation process. Therefore, combination therapy with antiplatelet agents and antithrombins are effective in the prevention and treatment of arterial thrombosis.

UFH is a glycosaminoglycan composed of heterogeneous chains with different molecular weights. UFH indirectly inhibits factor IIa (thrombin) and factor Xa, activating antithrombin III. It is perceived that thrombin inhibition with heparin should provide platelet inhibition. However, a small but finite interaction of heparin with platelets is complex and may result in their activation directly and indirectly. Heparin is inactive on fibrin-bound or cell-bound thrombin and itself is inactivated by platelet factor 4 (PF4), large quantities of which are released from platelets at the site of plaque rupture.

While UFH inhibits thrombin-induced platelet aggregation, it conversely potentiates platelet aggregation induced by a range of platelet agonists, including adenosine diphosphate (ADP), thrombin receptor activating peptide, platelet-activating factor and epinephrine; and these potentiating effects are detectable at therapeutic concentrations of heparin. These effects were demonstrated for patients with ACS and healthy volunteers [13].

The mechanism whereby UFH potentiates platelet aggregation is unknown. However, this "paradoxical" effect of UFH is not evident with enoxaparin or DTIs [14]. Heparin-associated platelet activation can be attenuated by ADP receptor antagonists and GPIs, and is not affected by aspirin [15].

One of the potentially most devastating complications of UFH therapy is its propensity to cause thrombocytopenia (heparin-induced thrombocytopenia, HIT) with associated thrombosis. With the almost ubiquitous use of heparin in recent years, the prevalence of this potentially catastrophic complication has prominently increased. While ordinarily thrombocytopenia is associated with an increased risk of bleeding, in patients with HIT it is associated with a tendency towards intravascular thrombosis, including deep venous thrombosis, disseminated intravascular coagulation, pulmonary embolism, cerebral thrombosis, myocardial infarction and ischemic injury to the legs or arms, and can produce severe morbidity and mortality [16].

HIT and its associated thrombotic disorders, known as heparin-induced thrombocytopenia and thrombosis syndrome (HITTS), typically occur after 5 to 10 days of heparin therapy, but they can appear sooner in patients previously treated with heparin. HIT is an immune-mediated reaction, most commonly caused by an IgG antibody that binds to a complex formed between heparin and platelet factor 4 (PF4), a heparin-binding protein normally found in the alpha granules of platelets [17].

Heparins and antiplatelet agents in patients with ACS

Several clinical studies showed that administration of UFH alone and especially combined with aspirin in patients with UA is associated with a decreased risk of death and MI. A meta-analysis of these trials showed a statistically borderline 33% relative risk reduction of death or MI in patients treated with UFH and aspirin comparing to aspirin alone during randomized treatment; however, the same end-points were decreased by 18% only when analyzed 2–12 weeks following randomization [18].

Anticoagulation with UFH or LMWH (primarily enoxaparin) is a Class I (Level A) indication for patients with UA/NSTEMI. UFH given intravenously (i.v.) is also a Class I (Level C) indication for the treatment of patients with STEMI with high risk for systemic emboli and Class IIA for treatment of all other patients with STEMI. Recently, the Food and Drug Administration approved enoxaparin as an alternative to UFH anticoagulation for STEMI. Historically, UFH has become a standard antithrombotic therapy to which other newly developed antithrombins are compared.

Presently, LMWHs are gradually replacing UFH for the treatment of patients with ACS. They have shown superior or the same efficacy and are more convenient and cost effective [19]. LMWH is produced by cleavage of UFH to yield smaller chains. As a result, LMWH has more anti-factor Xa activity, and thus better inhibition of both the generation and activity of thrombin. LMWHs have high bioavailability, allowing their subcutaneous use, are less bound to plasma proteins and, as a result, have predictable dose-dependant anticoagulation activity. The major advantage of LMWH over UFH is that it does not require routine laboratory monitoring. Several LMWHs are available worldwide; however, they are not proven interchangeable. Comparison of different preparations was performed to UFH or other antithrombotics, but not within the group (Table 9.3).

Several studies have answered the question of whether LMWHs provide additional benefit in patients with ACS treated with different antiplatelet regimens. The Fragmin during Instability in Coronary Artery Disease (FRISC) trial demonstrated 48% risk reduction of death, MI and need for urgent revascularization in patients with unstable coronary artery disease treated with dalteparin in addition to aspirin during the first 6 days. However, this effect became non-significant within 4–5 months after treatment [20]. This was confirmed in the Fragmin in Unstable Coronary Artery Disease Study (FRIC) trial, in which continuation of treatment with dalteparin over the initial 6 days at a lower once-daily dose did not confer any additional benefit over ASA (75 to 165 mg) alone [21].

Tirofiban compared to UFH was studied in PRISM and PRISM-PLUS trials. The PRISM trial randomized 3232 patients with non-ST-elevation ACS to either tirofiban or heparin. Patients receiving tirofiban had a 32% reduction in the likelihood of death, MI or refractory ischemia at 48 hours and a 36%

Table 9.3 Comparative properties of UFH, LMWHs.

Features	UFH	Dalteparin	Enoxaparin	Tinzaparin	Danaparoid
Route of administration	s.c. or i.v.	s.c. or i.v.	s.c. or i.v.	s.c.	s.c.
Target	Factor Xa = Factor IIa	Factor Xa > Factor IIa	Factor Xa > Factor IIa	Factor Xa > Factor IIa	Factor Xa >> Factor IIa
Bioavailability	variable	90%	100%	87%	90%
Half-life	1.5 hours	2–5 hours	4.5–7 hours	3–4 hours	25 hours
Risk of HIT	Yes	Yes	Yes	Yes	Minimal
Protein binding	Yes	Low	Low	Low	No
Neutralized by protamine sulfate	Yes	Partial	Partial	Partial	No
Structure	Heterogeneous	Heterogeneous	Heterogeneous	Heterogeneous	Heterogeneous
Excretion	Reticuloendothelial, renal	Renal	Renal	Renal	Renal

UFH, unfractionated heparin; LMWH, low molecular weight heparin; i.v., intravenous; s.c., subcutaneous; HIT, heparin induced thrombocytopenia.

reduction in death at 30 days [22]. The PRISM-PLUS trial randomized 1915 patients with severe non-ST-elevation ACS to either tirofiban alone, heparin alone or a combination of tirofiban and heparin. Patients treated with the combination of tirofiban and heparin had a 27% reduction in death or non-fatal MI at 30 days [23]. Of interest is that results of the PRISM-PLUS study were actually contradictory to those of PRISM with regards to the efficacy of tirofiban alone, as compared to UFH. The tirofiban alone treatment arm was stopped prematurely in the PRISM-PLUS trial because of excess mortality. This data again proved that despite advances in antiplatelet therapy, anticoagulation with heparins is adding additional benefits to patients with ACS.

Compared to other LMWHs, enoxaparin was shown to be superior to UFH in patients with UA/NSTEMI and STEMI. Enoxaparin was studied in UA/NSTEMI in several large studies. The first two were published in the late 1990s: ESSENCE trial randomized 3171 patients with UA/NSTEMI receiving aspirin to enoxaparin or UFH for 2–8 days. At 14 and 30 days the composite risk of death, MI or recurrent angina with electrocardiographic changes or prompting intervention was significantly lower in patients assigned to enoxaparin compared with UFH. The incidence of minor bleeding was significantly higher in the enoxaparin group [24]. The TIMI 11B study randomized 3910 patients to enoxaparin or UFH, including an out-patient study arm with enoxaparin. The results were similar to the ESSENCE trial. Enoxaparin was superior to UFH in reducing the composite of death and serious cardiac ischemic events during the acute management of UA/NSTEMI patients without a significant increase in the rate of major hemorrhage. No further relative decrease in events occurred with out-patient enoxaparin treatment, but there was an increase in the rate of major hemorrhage [25].

The meta-analysis of both studies showed that enoxaparin in UA/NSTEMI was associated with a 20% reduction in death and serious cardiac ischemic events that appeared within the first few days of treatment, and this benefit was sustained through 43 days. There was an increase in the rate of minor, but not major, hemorrhage during the acute phase of therapy [26]. As a result of these data, according to the 2002 ACC/AHA guideline update enoxaparin is preferable to UFH in patients with UA/NSTEMI (Class IIa, Level A).

However, there was no obvious advantage of enoxaparin over UFH in 10,027 high-risk patients with non-ST-segment elevation ACS included in SYNERGY trial. The primary end-point of all-cause death or non-fatal myocardial infarction during the first 30 days after randomization occurred in 14.0% of patients assigned to enoxaparin and 14.5% of patients assigned to UFH. No differences in ischemic events during PCI were observed between enoxaparin and UFH groups. More bleeding was observed with enoxaparin, with a statistically significant increase in TIMI (9.1% vs. 7.6%) but non-significant excess in GUSTO severe bleeding (2.7% vs. 2.2%) and transfusions (17.0% vs. 16.0%) [27]. After subgroup analysis it was evident that about two thirds of the patients received prerandomization antithrombotic therapy. This treatment with antithrombins before randomization had potential impact on comparison of study drug effects. After adjustment for differences in baseline characteristics between subgroups, consistent therapy with enoxaparin might be superior to UFH in reducing death or non-fatal MI, with a modest excess in bleeding [28].

Further evidence was obtained from compiled analysis of the six large randomized trials, including: ESSENCE, TIMI 11B, ACUTE II, INTERACT, A to Z and SYNERGY. Systematic evaluation of the outcomes for 21,946 patients with UA/NSTEMI was performed. No significant difference was found in death at 30 days for enoxaparin compared to UFH. A statistically significant reduction in the combined end-point of death or non-fatal MI at 30 days was observed for enoxaparin compared to UFH in the overall trial populations (10.1% vs. 11.0%). No significant difference was found in the rate of blood transfusion or major bleeding [29]. The observed increased rate of bleeding with enoxaparin was found to be largely related to relative overdosing in the patients with decreased creatinine clearance, which led to dose adjustment of enoxaparin in patients with creatinine clearance less than 30 ml/min; also measurment of anti-factor Xa activity may be required [30].

Enoxaparin was compared to UFH as an adjunctive therapy with fibrinolysis in 20,506 patients with ST-elevation myocardial infarction in Enoxaparin and Thrombolysis Reperfusion for Acute Myocardial Infarction Treatment-Thrombolysis In Myocardial Infarction study 25 (ExTRACT-TIMI 25). The composite of death, non-fatal reinfarction or urgent revascularization occurred in 14.5% of patients given UFH and 11.7% of those given enoxaparin. Major bleeding occurred in 1.4% and 2.1%, respectively. The net clinical benefit was in favor of enoxaparin with 10.1% vs. 12.2% of events in the UFH group. Interestingly, the superiority of enoxaparin over UFH in this trial was shown with ASA equally used in about 95% of patients, and clopidogrel more frequently used in the UFH group [31].

Another LMWH, reviparin, was studied versus placebo in the Clinical Trial of Reviparin and Metabolic Modulation in Acute Myocardial Infarction Treatment Evaluation (CREATE), which included 15,570 patients with STEMI at 341 hospitals in India and China. Primary composite outcome of death, myocardial reinfarction or stroke at 30 days benefited reviparin (11.8% vs. 13.6%); also a significant reduction in 30-day mortality (9.8% vs. 11.3%) was observed. There was a small absolute excess of life-threatening bleeding but the benefits outweighed the risks. The benefits of adding LMWH for treatment of patients with STEMI were obtained on top of ASA and clopidogrel/ticlopidine use in 97% and 55% of patients respectively [32].

Platelets and direct thrombin inhibitors

Direct thrombin inhibitors (DTI), as compared to heparins, appear to lack an activating effect on platelets. DTIs have been extensively studied in patients

Table 9.4 Comparative properties of direct thrombin inhibitors.

Features	Hirudin (Recombinant)	Bivalirudin	Argatroban
Route of administration	i.v., s.c.	i.v.	i.v.
Target	Factor IIa	Factor IIa	Factor IIa
Molecular mass (Daltons)	7000	1980	527
Half-life (minutes)	i.v.,60, s.c.-120	25	45
Risk of HIT	No	No	No
Protein binding	No*	No*	Yes
Main site of clearance	Renal	Liver, other sites Renal(minor)	Liver

Recombinant includes Lepirudin (Refludin) and Desirudin (Iprivask)
*Except binds to thrombin; i.v., intravenous; s.c., subcutaneous;
HIT, heparin induced thrombocytopenia

with ACS. Several agents have been developed: the prototype (hirudin), followed by lepirudin (recombinant hirudin), hirulog, followed by bivalirudin and argatroban (Table 9.4). These agents directly bind thrombin, independently from antithrombin III activity. They are not associated with HIT, and lepirudin and argatroban are approved for the treatment of HIT-associated thromboembolism.

Hirudin was first studied in the Global Use of Strategies to Open Occluded Coronary Arteries (GUSTO) IIb trial, involving 12,142 patients with ACS. Patients were randomly assigned to either UFH or hirudin. Hirudin provided a small advantage, as compared with heparin, principally related to a reduction in the risk of non-fatal MI, and was associated with a greater risk of moderate bleeding complications [33]. In the Organization to Assess Strategies for Ischemic Syndromes (OASIS-2) trial 10,141 patients with UA/NSTEMI were randomized to UFH or lepirudin. The primary end-point of death and MI at 7 days was not significantly different between the two groups, with rare but increased rate of major bleeding in the lepirudin group [34]. A newer agent, bivalirudin, is being intensively investigated. The Thrombolysis in Myocardial Infarction (TIMI) 8 trial was undertaken to compare the efficacy and safety of bivalirudin with UFH in patients with UA/NSTEMI and was terminated by the sponsor after enrollment of 133 of the planned 5320 patients. The trend toward a lower rate of death or non-fatal MI in the bivalirudin group was reported without an increased risk of bleeding [35]. A meta-analysis of 11 large, clinical, randomized trials of DTI compared to heparin in 35,970 patients with ACS showed that DTIs were associated with a lower risk of MI (2.8% vs. 3.5%; P <0.001) with no apparent effect on deaths (1.9% vs. 2.0%; P = 0.69). A reduction in death or MI was seen with hirudin and bivalirudin. Compared with heparin, there was an increased risk of major bleeding with hirudin, but a reduction with bivalirudin [36].

Bivalirudin was tested in 6010 patients undergoing urgent or elective PCI in REPLACE-2 trial. Of interest to our topic, is that one studied group included patients treated with bivalirudin and provisional GPIs (abciximab or eptifibatide) and another group included patients treated with UFH and planned GPIs. All patients were on ASA, 86% were pretreated with thienopyridine, while 92% were continued on thienopyridine. So, to some extent, triple antiplatelet therapy with ASA, thienopyridine and GPI combined with UFH was tested against dual antiplatelet therapy with ASA, thienopyridine combined with bivalirudin. The 30-day composite end-point rate of ischemic events in the bivalirudin group was non-inferior to the UFH plus GPI group (7.6% vs. 7.1% respectively). In-hospital major bleeding rates were significantly reduced in the bivalirudin group (2.4% vs. 4.1%). The subgroup analysis showed that bivalirudin was more effective in patients pretreated with thienopyridine and on the opposite UFH plus GPI was better in the no pretreatment group. These differences however did not reach statistical significance [37].

The regimen of bivalirudin used instead of heparins with GPIs was further tested in the Acute Catheterization and Urgent Intervention Triage Strategy (ACUITY) trial. The study included 13,819 patients with non-STEMI ACS undergoing an early invasive strategy. Patients were randomized to one of three antithrombotic regimens: UFH or enoxaparin plus GPI, bivalirudin plus GPI or bivalirudin alone. Three primary end-points were measured at 30 days: a composite ischemia end-point – death, myocardial infarction or unplanned revascularization for ischemia; major bleeding; and the net clinical outcome, defined as the combination of composite ischemia or major bleeding. Bivalirudin plus GPI, as compared with heparin plus GPI demonstrated the same rate of ischemia, bleeding, and net outcome end-points. Bivalirudin alone, as compared with heparin plus GPI, showed 7.8% composite ischemia end-point rate versus 7.3%. This difference met non-inferiority criteria. Rates of major bleeding were significantly reduced in the bivalirudin group (3.0% vs. 5.7%), contributing to the favorable net clinical outcome (10.1% vs. 11.7% of total events; P = 0.02). It is important to note that these results were obtained while 65% of randomized patients in all groups had been treated with UFH or enoxaparin before randomization, which could have influence the results. The same observation as in the Randomized Evaluation in PCI Linking Angiomax to Reduced Clinical Events (REPLACE)-2 trial was made in subgroup analysis. Patients not pretreated with thienopyridine benefited from heparin plus GPI compared to bivalirudin alone [38]. These data underscore the importance of early platelet blockade with dual ASA plus thienopyridine therapy in moderate–high risk ACS patients, especially those undergoing PCI. There is a necessity for early initiation of treatment with GPIs in the case of late thienopyridine use, an effect possibly independent from the type of anticoagulant used.

Summary

Management of cardiovascular diseases involves treatment and prevention of thrombotic events with combination therapy, including antiplatelet agents and antithrombins being a cornerstone of therapy of the arterial thrombosis. Effectiveness of single-agent or combined strategies in the prevention of ischemic events comes with the price of increased bleeding.

References

1 ISIS-2. ISIS-2 (Second International Study of Infarct Survival) Collaborative Group. Randomized trial of intravenous streptokinase, oral aspirin, both, or neither among 17,187 cases of suspected acute myocardial infarction. *J Am Coll Cardiol* 1988; **12** (6 Suppl. A): 3A–13A.

2 Fitzgerald DJ, Catella F, Roy L, FitzGerald GA. Marked platelet activation in vivo after intravenous streptokinase in patients with acute myocardial infarction. *Circulation* 1988; **77**: 142–150.

3 Piguet PF, Vesin C, Donati Y, Tacchini-Cottier F, Belin D, Barazzone C. Urokinase receptor (uPAR, CD87) is a platelet receptor important for kinetics and TNF-induced endothelial adhesion in mice. *Circulation* 1999; **99**: 3315–3321.

4 Lenich C, Liu JN, Gurewich V. Thrombin stimulation of platelets induces plasminogen activation mediated by endogenous urokinase-type plasminogen activator. *Blood* 1997; **90**: 3579–3586.

5 Moser M, Nordt T, Peter K, Ruef J, Kohler B, Schmittner M, *et al.* Platelet function during and after thrombolytic therapy for acute myocardial infarction with reteplase, alteplase, or streptokinase. *Circulation* 1999; **100**: 1858–1864.

6 Gurbel PA, Serebruany VL, Shustov AR, Bahr RD, Carpo C, Ohman EM, Topol EJ. Effects of reteplase and alteplase on platelet aggregation and major receptor expression during the first 24 hours of acute myocardial infarction treatment. GUSTO-III Investigators. Global Use of Strategies to Open Occluded Coronary Arteries. *J Am Coll Cardiol* 1998; **31**: 1466–1473.

7 Sabatine MS, Cannon CP, Gibson CM, López-Sendón JL, Montalescot G, Theroux P, *et al.* Addition of clopidogrel to aspirin and fibrinolytic therapy for myocardial infarction with ST-segment elevation. *New Engl J Med* 2005; **352**: 1179–1189.

8 Chen ZM, Jiang LX, Chen YP, Xie JX, Pan HC, Peto R, *et al.* Addition of clopidogrel to aspirin in 45,852 patients with acute myocardial infarction: randomised placebo-controlled trial. *Lancet* 2005; **366**: 1607–1621.

9 Antman EM, Giugliano RP, Gibson CM, McCabe CH, Coussement P, Kleiman NS, et al., for the TIMI 14 Investigators. Abciximab facilitates the rate and extent of thrombolysis. Results of the Thrombolysis in Myocardial Infarction (TIMI) 14 Trial. *Circulation* 1999; **99**: 2720–2732.

10 Topol EJ; GUSTO V Investigators. Reperfusion therapy for acute myocardial infarction with fibrinolytic therapy or combination reduced fibrinolytic therapy and platelet glycoprotein IIb/IIIa inhibition: the GUSTO V randomized trial. *Lancet* 2001; **357**: 1905–1914.

11 Assessment of the Safety and Efficacy of a New Thrombolytic Regimen (ASSENT)-3 Investigators. Efficacy and safety of tenecteplase in combination with enoxaparin, abciximab, or unfractionated heparin: the ASSENT-3 randomised trial in acute myocardial infarction. *Lancet* 2001; **358**: 605–613.

12 Antman EM, Anbe DT, Armstrong PW, Bates ER, Green LA, Hand M, et al. ACC/AHA guidelines for the management of patients with ST-elevation myocardial infarction; A report of the American College of Cardiology/American Heart Association Task Force on Practice Guidelines (Committee to Revise the 1999 Guidelines for the Management of Patients with Acute Myocardial Infarction). *J Am Coll Cardiol* 2004; **44**: E1–E211.

13 Xiao Z, Théroux P. Platelet activation with unfractionated heparin at therapeutic concentrations and comparisons with a low-molecular-weight heparin and with a direct thrombin inhibitor. *Circulation* 1998; **97**: 251–256.

14 Aggarwal A, Sobel BE, Schneider DJ. Decreased platelet reactivity in blood anticoagulated with bivalirudin or enoxaparin compared with unfractionated heparin: implications for coronary intervention. *J Thromb Thrombolysis* 2002; **13**: 161–165.

15 Storey RF, May JA, Heptinstall S. Potentiation of platelet aggregation by heparin in human whole blood is attenuated by P2Y12 and P2Y1 antagonists but not aspirin. *Thromb Res* 2005; **115**: 301–307.

16 Brieger DB, Mak KH, Kottke-Marchant K, Topol EJ. Heparin-induced thrombocytopenia. *J Am Coll Cardiol* 1998; **31**: 1449–1459.

17 Aster RH. Heparin-induced thrombocytopenia and thrombosis. *New Engl J Med* 1995; **332**: 1374–1376.

18 Oler A, Whooley MA, Oler J, Grady D. Adding heparin to aspirin reduces the incidence of myocardial infarction and death in patients with unstable angina. A meta-analysis. *JAMA* 1996; **276**: 811–815.

19 Fox KAA et al. Decline in death rates in ACS. *JAMA* 2007; **297**: 1892.

20 Fragmin during Instability in Coronary Artery Disease (FRISC) study group. Low-molecular-weight heparin during instability in coronary artery disease. *Lancet* 1996; **347**: 561–568.

21 Klein W, Buchwald A, Hillis SE, Monrad S, Sanz G, Turpie AG. Comparison of low-molecular-weight heparin with unfractionated heparin acutely and with placebo for 6 weeks in the management of unstable coronary artery disease. Fragmin in unstable coronary artery disease study (FRIC). *Circulation* 1997; **96**: 61–68. Erratum in: *Circulation* 1998; **97**: 413.

22 Platelet Receptor Inhibition in Ischemic Syndrome Management (PRISM) Study Investigators. A comparison of aspirin plus tirofiban with aspirin plus heparin for unstable angina. *New Engl J Med*. 1998; **338**: 1498–1505.

23 Platelet Receptor Inhibition in Ischemic Syndrome Management in Patients Limited by Unstable Signs and Symptoms (PRISM-PLUS) Study Investigators. Inhibition

of the platelet glycoprotein IIb/IIIa receptor with tirofiban in unstable angina and non-Q-wave myocardial infarction. *New Engl J Med.* 1998; **338**: 1488–1497. Erratum in: *New Engl J Med* 1998; **339**: 415.

24 Cohen M, Demers C, Gurfinkel EP, Turpie AG, Fromell GJ, Goodman S. Low-molecular-weight heparins in non-ST-segment elevation ischemia: the ESSENCE trial. Efficacy and safety of subcutaneous enoxaparin versus intravenous unfractionated heparin, in non-Q-wave coronary events.*Am J Cardiol.* 1998; **82**: 19L–24L.

25 Antman EM, McCabe CH, Gurfinkel EP, Turpie AG, Bernink PJ, Salein D. Enoxaparin prevents death and cardiac ischemic events in unstable angina/non-Q-wave myocardial infarction. Results of the thrombolysis in myocardial infarction (TIMI) 11B trial. *Circulation* 1999; **100**: 1593–1601.

26 Antman EM, Cohen M, Radley D, *et al.* Assessment of the treatment effect of enoxaparin for unstable angina/non-Q-wave myocardial infarction. TIMI 11B-ESSENCE meta-analysis. *Circulation* 1999; **100**: 1602–1608.

27 Ferguson JJ, Califf RM, Antman EM, Cohen M, Grines CL, Goodman S, *et al.* for SYNERGY Trial Investigators. Enoxaparin vs unfractionated heparin in high-risk patients with non-ST-segment elevation acute coronary syndromes managed with an intended early invasive strategy: primary results of the SYNERGY randomized trial. *JAMA* 2004; **292**: 45–54.

28 Cohen M, Mahaffey KW, Pieper K, Pollack CV Jr, Antman EM, Hoekstra J, *et al.* for SYNERGY Trial Investigators. A subgroup analysis of the impact of prerandomization antithrombin therapy on outcomes in the SYNERGY trial: enoxaparin versus unfractionated heparin in non-ST-segment elevation acute coronary syndromes. *J Am Coll Cardiol* 2006; **48**: 1346–1354.

29 Petersen JL, Mahaffey KW, Hasselblad V, *et al.* Efficacy and bleeding complications among patients randomized to enoxaparin or unfractionated heparin for antithrombin therapy in non-ST-Segment elevation acute coronary syndromes: a systematic overview. *JAMA* 2004; **292**: 89–96.

30 Chow SL, Zammit K, West K, *et al.* Correlation of antifactor Xa concentrations with renal function in patients on enoxaparin. *J Clin Pharmacol* 2003; **43**: 586–90.

31 Antman EM, Morrow DA, McCabe CH, Murphy SA, Ruda M, Sadowski Z. Enoxaparin versus unfractionated heparin with fibrinolysis for ST-elevation myocardial infarction. *New Engl J Med* 2006; **354**: 1477–1488.

32 Yusuf S, Mehta SR, Xie C, Ahmed RJ, Xavier D, Pais P, *et al.* Effects of reviparin, a low-molecular-weight heparin, on mortality, reinfarction, and strokes in patients with acute myocardial infarction presenting with ST-segment elevation. *JAMA* 2005; **293**: 427–435.

33 Global Use of Strategies to Open Occluded Coronary Arteries (GUSTO) IIb investigators. A comparison of recombinant hirudin with heparin for the treatment of acute coronary syndromes. *New Engl J Med* 1996; **335**: 775–782.

34 Organisation to Assess Strategies for Ischemic Syndromes (OASIS-2) Investigators. Effects of recombinant hirudin (lepirudin) compared with heparin on death, myocardial infarction, refractory angina, and revascularisation procedures in patients with acute myocardial ischaemia without ST elevation: a randomised trial. *Lancet* 1999; **353**: 429–438.

35 Antman EM, McCabe CH, Braunwald E. Bivalirudin as a replacement for unfractionated heparin in unstable angina/non-ST-elevation myocardial infarction: observations from the TIMI 8 trial. The thrombolysis in myocardial infarction. *Am Heart J* 2002; **143**: 229–234.

36 Direct Thrombin Inhibitor Trialists' Collaborative Group. Direct thrombin inhibitors in acute coronary syndromes: principal results of a meta-analysis based on individual patients' data. *Lancet* 2002; **359**: 294–302.

37 Lincoff AM, Bittl JA, Harrington RA, Feit F, Kleiman NS, Jackman JD, *et al.* Bivalirudin and provisional glycoprotein IIb/IIIa blockade compared with heparin and planned glycoprotein IIb/IIIa blockade during percutaneous coronary intervention: REPLACE-2 randomized trial. *JAMA* 2003; **289**: 853–863. Erratum in: *JAMA* 2003; **289**: 1638.

38 Stone GW, McLaurin BT, Cox DA, Bertrand ME, Lincoff AM, Moses JW, *et al.* Bivalirudin for patients with acute coronary syndromes. *New Engl J Med* 2006; **355**: 2203–2216.

PART IV

Clinical Use of Antiplatelet Agents in Cardiovascular Disease

Chapter 10

Antiplatelet therapy in acute coronary syndrome without ST elevation

Christian W. Hamm

Platelet activation and aggregation plays a key pathophysiological role in acute coronary syndromes (ACS). Therefore, effective antiplatelet therapy is of paramount importance, once the diagnosis is established. However, platelets need to be seen not only in the frame of the acute plaque rupture, but also as a contributor to subsequent atherothrombotic events.

Three complementary strategies provide effective antiplatelet action: cyclooxygenase-1 inhibition (acetylsalicylic acid, aspirin), inhibition of ADP mediated platelet activation with thienopyridines (clopidogrel, ticlopidine) and glycoprotein IIb/IIIa receptor inhibition (tirofiban, eptifibatide, abciximab).

Acetylsalicylic acid (aspirin)

Acetylsalicylic acid, commonly named aspirin, inhibits platelet activation by irreversible inhibition of platelet-derived cyclooxygenase-1, thereby limiting the formation of thromboxane A_2. Three trials have consistently shown that aspirin decreases death or myocardial infarction (MI) in patients with unstable angina [1–3]. In the meta-analysis by the Antithrombotic Trialists Collaboration, a 46% reduction in the rate of vascular events was evidenced [4]. This meta-analysis suggested that 75 to 150 mg aspirin is as effective as higher doses for chronic therapy. No robust relation between dose and efficacy has been demonstrated. An initial dose of non-enteric (chewed or intravenously administered) aspirin from 160 to 325 mg is recommended to minimize delay before platelet inhibition occurs [4]. In another meta-analysis, including four

Antiplatelet Therapy in Ischemic Heart Disease, 1st edition. Edited by Stephen D. Wiviott.
© 2009 American Heart Association, ISBN: 9-781-4051-7626-2

studies, the reduction in the rate of vascular events was 53%, with a number-needed-to-treat of 17 (Figure 10.1) [5].

The most common side effect of aspirin is gastrointestinal intolerance, which occurs in 5 to 40% of aspirin-treated patients. Gastrointestinal bleeding increases with higher doses. In the CAPRIE study, the rate of gastrointestinal bleeding leading to aspirin discontinuation was 0.93% [6]. In the CURE trial, aspirin was given in combination with clopidogrel at doses ranging from 75 to 325 mg [7]. The incidence of major bleeding increased as a function of the aspirin dose, both in patients treated with aspirin alone, and patients treated with the combination. The risk of bleeding was lowest with doses up to 100 mg of aspirin and there was no evidence of higher efficacy with higher doses of aspirin [8].

Proven hypersensitivity ("allergy") to aspirin is rare, as its prevalence depends on the clinical manifestation. More serious reactions, such as anaphylactic shock, are extremely rare [9,10]. Desensitization may be an option in selected patients [11]. Rarely, aspirin-exacerbated asthma is observed. Aspirin-induced rash or skin manifestations occur in 0.2–0.7% of the general population.

Aspirin resistance

Aspirin resistance describes partial or total failure to achieve the expected *in vitro* inhibition of platelet function and is therefore may be more aptly termed low- or hyporesponsiveness. Resistance to antiplatelet agents should not be confused with recurrence of events despite antiplatelet treatment. The term refers to the variability in the magnitude of platelet aggregation inhibition measured *ex vivo* achieved in a treated population. Up to 50% of

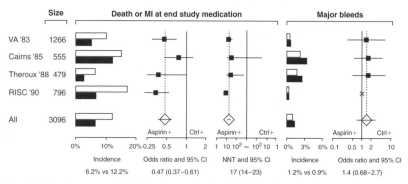

Fig. 10.1 Death, myocardial infarction and major bleeds at the end of study medication in four randomized trials of aspirin (dark bars) vs. control (open bars). NNT = number of patients who needed to be treated to avoid one event. (From reference [5] with permission.)

individuals exhibit a relative aspirin resistance in *ex vivo* tests. Some patients may develop treatment failure over time, even with increasing doses resulting in different degrees of thromboxane A_2 inhibition and a difference in event rates [12]. In addition, aspirin resistance may partially also be related to pharmacodynamic interaction with other drugs.

Drug interactions

Concomitant administration of NSAIDs, such as ibuprofen, may interfere with the inactivation of COX-1 due to a competitive action on the docking site of aspirin in the COX channel [13]. This possible interaction is not observed with selective COX-2 inhibitors or other anti-inflammatory drugs such as diclofenac. Nevertheless, it has been shown that more events occur in patients treated with the combination of aspirin and NSAIDs than with aspirin alone [14,15] and a retrospective analysis of a large cohort of patients discharged from hospital after MI, showed that the use of selective COX-2 inhibitors and non-selective NSAIDs are associated with a higher risk of death with any of these agents [16]. Therefore, anti-inflammatory drugs should be avoided in the post-MI period.

Summary

Aspirin is recommended for all patients presenting with acute coronary syndromes without known contraindications at an initial loading dose of 160–325 mg (non-enteric), and at an unlimited maintenance dose of 75 to 100 mg.

Thienopyridines

Clopidogrel and ticlopidine are adenosine diphosphate (ADP) receptor antagonists, which block the ADP-induced pathway of platelet activation by specific inhibition of the $P2Y_{12}$ receptor. New antiplatelet agents that block the $P2Y_{12}$ receptor with more potent receptor affinity and more rapid onset of action are currently under evaluation in large clinical trials (e.g. AZD6240, prasugrel, cangrelor).

Ticlopidine has been investigated in the setting of unstable angina in a single study, in which a significant 46% risk reduction of death and myocardial infarction at 6 months has been observed [17]. Meanwhile, ticlopidine was replaced by clopidogrel because of potentially serious side effects, such as the risk of neutropenia or thrombocytopenia, as well as slower onset of action.

Randomized evidence

In the CURE trial clopidogrel was compared on top of aspirin (75 to 325 mg) versus aspirin alone in 12,562 patients presenting with ACS. Patients received placebo or a loading dose of 300 mg clopidogrel followed by 75 mg daily in addition to conventional therapy [7]. A 20% risk reduction at 12 months for death from cardiovascular causes, non-fatal MI or stroke was observed in the treatment arm (9.3% vs. 11.4%, RR 0.80, 95% CI 0.72–0.90, p < 0.001). The risk reduction was significant for myocardial infarction, and there was a trend towards reduction of death and stroke. The risk reduction was consistent across all risk groups as well as various subsets of patients (elderly, ST deviation, with or without elevated cardiac biomarkers, diabetic patients) [18]. The benefit was obtained early, with a significant 34% risk reduction of cardiovascular death, myocardial infarction, stroke or severe ischemia at 24 hours in the clopidogrel group (1.4% vs. 2.1%, OR 0.66, 95% CI 0.51–0.86, p < 0.01) and was maintained throughout the 12 months of the study period (Figure 10.2). The need for GP IIb/IIIa inhibitors was 5.9% in conjunction with clopidogrel as compared with 7.2% in the placebo group (RR 0.82, 95% CI 0.72–0.93, p = 0.003).

In less acute settings, two other large trials investigated clopidogrel against aspirin, and clopidogrel plus aspirin against placebo plus aspirin. In CAPRIE, clopidogrel 75 mg once daily was compared to 325 mg of aspirin once daily in a population of 19,185 patients with documented atherosclerotic disease, manifested as either recent ischemic stroke, recent MI or symptomatic peripheral arterial disease [6]. A significant relative-risk reduction of 8.7% in favour of clopidogrel was observed versus aspirin (95% CI 0.3–16.5, p = 0.043) after a mean follow-up of 23 months. There was no significant difference in the rate of major bleeding, particularly intracranial or gastrointestinal hemorrhage.

The TRITON-TIMI 38 trial compared the third generation thienopyridine, prasugrel, which is more rapid in onset, more consistent and more potent, with clopidogrel in patients with ACS undergoing PCI [19]. Patients were followed for 6 to 15 months. In the population of patients with unstable angina/non

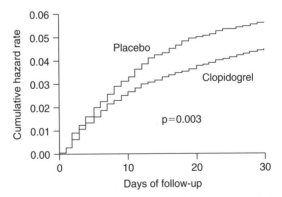

Figure 10.2 Early effect of adding clopidogrel to aspirin in the CURE trial. Cumulative hazard rates during the first 30 days for the end-point cardiovascular death, non-fatal myocardial infarction or stroke. (from reference [7] with permission)

ST elevation myocardial infarction (UA/NSTEMI), a 18% reduction in the primary endpoint of cardiovascular death, non-fatal MI or non-fatal stroke was observed with prasugrel (12.1% vs. 9.9%, HR 0.82 [0.73–0.93], p = 0.002) [19].

Bleeding risk

A major concern is the risk of bleeding of dual antiplatelet treatment, because there is no known antidote to clopidogrel or other ADP receptor antagonists. In CURE, an increased rate of major bleedings was observed in clopidogrel, plus aspirin, treated patients (3.7% vs. 2.7%, RR 1.38, 95% CI 1.13–1.67, p = 0.001), but with a non-significant increase in life-threatening and fatal bleeds [7]. Bleeding rates were higher in patients who underwent CABG, but this reached only borderline significance in 912 patients submitted to surgery less than 5 days after cessation of clopidogrel treatment (9.6% vs. 6.3%, RR 1.53, 95% CI 0.97–2.40, p = 0.06). For those treated more than 5 days after interruption of clopidogrel there was no significant increase in bleeding [20]. However, in the entire cohort, the benefit of clopidogrel treatment, including among patients submitted to revascularization by both PCI and CABG, outweighed the risk of bleeding. In total, treating 1000 patients resulted in 21 fewer cardiovascular deaths, MI or stroke, at the cost of an excess of seven patients requiring transfusions, and a trend for four patients to experience life-threatening bleeds [21]. The excess bleeding risk in patients submitted to surgery can be attenuated or eliminated by stopping clopidogrel 5 days before surgery. However, it is not known whether this results in increased complication rates during wash-out.

In the TRITON-TIMI 38 study, treatment with prasugrel also resulted in more bleeding than with standard dose clopidogrel. The key safety endpoint of TIMI major bleeding was increased from 1.8 to 2.4% over 15 months (HR 1.32 [1.03–1.68], p = 0.03). This increase in bleeding was also observed for life-threatening and fatal bleeding.

Dose and timing of clopidogrel

In patients with ACS it is recommended that clopidogrel be given at first contact both to prevent events prior to PCI and to allow adequate time for drug effect prior to PCI. It was shown in several trials that pretreatment of unselected patients with clopidogrel before angiography results in better outcome of PCI [21–23]. Accordingly, postponing clopidogrel administration until coronary anatomy is known by angiography is discouraged, as the highest rates of events are observed in the early phase of ACS. The only potential advantage of this approach is to reduce higher bleeding risk in patients requiring immediate surgery. However, this situation is rare and frequently surgery can be deferred safely by 5 days. In patients who cannot be given clopidogrel before PCI, GP IIb/IIIa inhibitors may be chosen alternatively.

Multiple smaller studies have tested higher loading doses of clopidogrel (600 or 900 mg) demonstrating a more rapid inhibition of platelet aggregation than achieved with 300 mg. However, no large-scale outcome clinical trials are yet available in the setting of ACS. Nevertheless, first clinical experience suggests that faster platelet inhibition with higher loading doses (600 mg, ~2 hours) may be more effective in reducing clinical end-points [24–27]. The definitive answer to the risk versus benefit will be provided by ongoing large-scale clinical trials.

Clopidogrel resistance

Clopidogrel is an inactive compound, which needs oxidation by hepatic cyto-chrome P450 to generate an active metabolite. CYP3A4 and CYP3A5 are the P450 isoforms responsible for the oxidation of clopidogrel, which produce the active form of the drug. The standard dose of clopidogrel achieves approximately 30 to 50% inhibition of ADP-induced platelet aggregation through antagonism to the $P2Y_{12}$ platelet ADP receptor [28].

Clopidogrel resistance, or more aptly termed variability in response, is not clearly defined and depends on the *in vitro* test system used. With these limitations, clopidogrel resistance has been reported to occur in 4% to 30% of patients [14,29]. The mechanism of clopidogrel resistance is still under investigation. Despite small studies that have shown higher rate of events associated with low inhibition of platelet aggregation [29–31], the clinical importance of this phenomenon remains uncertain.

Drug interaction

Reduced bioavailability through drug interactions has recently been discussed, particularly with certain statins that are metabolized by CYP3A4 and CYP3A5 and have been shown from *in vitro* studies to limit by 90% the degradation of clopidogrel into its active metabolite form [29]. However, this has not been translated into any demonstrable negative clinical effect [32]. Indeed, in the GRACE registry, the combination of clopidogrel and statins is suggestive of an additive beneficial effect [33].

The combination of clopidogrel with oral vitamin K antagonists (warfarin, phencoumon) is recommended only after careful benefit risk assessment, since it may potentially increase the risk of bleeding. This combination can be necessary in the context of mechanical heart valves or in the case of high risk of thromboembolic events. Under these circumstances the lowest efficacious INR and shortest duration of clopidogrel treatment should be targeted.

Withdrawal of oral antiplatelet agents

Some reports have shown that in patients with coronary artery disease, withdrawal of antiplatelet agents may result in an increased rate of recurrence of events [34,35]. Similar to after coronary stenting, interruption of dual antiplatelet treatment soon after the acute phase of ACS may expose patients to a high risk of recurrence of events, even though only few data are available to support this notion. However, the interruption of dual antiplatelet therapy in case of necessary surgical procedures more than 1 month after ACS in patients without drug eluting stents may be reasonable. If during the early phase interruption of dual antiplatelet therapy becomes mandatory, such as the need for urgent surgery or major bleeding that cannot be controlled by local treatment, no proven effective alternative therapy can currently be recommended as a substitute. Low molecular weight heparins have been advocated but without tangible proof of efficacy and safety.

Summary

A 300-mg loading dose of clopidogrel is recommended, followed by 75 mg clopidogrel daily for patients with ACS. Clopidogrel should be maintained for at least 12 months unless there is an excessive risk of bleeding. Prolonged or permanent withdrawal of aspirin, clopidogrel or both is discouraged unless strongly clinically indicated. For all patients with aspirin contraindication clopidogrel should be given as substitute. In patients considered for an invasive procedure/PCI, a loading dose of 600 mg of clopidogrel may be used to achieve more rapid inhibition of platelet function, although randomized evidence is not yet available. In patients pretreated with clopidogrel who need to undergo CABG, surgery should be postponed for 5 days for clopidogrel withdrawal, if clinically feasible. The triple combination of aspirin, clopidogrel and vitamin K antagonists (warfarin) should be restricted to compelling indications, in which case the lowest efficacious INR and shortest duration of triple treatment should be anticipated.

Glycoprotein IIb/IIIa receptor inhibitors

Three glycoprotein (GP) IIb/IIIa inhibitors are approved for clinical use, namely abciximab, and the small molecules eptifibatide and tirofiban. They block the final common pathway of platelet activation by binding to the fibrinogen and, under high shear conditions, to the von Willebrand factor, and thereby inhibiting the bridging between activated platelets. Abciximab is a monoclonal antibody fragment, eptifibatide is a cyclic peptide and tirofiban a peptidomimetic inhibitor. The results in randomized trials obtained with GP IIb/IIIa inhibitors differ according to their use in a conservative or an invasive strategy of ACS.

Conservative strategy

GP IIb/IIIa inhibitors have only a modest beneficial effect in a conservative strategy (Figure 10.3), without routine cardiac catheterization and PCI. A meta-analysis including 31,402 ACS patients treated in clinical trials using GP IIb/IIIa inhibitors showed only a 9% risk reduction for death and MI at 30 days with GP IIb/IIIa inhibitors (11.8% vs. 10.8%, OR 0.91, 95% CI 0.84–0.98,

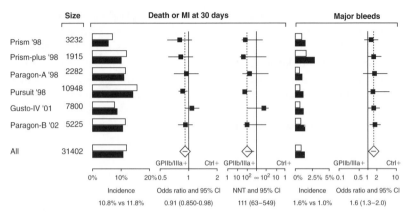

Fig. 10.3 Death, MI and major bleeds at 30 days in randomized trials of GP IIb/IIIa inhibitors (dark bars) vs. control (open bars) in conservative strategy. NNT = number of patients who needed to be treated to avoid one event. (From reference [5] with permission.)

p = 0.015) [36]. This risk reduction was consistent across multiple subgroups, and was evident particularly in high-risk patients (diabetic patients, ST segment depression, troponin-positive patients) and in patients submitted to PCI during initial hospitalization. GP IIb/IIIa inhibitors had no effects in troponin-negative patients and in women. However, women with troponin release derived the same benefit as men. The use of GP IIb/IIIa inhibitors was associated with an increase in major bleeding complications, but intracranial bleeding was not significantly increased [37] (Figure 10.3).

The outcome as a function of the utilization of GP IIb/IIIa inhibitors in patients initially medically managed, and submitted to PCI, was explored in a further meta-analysis involving 29,570 patients [37]. A 9% risk reduction overall was confirmed, but the benefit was non-significant in purely medically managed patients receiving GP IIb/IIIa inhibitors versus placebo, with a rate of death and MI at 30 days of 9.3% versus 9.7% (OR 0.95, 95% CI 0.86–1.04, p = 0.27). The only significant beneficial effect was observed when GP IIb/IIIa inhibitors were maintained during PCI (10.5% vs. 13.6%, OR 0.74, 95% CI 0.57–0.96, p = 0.02). These data confirm previous reports showing a risk reduction for ischemic events in patients pretreated with GP IIb/IIIa inhibitors before PCI [38,39]. In diabetic patients, a meta-analysis showed a highly significant risk reduction for death at 30 days with the use of GP IIb/IIIa inhibitors [40], which was particularly pronounced when submitted to PCI.

Abciximab was tested in the GUSTO-4-ACS trial [41] in 7800 patients randomized to one of three drug regimens: placebo, abciximab bolus plus 24 hours infusion or abciximab bolus plus 48 hours infusion. No significant benefit was demonstrated for the two groups treated with abciximab, and an increased bleeding risk was observed. Thrombocytopenia (defined as platelet count <50,000/μL) was observed in 1.5% of patients receiving abciximab, versus 1% in the placebo group.

Eptifibatide was investigated in the PURSUIT trial [42], which enrolled 10,948 patients. In addition to conventional therapy including aspirin and unfractionated heparin (UFH), patients were randomized to placebo or two different regimens of eptifibatide infusion, after the same initial bolus. The arm with lower dose of eptifibatide was stopped because of lack of efficacy. A significant reduction of the 30-day composite end-point of death or non-fatal MI was observed (14.2 vs. 15.7%, eptifibatide high dose vs. placebo, p = 0.04). The benefit was maintained over 6 months. There was an excess risk of TIMI major bleeding (10.6 vs. 9.1%, p = 0.02), but no excess of intracranial bleedings. The rate of mild or severe thrombocytopenia was not statistically different in both treatment arms.

Tirofiban has been tested in two separate, randomized trials [43,44]. In the PRISM trial, 3231 patients presenting with NSTE-ACS were randomized to receive either tirofiban or UFH for 48 hours. A significant reduction in the composite end-point of death, MI or refractory ischemia was observed at 48 hours and maintained at 30 days, but not thereafter (3.8 vs. 5.6%, RR 0.67, 95% CI 0.48–0.92, p = 0.01 at 48 hours). However, the benefit was highly significant throughout follow-up in troponin-positive patients [45]. The rate of thrombocytopenia (defined as platelet count <90,000/mm^3) was significantly more frequent with tirofiban than with UFH (1.1% vs. 0.4%, p = 0.04).

In the PRISM-PLUS trial, 1915 patients at higher risk than in the PRISM trial, were randomized to three different arms: tirofiban alone, tirofiban plus UFH or UFH alone. The tirofiban-alone arm was prematurely stopped, because of an excess of adverse events. A significant reduction of the risk of death, MI and refractory ischemia was obtained at 7 days (12.9% vs. 17.9%, RR 0.68, 95% CI 0.53–0.88, p = 0.004) and maintained at 30 days and 6 months in the tirofiban plus UFH group, as compared to UFH alone. Major bleeding complications were statistically not more frequent in the tirofiban group (1.4% vs. 0.8%, p = 0.23).

Invasive strategy

GP IIb/IIIa inhibitors exert their beneficial potential best in patients with ACS scheduled for invasive management. Consistent results have been obtained in three different meta-analyses exploring the impact of the use of GP IIb/IIIa inhibitors in the setting of PCI. Two meta-analyses showed that a significant risk reduction for death and MI at 30 days could be achieved when GP IIb/IIIa inhibitors were administered before taking patients to the catheterization laboratory, and maintained during PCI [38,39]. Another meta analysis demonstrated a significant risk reduction in 30-day mortality among a total of 20,186

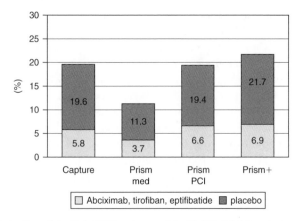

Fig. 10.4 Reduction of death/ AMI by glycoprotein IIb/IIIa inhibitors in troponin-positive patients.

patients (0.9% vs. 1.3%, OR 0.73, 95% CI 0.55–0.96, p = 0.024) [46]. However, thienopyridines and stents were not routinely used in these trials.

Abciximab was the first drug to be tested in three trials as an adjunct to PCI in the setting of ACS [47–49]. In total, 7290 patients were included, revealing a significant reduction in the combination of death and MI or need for urgent revascularization at 30 days. Pooled data from these three trials showed also a significant late mortality benefit (HR 0.71, 95% CI 0.57–0.89, p = 0.003) [50].

In the CAPTURE trial, abciximab has been tested in patients with NSTE-ACS with planned single-vessel PCI without routine use of stents and clopidogrel. Treatment with abciximab for 24 hours before and 12 after the intervention significantly reduced the rate of death, MI and need for urgent intervention for recurrent ischemia as compared to placebo at 30 days (11.3% vs. 15.9%, p = 0.012) [51]. The benefit, as in other trials, was restricted to patients with elevated troponin levels [46,52] (Figure 10.4).

In the more recent ISAR-REACT-2 study, 2022 high-risk NSTE-ACS patients were randomized following pretreatment with aspirin and 600 mg of clopidogrel to either abciximab or placebo [53]. There was a similar rate of diabetic patients in each group (average 26.5%); 52% of patients had elevated troponins, and 24.1% had previous MI. The 30-day composite end-point of death, MI or urgent target vessel revascularization was significantly reduced in abciximab-treated patients versus placebo (8.9% vs. 11.9%, RR 0.75, 95% CI 0.58–0.97, p = 0.03). Most of the risk reduction generated by abciximab resulted from a reduction in the occurrence of death and MI. The effect was more pronounced in certain prespecified subgroups, particularly troponin-positive patients (13.1% vs. 18.3%, RR 0.71, 95% CI 0.54–0.95, p = 0.02) (Figure 10.5). The duration of pretreatment with clopidogrel had no influence on outcome, and there was no beneficial effect in troponin-negative patients or among

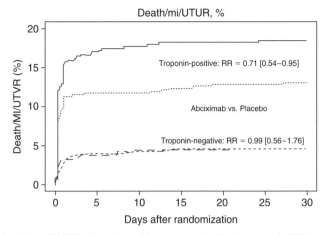

Fig. 10.5 Results of ISAR REACT 2 according to troponin T status [54]. (UTVR = urgent target vessel revascularization). Triple antiplatelet therapy reduces events only in patients with elevated troponins.

diabetic patients. However, the number of diabetic patients in this trial was too low to provide robust statistical power.

The TARGET trial is the only larger head-to-head comparison of abciximab versus tirofiban, in which two-thirds of the patients had recent or ongoing NSTE-ACS. Abciximab was shown to be superior to tirofiban in standard doses in reducing the risk of death, MI and urgent revascularization at 30 days, but the difference was not significant at 6 months and 1 year [54].

Eptifibatide was first tested in patients undergoing PCI, including 38% with unstable angina (IMPACT-2) and exhibited no significant benefit as compared to placebo [55]. Subsequently, eptifibatide was tested in the ESPRIT trial with an increased dose of eptifibatide and including 46% of patients with acute coronary syndrome [56]. Compared to placebo a significant reduction in the risk of death, MI, urgent target vessel revascularization and bail-out use of GP IIb/IIIa inhibitors was revealed at 48 hours, maintained at 30 days, and at 6 months (6.6% vs. 10.5%, RR 0.63, 95% CI 0.47–0.84, p = 0.0015 at 48 hours). The secondary composite end-point of death, MI or urgent target vessel revascularization was also significantly reduced at this time point (6.0% vs. 9.3%, RR 0.65, 95% CI 0.47–0.87, p = 0.0045).

Tirofiban was tested in the RESTORE trial, in 2139 patients with recent acute coronary syndrome. A significant 38% relative-risk reduction in the primary composite endpoint of death, MI, repeat revascularization or recurrent ischemia at 48 hours was observed at 7 days but not at 30 days [57]. Tirofiban was used at the same dose in the TARGET and RESTORE trials. In retrospect, the dose may have been too low.

Recent, smaller trials explored higher doses of tirofiban (bolus $25\mu g/kg$ and infusion $0.15\mu g/kg/min$ for 24–48 hours) in various clinical settings. In a trial of 202 patients, the high dose was shown to reduce the incidence of ischemic thrombotic complications versus placebo during high-risk PCI [58]. TENACITY, designed as a large-scale study testing high-dose tirofiban against abciximab was stopped for non-scientific reasons after inclusion of 383 patients.

Upstream use of GP IIb/IIIa inhibitors prior to revascularization

It has been discussed whether so called upstream use of glycoprotein IIb/IIIa inhibitors could be of benefit with the intention to reduce thrombus burden before PCI and to avoid complications in the waiting phase. This strategy has been shown in meta-analyses to further reduce the risk of death and MI at 30 days, if GP IIb/IIIa inhibitors are started upstream of, and maintained during, the PCI procedure [38,39]. This question will be further explored prospectively in upcoming trials (EARLY-ACS) [59].

In the ACUITY-TIMING study, deferred selective versus routine upstream administration of GP IIb/IIIa inhibitors was tested in a 2×2 factorial, open-label design [60]. GP IIb/IIIa inhibitors were used in 55.7% of patients for 13.1 hours in the deferred selective and in 98.3% of patients for 18.3 hours in the routine upstream strategy. The deferred selective strategy resulted in a reduced 30-day major bleeding rate (4.9% vs. 6.1%, RR 0.80, 95% CI 0.67–0.95). The rate of ischemic events did not meet the set criteria for non-inferiority, although a trend towards a higher rate was noted (7.9% vs. 7.1%, RR 1.12, 95% CI 0.97–1.29; p = 0.13). TIMI minor bleeding rate was significantly lower (5.4% vs. 7.1%, p <0.001; deferred selective vs. routine upstream), whereas TIMI major bleeding rate was not significantly different (1.6% vs. 1.9%, p = 0.20). The ischemic composite end-point was achieved more frequently in patients submitted to PCI with deferred selective versus routine upstream GP IIb/IIIa inhibitors (9.5% vs. 8.0%, RR 1.19, 95% CI 1.00–1.42, p = 0.05). From these results it can be concluded that more frequent and more prolonged use of GP IIb/IIIa inhibitors in an upstream strategy leads to an excess risk of bleedings; however, there is a potentially higher protection against ischemic events.

GP IIb/IIIa inhibitors and CABG

Inhibition of platelet aggregation increases bleeding complications associated with cardiac surgery. However, surgery in patients receiving GP IIb/IIIa inhibitors can safely be performed when appropriate measures are taken to ensure adequate hemostasis and the pharmacokinetics of the different compounds are understood. GP IIb/IIIa inhibitors should be discontinued at the time cardiac surgery starts. Eptifibatide and tirofiban have a short half-life (4 to 6 hours) allowing platelet function to recover by the end of CABG. Abciximab has a longer effective half-life (~6–12 hours) and earlier discontinuation is warranted. If excessive bleeding occurs, fresh platelet transfusions may be considered. Fibrinogen supplementation with fresh frozen plasma or cryoprecipitate either alone or in combination with platelet transfusion can also be used for restoring the haemostatic potential after the administration of small-molecule GP IIb/IIIa inhibitors [61].

Adjunctive therapy

GP IIb/IIIa inhibitors must be used in combination with an anticoagulant. Unfractionated heparin is safe, if the dose is adjusted. Several trials and observational studies in PCI have shown that LMWH, predominantly enoxaparin, can be safely used with GP IIb/IIIa inhibitors without compromising efficacy [62–64]. The combination with fondaparinux was shown to be safe in the OASIS-5 study. Bivalirudin and UFH/LMWH were shown to have equivalent safety and efficacy when used with triple antiplatelet therapy, including GP IIb/IIIa inhibitors in the ACUITY trial [65].

Bivalirudin alone was associated with a lower bleeding risk as compared to any combination with GP IIb/IIIa inhibitors and may therefore be used as an alternative in patients with high bleeding risk [66–67].

Summary

For patients at intermediate to high risk, namely patients with elevated troponins, ST-depression, or diabetes, either eptifibatide or tirofiban for initial early treatment are recommended in addition to dual oral antiplatelet treatment. The initial treatment with these drugs prior to angiography should be maintained during and after PCI. For high-risk patients not pretreated with tirofiban or eptifibatide proceeding to PCI, abciximab is the drug with the best evidence. The use of eptifibatide or tirofiban in this setting is less well established. Bivalirudin may be used as an alternative to GP IIb/IIIa inhibitors plus UFH/LMWH in patients with high risk of bleeding.

References

1 Theroux P, Ouimet H, McCans J, Latour JG, Joly P, Levy G, Pelletier E, Juneau M, Stasiak J, deGuise P, *et al*. Aspirin, heparin, or both to treat acute unstable angina. *New Engl J Med* 1988; **319**: 1105–1111.

2 Theroux P, Waters D, Qiu S, McCans J, de Guise P, Juneau M. Aspirin versus heparin to prevent myocardial infarction during the acute phase of unstable angina. *Circulation* 1993; **88**: 2045–2048.

3 Cairns JA, Singer J, Gent M, Holder DA, Rogers D, Sackett DL, Sealey B, Tanser P, Vandervoort M. One year mortality outcomes of all coronary and intensive care unit patients with acute myocardial infarction, unstable angina or other chest pain in Hamilton, Ontario, a city of 375,000 people. *Can J Cardiol* 1989; **5**: 239–246.

4 Antithrombotic Trialists Collaboration. Collaborative meta-analysis of randomised trials of antiplatelet therapy for prevention of death, myocardial infarction, and stroke in high risk patients. *BMJ* 2002; **324**: 71–86.

5 Bassand JP, Hamm CW, Ardissino D, et al. Guidelines for the diagnosis and treatment of non-ST-segment elevation acute coronary syndromes. The Task Force for the Diagnosis and Treatment of Non-ST-Segment Elevation Acute Coronary Syndromes of the European Society of Cardiology. *Eur Heart J* 2007; **28**(13): 1598–1660.

6 CAPRIE Steering Committee. A randomised, blinded, trial of clopidogrel versus aspirin in patients at risk of ischaemic events (CAPRIE). *Lancet* 1996; **348**: 1329–1339.

7 Yusuf S, Zhao F, Mehta SR, Chrolavicius S, Tognoni G, Fox KK. Effects of clopidogrel in addition to aspirin in patients with acute coronary syndromes without ST-segment elevation. *New Engl J Med* 2001; **345**: 494–502.

8 Peters RJ, Mehta SR, Fox KA, Zhao F, Lewis BS, Kopecky SL, Diaz R, Commerford PJ, Valentin V, Yusuf S. Effects of aspirin dose when used alone or in combination with clopidogrel in patients with acute coronary syndromes: observations from the Clopidogrel in Unstable angina to prevent Recurrent Events (CURE) study. *Circulation* 2003; **108**: 1682–1687.

9 Gollapudi RR, Teirstein PS, Stevenson DD, Simon RA. Aspirin sensitivity: implications for patients with coronary artery disease. *JAMA* 2004; **292**: 3017–3023.

10 Ramanuja S, Breall JA, Kalaria VG. Approach to "aspirin allergy" in cardiovascular patients. *Circulation* 2004; **110**: e1–4.

11 Silberman S, Neukirch-Stoop C, Steg PG. Rapid desensitization procedure for patients with aspirin hypersensitivity undergoing coronary stenting. *Am J Cardiol* 2005; **95**: 509–510.

12 Eikelboom JW, Hirsh J, Weitz JI, Johnston M, Yi Q, Yusuf S. Aspirin-resistant thromboxane biosynthesis and the risk of myocardial infarction, stroke, or cardiovascular death in patients at high risk for cardiovascular events. *Circulation* 2002; **105**: 1650–1655.

13 Catella-Lawson F, Reilly MP, Kapoor SC, Cucchiara AJ, DeMarco S, Tournier B, Vyas SN, FitzGerald GA. Cyclooxygenase inhibitors and the antiplatelet effects of aspirin. *New Engl J Med* 2001; **345**: 1809–1817.

14 Patrono C, Coller B, FitzGerald GA, Hirsh J, Roth G. Platelet-active drugs: the relationships among dose, effectiveness, and side effects: the Seventh ACCP Conference on Antithrombotic and Thrombolytic Therapy. *Chest* 2004; **126**: 234S–264S.

15 Kurth T, Glynn RJ, Walker AM, Chan KA, Buring JE, Hennekens CH, Gaziano JM. Inhibition of clinical benefits of aspirin on first myocardial infarction by nonsteroidal antiinflammatory drugs. *Circulation* 2003; **108**: 1191–1195.

16 Gislason GH, Jacobsen S, Rasmussen JN, Rasmussen S, Buch P, Friberg J, Schramm TK, Abildstrom SZ, Kober L, Madsen M, Torp-Pedersen C. Risk of death or reinfarction associated with the use of selective cyclooxygenase-2 inhibitors and nonselective nonsteroidal antiinflammatory drugs after acute myocardial infarction. *Circulation* 2006; **113**: 2906–2913.

17 Balsano F, Rizzon P, Violi F, Scrutinio D, Cimminiello C, Aguglia F, Pasotti C, Rudelli G. Antiplatelet treatment with ticlopidine in unstable angina. A controlled multicenter clinical trial. The Studio della Ticlopidina nell'Angina Instabile Group. *Circulation* 1990; **82**: 17–26.

18 Budaj A, Yusuf S, Mehta SR, Fox KA, Tognoni G, Zhao F, Chrolavicius S, Hunt D, Keltai M, Franzosi MG. Benefit of clopidogrel in patients with acute coronary syndromes without ST-segment elevation in various risk groups. *Circulation* 2002; **106**: 1622–1626.

19 Wiviott SD, Braunwald E, McCabe CH, Montalescot G, Ruzyllo W, Gottlieb S, Neumann FJ, Ardissino D, De Servi S, Murphy SA, Riesmeyer J, Weerakkody G, Gibson CM Antman EM. Prasugrel versus clopidogrel in patients with acute coronary syndromes. *N Eng J Med* 2007; **357**: 2001–2015.

20 Fox KA, Mehta SR, Peters R, Zhao F, Lakkis N, Gersh BJ, Yusuf S. Benefits and risks of the combination of clopidogrel and aspirin in patients undergoing surgical revascularization for non-ST-elevation acute coronary syndrome: the Clopidogrel in Unstable angina to prevent Recurrent ischemic Events (CURE) Trial. *Circulation* 2004; **110**: 1202–1208.

21 Chan AW, Moliterno DJ, Berger PB, Stone GW, DiBattiste PM, Yakubov SL, Sapp SK, Wolski K, Bhatt DL, Topol EJ. Triple antiplatelet therapy during percutaneous coronary intervention is associated with improved outcomes including one-year survival: results from the Do Tirofiban and ReoProGive Similar Efficacy Outcome Trial (TARGET). *J Am Coll Cardiol* 2003; **42**: 1188–1195.

22 Steinhubl SR, Berger PB, Mann JT, 3rd, Fry ET, DeLago A, Wilmer C, Topol EJ. Early and sustained dual oral antiplatelet therapy following percutaneous coronary intervention: a randomized controlled trial. *JAMA* 2002; **288**: 2411–2420.

23 Szuk T, Gyongyosi M, Homorodi N, Kristof E, Kiraly C, Edes IF, Facsko A, Pavo N, Sodeck G, Strehblow C, Farhan S, Maurer G, Glogar D, Domanovits H, Huber K, Edes I. Effect of timing of clopidogrel administration on 30-day clinical outcomes: 300-mg loading dose immediately after coronary stenting versus pretreatment 6 to 24 hours before stenting in a large unselected patient cohort. *Am Heart J* 2007; **153**: 289–295.

24 Kandzari DE, Berger PB, Kastrati A, Steinhubl SR, Mehilli J, Dotzer F, Ten Berg JM, Neumann FJ, Bollwein H, Dirschinger J, Schomig A. Influence of treatment duration with a 600-mg dose of clopidogrel before percutaneous coronary revascularization. *J Am Coll Cardiol* 2004; **44**: 2133–2136.

25 Montalescot G, Sideris G, Meuleman C, Bal-dit-Sollier C, Lellouche N, Steg PG, Slama M, Milleron O, Collet JP, Henry P, Beygui F, Drouet L. A randomized comparison of high clopidogrel loading doses in patients with non-ST-segment elevation acute coronary syndromes: the ALBION (Assessment of the Best Loading Dose of Clopidogrel to Blunt Platelet Activation, Inflammation and Ongoing Necrosis) trial. *J Am Coll Cardiol* 2006; **48**: 931–938.

26 Patti G, Colonna G, Pasceri V, Pepe LL, Montinaro A, Di Sciascio G. Randomized trial of high loading dose of clopidogrel for reduction of periprocedural myocardial infarction in patients undergoing coronary intervention: results from the ARMYDA-2 (Antiplatelet therapy for Reduction of MYocardial Damage during Angioplasty) study. *Circulation* 2005; **111**: 2099–2106.

27 von Beckerath N, Taubert D, Pogatsa-Murray G, Schomig E, Kastrati A, Schomig A. Absorption, metabolization, and antiplatelet effects of 300-, 600-, and 900-mg loading doses of clopidogrel: results of the ISAR-CHOICE (Intracoronary Stenting and Antithrombotic Regimen: Choose Between 3 High Oral Doses for Immediate Clopidogrel Effect) Trial. *Circulation* 2005; **112**: 2946–2950.

28 Nguyen TA, Diodati JG, Pharand C. Resistance to clopidogrel: a review of the evidence. *J Am Coll Cardiol* 2005; **45**: 1157–1164.

29 Geisler T, Langer H, Wydymus M, Gohring K, Zurn C, Bigalke B, Stellos K, May AE, Gawaz M. Low response to clopidogrel is associated with cardiovascular outcome after coronary stent implantation. *Eur Heart J* 2006; **27**: 2420–2425.

30 Gurbel PA, Bliden KP, Hiatt BL, O'Connor CM. Clopidogrel for coronary stenting: response variability, drug resistance, and the effect of pretreatment platelet reactivity. *Circulation* 2003; **107**: 2908–2913.

31 Matetzky S, Shenkman B, Guetta V, Shechter M, Bienart R, Goldenberg I, Novikov I, Pres H, Savion N, Varon D, Hod H. Clopidogrel resistance is associated with increased risk of recurrent atherothrombotic events in patients with acute myocardial infarction. *Circulation* 2004; **109**: 3171–3175.

32 Saw J, Steinhubl SR, Berger PB, Kereiakes DJ, Serebruany VL, Brennan D, Topol EJ. Lack of adverse clopidogrel-atorvastatin clinical interaction from secondary analysis of a randomized, placebo-controlled clopidogrel trial. *Circulation* 2003; **108**: 921–924.

33 Lim MJ, Spencer FA, Gore JM, Dabbous OH, Agnelli G, Kline-Rogers EM, Dibenedetto D, Eagle KA, Mehta RH. Impact of combined pharmacologic treatment with clopidogrel and a statin on outcomes of patients with non-ST-segment elevation acute coronary syndromes: perspectives from a large multinational registry. *Eur Heart J* 2005; **26**: 1063–1069.

34 Collet JP, Montalescot G, Blanchet B, Tanguy ML, Golmard JL, Choussat R, Beygui F, Payot L, Vignolles N, Metzger JP, Thomas D. Impact of prior use or recent withdrawal of oral antiplatelet agents on acute coronary syndromes. *Circulation* 2004; **110**: 2361–2367.

35 Ho MP, Peterson ED, Wang, L, Magid DJ, Fihn SD, Larsen GC, Jesse RA, Rumsfeld JS. Incidence of death and acute myocardial infarction associated with stopping clopidogrel after acute coronary syndrome. *JAMA* 2008; **299**: 532–539.

36 Boersma E, Harrington RA, Moliterno DJ, White H, Theroux P, Van de Werf F, de Torbal A, Armstrong PW, Wallentin LC, Wilcox RG, Simes J, Califf RM, Topol EJ, Simoons ML. Platelet glycoprotein IIb/IIIa inhibitors in acute coronary syndromes: a meta-analysis of all major randomised clinical trials. *Lancet* 2002; **359**: 189–198.

37 Roffi M, Chew DP, Mukherjee D, Bhatt DL, White JA, Moliterno DJ, Heeschen C, Hamm CW, Robbins MA, Kleiman NS, Theroux P, White HD, Topol EJ. Platelet glycoprotein IIb/IIIa inhibition in acute coronary syndromes. Gradient of benefit related to the revascularization strategy. *Eur Heart J* 2002; **23**: 1441–1448.

38 Boersma E, Akkerhuis KM, Theroux P, Califf RM, Topol EJ, Simoons ML. Platelet glycoprotein IIb/IIIa receptor inhibition in non-ST-elevation acute coronary syndromes: early benefit during medical treatment only, with additional protection during percutaneous coronary intervention. *Circulation* 1999; **100**: 2045–2048.

39 Kong DF, Califf RM, Miller DP, Moliterno DJ, White HD, Harrington RA, Tcheng JE, Lincoff AM, Hasselblad V, Topol EJ. Clinical outcomes of therapeutic agents that block the platelet glycoprotein IIb/IIIa integrin in ischemic heart disease. *Circulation* 1998; **98**: 2829–2835.

40 Roffi M, Chew DP, Mukherjee D, Bhatt DL, White JA, Heeschen C, Hamm CW, Moliterno DJ, Califf RM, White HD, Kleiman NS, Theroux P, Topol EJ. Platelet glycoprotein IIb/IIIa inhibitors reduce mortality in diabetic patients with non-ST-segment-elevation acute coronary syndromes. *Circulation* 2001; **104**: 2767–2771.

41 Simoons ML. Effect of glycoprotein IIb/IIIa receptor blocker abciximab on outcome in patients with acute coronary syndromes without early coronary revascularisation: the GUSTO IV-ACS randomised trial. *Lancet* 2001; **357**: 1915–1924.

42 PURSUIT Investigators. Inhibition of platelet glycoprotein IIb/IIIa with eptifibatide in patients with acute coronary syndromes. Platelet Glycoprotein IIb/IIIa in Unstable

Angina: Receptor Suppression Using Integrilin Therapy. *New Engl J Med* 1998; **339**: 436–443.

43 Platelet Receptor Inhibition in Ischemic Syndrome Management (PRISM) Study Investigators. A comparison of aspirin plus tirofiban with aspirin plus heparin for unstable angina. *New Engl J Med* 1998; **338**: 1498–1505.

44 Platelet Receptor Inhibition in Ischemic Syndrome Management in Patients Limited by Unstable Signs and Symptoms (PRISM-PLUS) Study Investigators. Inhibition of the platelet glycoprotein IIb/IIIa receptor with tirofiban in unstable angina and non-Q-wave myocardial infarction. *New Engl J Med* 1998; **338**: 1488–1497.

45 Heeschen C, Hamm CW, Goldmann B, Deu A, Langenbrink L, White HD. Troponin concentrations for stratification of patients with acute coronary syndromes in relation to therapeutic efficacy of tirofiban. PRISM Study Investigators. Platelet Receptor Inhibition in Ischemic Syndrome Management. *Lancet* 1999; **354**: 1757–1762.

46 Kong DF, Hasselblad V, Harrington RA, White HD, Tcheng JE, Kandzari DE, Topol EJ, Califf RM. Meta-analysis of survival with platelet glycoprotein IIb/IIIa antagonists for percutaneous coronary interventions. *Am J Cardiol* 2003; **92**: 651–655.

47 EPILOG Investigators. Platelet glycoprotein IIb/IIIa receptor blockade and low-dose heparin during percutaneous coronary revascularization. *New Engl J Med* 1997; **336**: 1689–1696.

48 EPISTENT Investigators. Randomised placebo-controlled and balloon-angioplasty-controlled trial to assess safety of coronary stenting with use of platelet glycoprotein-IIb/IIIa blockade. Evaluation of Platelet IIb/IIIa Inhibitor for Stenting. *Lancet* 1998; **352**: 87–92.

49 Lincoff AM, Califf RM, Anderson KM, Weisman HF, Aguirre FV, Kleiman NS, Harrington RA, Topol EJ. Evidence for prevention of death and myocardial infarction with platelet membrane glycoprotein IIb/IIIa receptor blockade by abciximab (c7E3 Fab) among patients with unstable angina undergoing percutaneous coronary revascularization. EPIC Investigators. Evaluation of 7E3 in Preventing Ischemic Complications. *J Am Coll Cardiol* 1997; **30**: 149–156.

50 Anderson KM, Califf RM, Stone GW, Neumann FJ, Montalescot G, Miller DP, Ferguson JJ, 3rd, Willerson JT, Weisman HF, Topol EJ. Long-term mortality benefit with abciximab in patients undergoing percutaneous coronary intervention. *J Am Coll Cardiol* 2001; **37**: 2059–2065.

51 CAPTURE Investigators. Randomised placebo-controlled trial of abciximab before and during coronary intervention in refractory unstable angina: the CAPTURE Study. *Lancet* 1997; **349**: 1429–1435.

52 Hamm CW, Heeschen C, Goldmann B, Vahanian A, Adgey J, Miguel CM, Rutsch W, Berger J, Kootstra J, Simoons ML. Benefit of abciximab in patients with refractory unstable angina in relation to serum troponin T levels. c7E3 Fab Antiplatelet Therapy in Unstable Refractory Angina (CAPTURE) Study Investigators. *New Engl J Med* 1999; **340**: 1623–1629.

53 Kastrati A, Mehilli J, Neumann FJ, Dotzer F, ten Berg J, Bollwein H, Graf I, Ibrahim M, Pache J, Seyfarth M, Schuhlen H, Dirschinger J, Berger PB, Schomig A. Abciximab in patients with acute coronary syndromes undergoing percutaneous coronary intervention after clopidogrel pretreatment: the ISAR-REACT 2 randomized trial. *JAMA* 2006; **295**: 1531–1538.

54 Moliterno DJ, Yakubov SJ, DiBattiste PM, Herrmann HC, Stone GW, Macaya C, Neumann FJ, Ardissino D, Bassand JP, Borzi L, Yeung AC, Harris KA,

Demopoulos LA, Topol EJ. Outcomes at 6 months for the direct comparison of tirofiban and abciximab during percutaneous coronary revascularisation with stent placement: the TARGET follow-up study. *Lancet* 2002; **360**: 355–360.

55 IMPACT-II Investigators. Randomised placebo-controlled trial of effect of eptifibatide on complications of percutaneous coronary intervention: IMPACT-II. Integrilin to Minimise Platelet Aggregation and Coronary Thrombosis-II. *Lancet* 1997; **349**: 1422–1428.

56 ESPRIT Investigators. Novel dosing regimen of eptifibatide in planned coronary stent implantation (ESPRIT): a randomised, placebo-controlled trial. *Lancet* 2000; **356**: 2037–2044.

57 RESTORE Investigators. Effects of platelet glycoprotein IIb/IIIa blockade with tirofiban on adverse cardiac events in patients with unstable angina or acute myocardial infarction undergoing coronary angioplasty. Randomized Efficacy Study of Tirofiban for Outcomes and REstenosis. *Circulation* 1997; **96**: 1445–1453.

58 Valgimigli M, Percoco G, Barbieri D, Ferrari F, Guardigli G, Parrinello G, Soukhomovskaia O, Ferrari R. The additive value of tirofiban administered with the high-dose bolus in the prevention of ischemic complications during high-risk coronary angioplasty: the ADVANCE Trial. *J Am Coll Cardiol* 2004; **44**: 14–19.

59 Giugliano RP, Newby LK, Harrington RA, Gibson CM, Van de Werf F, Armstrong P, Montalescot G, Gilbert J, Strony JT, Califf RM, Braunwald E. The early glycoprotein IIb/IIIa inhibition in non-ST-segment elevation acute coronary syndrome (EARLY ACS) trial: a randomized placebo-controlled trial evaluating the clinical benefits of early front-loaded eptifibatide in the treatment of patients with non-ST-segment elevation acute coronary syndrome – study design and rationale. *Am Heart J* 2005; **149**: 994–1002.

60 Stone GW, Bertrand ME, Moses JW, Ohman EM, Lincoff AM, Ware JH, Pocock SJ, McLaurin BT, Cox DA, Jafar MZ, Chandna H, Hartmann F, Leisch F, Strasser RH, Desaga M, Stuckey TD, Zelman RB, Lieber IH, Cohen DJ, Mehran R, White HD. Routine upstream initiation vs deferred selective use of glycoprotein IIb/IIIa inhibitors in acute coronary syndromes: The ACUITY Timing Trial. *JAMA* 2007; **297**: 591–602.

61 Li YF, Spencer FA, Becker RC. Comparative efficacy of fibrinogen and platelet supplementation on the in vitro reversibility of competitive glycoprotein IIb/IIIa receptor-directed platelet inhibition. *Am Heart J* 2002; **143**: 725–732.

62 Cohen M, Theroux P, Borzak S, Frey MJ, White HD, Van Mieghem W, Senatore F, Lis J, Mukherjee R, Harris K, Bigonzi F. Randomized double-blind safety study of enoxaparin versus unfractionated heparin in patients with non-ST-segment elevation acute coronary syndromes treated with tirofiban and aspirin: the ACUTE II study. The Antithrombotic Combination Using Tirofiban and Enoxaparin. *Am Heart J* 2002; **144**: 470–477.

63 Petersen JL, Mahaffey KW, Hasselblad V, Antman EM, Cohen M, Goodman SG, Langer A, Blazing MA, Le-Moigne-Amrani A, de Lemos JA, Nessel CC, Harrington RA, Ferguson JJ, Braunwald E, Califf RM. Efficacy and bleeding complications among patients randomized to enoxaparin or unfractionated heparin for antithrombin therapy in non-ST-Segment elevation acute coronary syndromes: a systematic overview. *JAMA* 2004; **292**: 89–96.

64 Ferguson JJ, Antman EM, Bates ER, Cohen M, Every NR, Harrington RA, Pepine CJ, Theroux P. Combining enoxaparin and glycoprotein IIb/IIIa antagonists for the treatment of acute coronary syndromes: final results of the National Investigators Collaborating on Enoxaparin-3 (NICE-3) study. *Am Heart J* 2003; **146**: 628–634.

65 de Lemos JA, Blazing MA, Wiviott SD, Brady WE, White HD, Fox KA, Palmisano J, Ramsey KE, Bilheimer DW, Lewis EF, Pfeffer M, Califf RM, Braunwald E. Enoxaparin versus unfractionated heparin in patients treated with tirofiban, aspirin and an early conservative initial management strategy: results from the A phase of the A-to-Z trial. *Eur Heart J* 2004; **25**: 1688–1694.

66 Stone GW, McLaurin BT, Cox DA, Bertrand ME, Lincoff AM, Moses JW, White HD, Pocock SJ, Ware JH, Feit F, Colombo A, Aylward PE, Cequier AR, Darius H, Desmet W, Ebrahimi R, Hamon M, Rasmussen LH, Rupprecht HJ, Hoekstra J, Mehran R, Ohman EM. Bivalirudin for patients with acute coronary syndromes. *New Engl J Med* 2006; **355**: 2203–2216.

67 Stone GW, McLaurin BT, Cox DA, Bertrand ME, Lincoff AM, Moses JW, White HD, Pocock SJ, Ware JH, Feit F, Colombo A, Aylward P, Cequier AR, Darius H, Desmet W, Ebrahimi R, Hamon M, Rasmussen LH, Rupprecht HJ, Hoekstra JW, Mehran R, Ohman EM, For the ACUITY Investigators. Bivalirudin for patients with acute coronary syndromes. *N Engl J Med* 2006; **355**: 2203–2216.

Chapter 11

Antiplatelet therapy in ST-elevation myocardial infarction

Michelle O'Donoghue and Marc S. Sabatine

Introduction

The past two decades have marked several key advances in the management of patients with ST-elevation myocardial infarction (STEMI). The combination of aspirin, heparin and fibrinolytic drugs became well established in the 1980s as the basis for pharmacologic reperfusion. In the late 1990s, primary percutaneous coronary intervention (PCI) emerged as an invasive approach to reperfusion that offered improved outcomes over fibrinolytic therapy. Regardless of the primary treatment strategy, platelets play a central role in the initiation and propagation of pathologic thrombosis after spontaneous and/or mechanical plaque rupture. As such, antiplatelet therapies are a key component in the pharmacotherapy of acute coronary syndromes (ACS), particularly STEMI [1]. Not surprisingly, therefore, advances in adjunctive antiplatelet therapies have improved outcomes in patients receiving pharmacologic or catheter-based reperfusion strategies in STEMI.

STEMI treated with pharmacologic reperfusion

Aspirin

The first trial to demonstrate a clear benefit for aspirin therapy in the setting of acute MI was ISIS-2 (Second International Study of Infarct Survival) in 1988 [2]. The trial randomized 17,187 patients with STEMI to treatment with streptokinase, aspirin, aspirin and streptokinase in combination, or placebo. Treatment with aspirin reduced vascular mortality by 23% when compared

Antiplatelet Therapy in Ischemic Heart Disease, 1st edition. Edited by Stephen D. Wiviott.
© 2009 American Heart Association, ISBN: 9-781-4051-7626-2

to placebo therapy (9.4% vs. 11.8%, p < 0.001). In addition, aspirin reduced non-fatal MI by 49% and stroke by 46%, with no apparent increase in major bleeding after 5 weeks' follow-up. Moreover, the combination of aspirin and thrombolytic was shown to provide incremental benefit to either therapy alone, with a 42% reduction in mortality with both drugs compared to neither (8% vs. 13.2%, p < 0.001, Figure 11.1). Subsequent long-term follow-up data have demonstrated that the early survival advantage of streptokinase and short-term aspirin therapy are maintained over 10 years [3].

Additional data from the Antiplatelet Trialists' Collaboration further support the efficacy of aspirin as an adjunct to fibrinolytic therapy and in the management of patients following MI [4]. Among approximately 20,000 patients with acute MI pooled from several trials, a 30% reduction in the odds of stroke, recurrent MI or vascular death (10.4% vs. 14.2%, p < 0.001) was observed when antiplatelet therapy (primarily aspirin) was used in the acute management of MI and continued for a mean of 1 month after the acute event.

Thienopyridines

A greater understanding of the biochemistry of plaque rupture and clot formation has led to growing interest in the addition of more potent antiplatelet agents to existing therapies. Clopidogrel is an oral antiplatelet agent that inhibits platelet activation and aggregation by targeting the $P2Y_{12}$ component of the adenosine diphosphate (ADP) receptor on the platelet cell surface [5]. It is absorbed into the circulation as a prodrug and requires metabolism via the hepatic cytochrome P450 enzyme system to form its active metabolite.

The CLARITY-TIMI 28 (Clopidogrel as Adjunctive Reperfusion Therapy-Thrombolysis in Myocardial Infarction 28) trial was a placebo-controlled, double-blinded trial that enrolled 3491 patients with STEMI within 12 hours of symptom

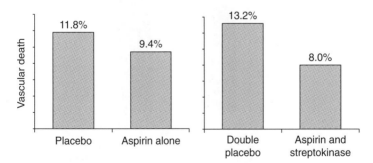

Fig. 11.1 Incidence of vascular death for patients in the ISIS-2 trial randomized to treatment with placebo, aspirin or a combination of streptokinase and aspirin after 5 weeks' follow-up. Reproduced with permission from [2].

onset [6]. Patients enrolled in the trial were randomized to treatment with clopidogrel (300 mg loading dose, followed by 75 mg once daily) or placebo. All patients were to be treated with aspirin (150–325 mg on the first day and 75–162 mg daily thereafter) and the physician's choice of fibrinolytic drug. Patients who were administered a fibrin-specific lytic were required to receive 48 hours of unfractionated or low-molecular-weight heparin.

All patients were to undergo coronary angiography during the index hospitalization (2–8 days after randomization) in order to assess late patency of the infarct-related artery. Patients were treated with either clopidogrel or placebo up to and including the day of angiography.

The rates of the primary efficacy end-point, a composite of an occluded infarct-related artery (TIMI flow grade 0 or 1), or death or recurrent MI prior to angiography, were 21.7% in the placebo group and 15.0% in the clopidogrel group, representing a 36% reduction in the odds or an absolute reduction of 6.7% in favor of treatment with clopidogrel (p < 0.001; Figure 11.2). Among the individual components of the primary end-point, clopidogrel had the greatest effect on reducing the incidence of an occluded infarct-related artery (18.4% to 11.7%; p < 0.001) and reducing recurrent MI prior to angiography (3.6% to 2.5%; p = 0.08). The benefit of clopidogrel on the risk of the primary end-point was observed across all prespecified subgroups.

Treatment with clopidogrel also reduced the odds of cardiovascular death, recurrent MI or recurrent ischemia leading to urgent revascularization by 20% at 30 days' follow-up (14.1% to 11.6%; p = 0.03; Figure 11.3). Importantly, the addition of clopidogrel to aspirin and fibrinolytic therapy did not result in a

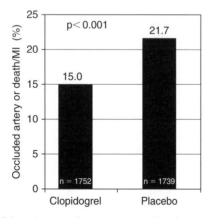

Fig. 11.2 Incidence of the primary end-point, a composite of an occluded infarct-related artery (defined as a TIMI flow grade of 0 or 1), or death or recurrent MI prior to coronary angiography, in the CLARITY–TIMI 28 trial. Patients were randomized to treatment with clopidogrel or placebo in the setting of fibrinolytic therapy for STEMI. Reproduced with permission from [6].

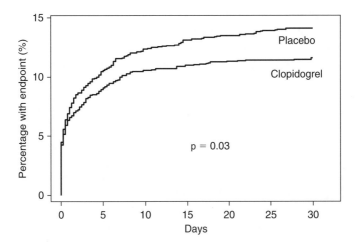

Fig. 11.3 Cumulative incidence curves for the end-point of death from cardiovascular causes, recurrent myocardial infarction or recurrent ischemia leading to need for urgent revascularization through 30 days' follow-up in the CLARITY-TIMI 28 trial. Reproduced with permission from [6].

significant increase in the risk of major bleeding (1.3% with clopidogrel vs. 1.1% with placebo; p = 0.64), nor intracranial hemorrhage (0.5% with clopidogrel vs. 0.7% with placebo; p = 0.38).

Electrocardiographic analyses from the trial have provided insights into the mechanism of clopidogrel's benefit in the setting of fibrinolytic therapy. Clopidogrel therapy did not significantly improve the degree of resolution of ST-segment elevation (a non-invasive marker of early reperfusion) at 180 minutes. However, clopidogrel offered a greater treatment benefit in patients who achieved initial vessel reperfusion, as suggested by either partial (30–70%) or complete (>70%) ST-segment resolution at 90 minutes, than in those with no ST-segment resolution [7]. These data suggest that clopidogrel improved outcomes in patients receiving fibrinolytic therapy by preventing reocclusion of the infarct-related artery rather than by facilitating early reperfusion.

The COMMIT/CCS-2 (Clopidogrel and Metoprolol in Myocardial Infarction Trial/the Second Chinese Cardiac Study) trial was another landmark study that evaluated the role of clopidogrel in patients with STEMI [8]. The trial enrolled 45,852 patients in China and used a 2 × 2 factorial design to randomize subjects to treatment with clopidogrel (75 mg daily without a loading dose) or placebo, and metoprolol or placebo, within 24 hours of symptom onset. All subjects were to be treated with aspirin. A total of 93% of patients had evidence of ST-segment elevation or left bundle branch block on their electrocardiogram at the time of randomization, 54% were treated with fibrinolytic therapy, 75% received an anticoagulant, and fewer than 5% of patients underwent PCI. In addition, there was no upper age limit to the trial and more than a quarter of subjects were older than 70 years old.

COMMIT/CCS-2 examined two prespecified co-primary clinical end-points: all-cause mortality, and the composite of death, reinfarction or stroke. Patients were followed until hospital discharge or day 28, whichever occurred sooner. Treatment with clopidogrel resulted in a statistically significant 7% relative reduction in the risk of death (8.1% to 7.5%; p = 0.03; Figure 11.4) and a 9% reduction in the incidence of death, reinfarction or stroke (10.1% vs. 9.2%; p = 0.002). The benefit of clopidogrel on the incidence of the composite primary end-point was seen irrespective of age, sex and the use of fibrinolytic therapy.

Despite the absence of a loading dose, the clinical benefit of clopidogrel emerged early following initiation of treatment, with a significant 11% reduction in the incidence of death, reinfarction or stroke by the end of the second hospital day (p = 0.014), due largely to a reduction in the risk of death (3.6% to 3.2%; p = 0.019).

The incidence of major bleeding was low in both treatment arms. Clopidogrel did not significantly increase the risk of major bleeding (0.58% with clopidogrel vs. 0.55% with placebo; p = 0.59) and the rates of intracranial hemorrhage were identical across treatment arms (0.2%), including those participants who received concomitant fibrinolytic therapy and irrespective of patient age. Treatment with clopidogrel was associated with a significant increase in minor bleeding, including bruising and dental bleeding (3.6% vs. 3.1%; p = 0.005).

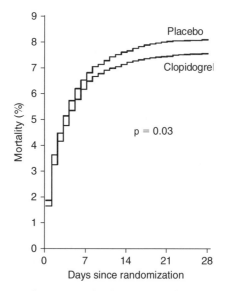

Fig. 11.4 Cumulative incidence curves for the end-point of death prior to discharge in COMMIT/CCS-2. Reproduced with permission from [8].

Glycoprotein IIb/IIIa inhibitors

Glycoprotein (GP) IIb/IIIa inhibitors are potent inhibitors of platelet aggregation that act by targeting the GP IIb/IIIa receptor on the activated platelet cell surface. As the drug provides both rapid and potent platelet inhibition, it has been hypothesized that the addition of a GP IIb/IIIa inhibitor to fibrinolytic therapy might improve clinical outcomes and reduce bleeding complications by allowing for a reduction in the dose of co-administered thrombolytic. Early angiographic studies suggested this combination might offer incremental benefit and improve infarct-related artery patency [9–12]. However in phase III trials, the combination of a GP IIb/IIIa and half-dose lytic failed to improve mortality. Although combination therapy reduced the risk of recurrent MI, it came at the cost of increased risk of bleeding, including a doubling in the rate of intracranial hemorrhage in the elderly [13,14].

STEMI treated with primary PCI

Despite advances in fibrinolytic therapy, one-fifth of patients fail to reperfuse and fewer than 60% of patients achieve optimal epicardial flow [15]. Moreover, reocclusion of the culprit vessel may occur in up to one-quarter of patients treated with fibrinolytic therapy [16]. In the 1990s, primary PCI emerged as a mechanical reperfusion approach that offers improved outcomes as compared to fibrinolytic therapy, including a significant reduction in short-term death, reinfarction and stroke [17]. The use of coronary stenting has since been shown to result in lower rates of restenosis and need for target vessel revascularization as compared to balloon angioplasty alone [18–20].

Thienopyridines

The combination of aspirin and a thienopyridine has been shown to reduce the risk of cardiovascular events in patients undergoing elective and urgent PCI [21]. For this reason, combination therapy including aspirin and clopidogrel is considered the standard of care for patients receiving primary PCI for STEMI [22], despite a paucity of clinical trial data specific to this patient population.

Of note though, even when a 300-mg loading dose is used, clopidogrel requires at least 4–6 hours in order to attain its maximal effect [23]. To that end, a growing body of evidence suggests that pretreatment with clopidogrel several hours prior to PCI is necessary to confer a significant treatment benefit.

CLARITY-TIMI 28 provided an opportunity to examine the benefit of early administration of clopidogrel prior to PCI, as all patients were required to undergo coronary angiography 2–8 days after randomization to either clopidogrel or placebo. For patients who required PCI in the trial, it was recommended that all patients receive an open-label loading dose of ⩾300 mg clopidogrel after diagnostic angiography. As such, the PCI–CLARITY-TIMI 28 analysis evaluated the question of whether clopidogrel pretreatment initiated hours or days prior to PCI would reduce cardiovascular events following PCI, when compared with clopidogrel administration at the time of angiography [24]. Pretreatment with clopidogrel reduced the odds of death, MI or stroke by 46% following PCI through to 30 days from randomization (3.6% vs. 6.2%; adjusted p = 0.008), without a significant increase in bleeding. Of interest, the Kaplan–Meier estimated event rate curves for the two treatment groups separated soon after PCI and continued to diverge over time (Figure 11.5). A meta-analysis of studies of pretreatment prior to PCI including PCI-CLARITY [24], Clopidogrel in Unstable Angina to Prevent Recurrent Events (PCI-CURE) [25] and Clopidogrel for the Reduction of Events During Observation (CREDO) [26] showed clopidogrel pretreatment being associated with a 29% reduction in the odds of death or MI following PCI [24]. A consistent benefit has also been seen irrespective of GP IIb/IIIa inhibitor use at the time of PCI [27].

It should be noted, though, that some clinicians are reluctant to administer clopidogrel before angiography due to concerns for bleeding in patients who require coronary artery bypass graft (CABG) surgery within 5 days of receiving drug [28]. However, in CLARITY-TIMI 28 there was no excess in major bleeding for patients on clopidogrel who required CABG surgery during the index hospitalization, including those patients who required surgery sooner than 5 days after drug discontinuation [29].

The Trial to Assess Improvement in Therapeutic Outcomes by Optimizing Platelet Inhibition with Prasugrel (TRITON-TIMI 38) study compared

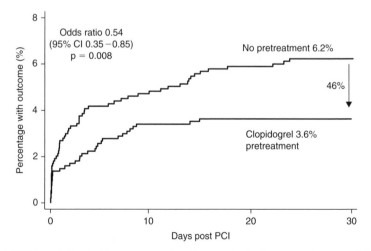

Fig. 11.5 Cumulative incidence curves of cardiovascular death, recurrent myocardial infarction or stroke following PCI through 30 days' follow-up in the PCI–CLARITY-TIMI 28 study. Reproduced with permission from [24].

prasugrel, a third generation thienopyridine, to clopidogrel in patients with ACS undergoing PCI. In this study, 3534 patients were enrolled with STEMI, including patients undergoing primary PCI and patients undergoing PCI following initial medical therapy for STEMI. Patients with primary PCI could receive study drug on first contact prior to coronary angiography; however, patients enrolled following medical treatment had to have coronary anatomy known to be suitable for PCI prior to study drug dosing [30]. Prasugrel was associated with a 21% reduction in the primary composite end-point of cardiovascular death, non-fatal MI and non-fatal stroke (12.4 vs. 10.0%, HR 0.79, p = 0.02) in the STEMI population [31]. In the overall trial cohort, prasugrel-treated patients had a higher rate of major hemorrhage; however, no significant difference was noted among the STEMI patients [32].

GP IIb/IIIa inhibitors

A growing body of evidence suggests that the adjunctive use of GP IIb/IIIa inhibitors, in particular abciximab, is associated with improved tissue reperfusion, recovery of left ventricular function and clinical outcomes in the setting of primary PCI [33–35]. By directly targeting the receptor on the activated cell surface, GP IIb/IIIa inhibitors may act by preventing distal embolization of platelet aggregates and inhibiting activated platelets from interacting with the endothelium.

Several trials have now demonstrated a consistent reduction in death, MI or urgent target vessel revascularization with the addition of abciximab in the setting of primary PCI (Figure 11.6) [19,35–39]. Moreover a recent, comprehensive meta-analysis demonstrated a significant reduction in mortality at 30 days in patients treated with abciximab and primary angioplasty that was maintained after 1 year of follow-up [40]. A second meta-analysis suggests that a reduction in death or recurrent MI may extend to 3 years [41], including a fivefold greater benefit in patients with diabetes mellitus. To date, there are few trials examining the utility of either tirofiban or eptifibatide in the setting of primary PCI, although there is growing evidence to suggest that eptifibatide is non-inferior to abciximab in this setting [42,43].

The optimal timing of GP IIb/IIIa inhibitor administration is an area under continued investigation. Pilot studies have shown that initiation of GP IIb/IIIa blockade while in the emergency department compared with at the time of catheterization may increase pre-PCI vessel patency at the time of angiography [34,44–46]. In turn, restoration of optimal epicardial flow prior to PCI has been shown to be associated with improved clinical outcomes [47]. In addition to the potential clinical benefit behind the "open artery" hypothesis, improved flow may allow for better visualization of the culprit lesion and in itself help facilitate PCI and improve microvascular perfusion. In the TITAN (Time to Integrilin Therapy in Acute Myocardial Infarction)-TIMI 34 trial, initiation of eptifibatide in the emergency department was shown to improve

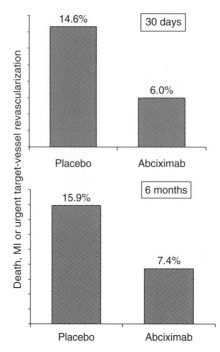

Fig. 11.6 Incidence of death, reinfarction and urgent target-vessel revascularization at 30 days and at 6 months after randomization to abciximab or placebo in patients with acute MI undergoing primary PCI in the ADMIRAL trial. Reproduced with permission from [34].

myocardial perfusion without a significant increase in major bleeding [48]. Similarly, in Randomized Early Versus Late Abciximab in Acute Myocardial Infarction Treated With Primary Coronary Intervention (RELAx-AMI), early initiation of abciximab resulted in improved epicardial and myocardial perfusion pre-PCI, as well as improved myocardial perfusion and ejection fraction post-PCI [49]. Finally, in a meta-analysis of six randomized trials, early administration of a GP IIb/IIIa inhibitor in STEMI was shown to improve vessel patency with a trend towards improved clinical outcomes [50]. However, the overall clinical benefit of this approach remains unproven. In a meta-analysis of randomized trials, "facilitation" with GP IIb/IIIa inhibitors or fibrinolytic therapy prior to PCI failed to improve clinical outcomes and was associated with an increased risk of bleeding [51]. Moreover, the more recently presented Facilitated Intervention With Enhanced Reperfusion Speed to Stop Events (FINESSE) trial failed to show any clinical benefit for either upstream abciximab or the combination of half-dose reteplase with abciximab prior to PCI, and at the cost of a higher risk of TIMI major or minor bleeding [52].

Summary, current guidelines and future directions

Antiplatelet therapies, in particular aspirin, play a central role in the management of patients with STEMI. To that end, the ACC/AHA Guidelines for the Treatment of STEMI, give aspirin a Class I recommendation. Since the publication of the guidelines in 2004, recent advances in adjunctive antiplatelet therapies have led to further improvement in cardiovascular outcomes after ACS. The results of the CLARITY–TIMI 28 and COMMIT/CCS-2 trials have shown that the addition of clopidogrel to aspirin in patients with STEMI receiving fibrinolytic therapy helps to maintain infarct-related artery patency and reduce ischemic complications, including mortality. Based on the available data, a clopidogrel loading dose of 300 mg is appropriate for patients aged ≤75 years receiving fibrinolytic therapy, followed by a daily dose of 75 mg. For patients aged >75 years, the addition of clopidogrel 75 mg daily (without a loading dose) to fibrinolytic therapy appears to be well tolerated and improves clinical outcomes without any significant excess in bleeding. At this time, there is no role for GP IIb/IIIa inhibitors in the setting of fibrinolytic therapy [1].

For patients with STEMI proceeding directly to primary PCI, the 2004 ACC/AHA Guidelines recommend a clopidogrel loading dose of 300 mg after diagnostic angiography and prior to PCI [22]. The 2005 ACC/AHA/SCAI Guidelines recommend a 300 mg loading dose of clopidogrel at least 6 hours before PCI and support a loading dose of >300 mg for patients undergoing PCI who need to achieve a greater degree of platelet inhibition more rapidly, as would be the case in primary PCI for STEMI [53]. Most recently, the 2007 guidelines from the European Society of Cardiology recommend a 600 mg loading dose of clopidogrel in patients with STEMI going for primary PCI [54]. Several point-of-care assays are now available to help assess the degree of platelet inhibition in response to drug therapy. However, at this time it remains unknown whether targeting a specific degree of platelet inhibition will translate into improved outcomes [5].

The current guidelines provide a Class IIa indication for abciximab to be initiated as early as possible for patients going directly to primary PCI and a Class IIb indication for the small molecule GP IIb/IIIa receptor antagonists.

References

1 Antman EM, Hand M, Armstrong PW, et al. 2007 Focused Update of the ACC/AHA 2004 Guidelines for the Management of Patients With ST-Elevation Myocardial Infarction: a report of the American College of Cardiology/American Heart Association Task Force on Practice Guidelines: developed in collaboration With the Canadian Cardiovascular Society endorsed by the American Academy of Family Physicians: 2007 Writing Group to Review New Evidence and Update the ACC/AHA 2004 Guidelines for the Management of Patients With ST-Elevation Myocardial Infarction, Writing on Behalf of the 2004 Writing Committee. *Circulation* 2008; **117**(2): 296–329.

2 ISIS-2 (Second International Study of Infarct Survival) Collaborative Group. Randomised trial of intravenous streptokinase, oral aspirin, both or neither among 17,187 cases of suspected acute myocardial infarction: ISIS-2. *Lancet* 1988; **ii**: 349–360.

3 Baigent C, Collins R, Appleby P, Parish S, Sleight P, Peto R. ISIS-2: 10 year survival among patients with suspected acute myocardial infarction in randomised comparison of intravenous streptokinase, oral aspirin, both, or neither. The ISIS-2 (Second International Study of Infarct Survival) Collaborative Group. *BMJ* 1998; **316**: 1337–1343.

4 Antiplatelet Trialists' Collaboration. Collaborative overview of randomised trials of antiplatelet therapy – I: Prevention of death, myocardial infarction, and stroke by prolonged antiplatelet therapy in various categories of patients. *BMJ* 1994; **308**: 81–106.

5 O'Donoghue M, Wiviott SD. Clopidogrel response variability and future therapies: clopidogrel: does one size fit all? *Circulation* 2006; **114**: e600–606.

6 Sabatine MS, Cannon CP, Gibson CM, *et al*. Addition of clopidogrel to aspirin and fibrinolytic therapy for myocardial infarction with ST-segment elevation. *New Engl J Med* 2005; **352**: 1179–1189.

7 Scirica BM, Sabatine MS, Morrow DA, *et al*. The role of clopidogrel in early and sustained arterial patency after fibrinolysis for ST-segment elevation myocardial infarction: the ECG CLARITY-TIMI 28 Study.*J Am Coll Cardiol* 2006; **48**: 37–42.

8 Chen ZM, Jiang LX, Chen YP, *et al*. Addition of clopidogrel to aspirin in 45,852 patients with acute myocardial infarction: randomised placebo-controlled trial. *Lancet* 2005; **366**: 1607–1621.

9 Antman EM, Giugliano RP, Gibson CM, *et al*. Abciximab facilitates the rate and extent of thrombolysis. Results of the Thrombolysis in Myocardial Infarction (TIMI) 14 trial. *Circulation* 1999; **99**: 2720–2732.

10 Giugliano RP, Roe MT, Harrington RA, *et al*. Combination reperfusion therapy with eptifibatide and reduced-dose tenecteplase for ST-elevation myocardial infarction: results of the integrilin and tenecteplase in acute myocardial infarction (INTEGRITI) Phase II Angiographic Trial.*J Am Coll Cardiol* 2003; **41**: 1251–1260.

11 Strategies for Patency Enhancement in the Emergency Department (SPEED) Group. Trial of abciximab with and without low-dose reteplase for acute myocardial infarction. *Circulation* 2000; **101**: 2788–2794.

12 Brener SJ, Zeymer U, Adgey AA, *et al*. Eptifibatide and low-dose tissue plasminogen activator in acute myocardial infarction: the integrilin and low-dose thrombolysis in acute myocardial infarction (INTRO AMI) trial. *J Am Coll Cardiol* 2002; **39**: 377–386.

13 GUSTO V Investigators. Reperfusion therapy for acute myocardial infarction with fibrinolytic therapy or combination reduced fibrinolytic therapy and platelet glycoprotein IIb/IIIa inhibition: the GUSTO V randomised trial. *Lancet* 2001; **357**: 1905–1914.

14 Assessment of the Safety and Efficacy of a New Thrombolytic Regimen (ASSENT)-3 Investigators. Efficacy and safety of tenecteplase in combination with enoxaparin, abciximab, or unfractionated heparin: the ASSENT-3 randomised trial in acute myocardial infarction. *Lancet* 2001; **358**: 605–613.

15 Smalling RW, Bode C, Kalbfleisch J, *et al*. More rapid, complete, and stable coronary thrombolysis with bolus administration of reteplase compared with alteplase infusion in acute myocardial infarction. RAPID Investigators. *Circulation* 1995; **91**: 2725–2732.

16 Gibson CM, Karha J, Murphy SA, *et al.* Early and long-term clinical outcomes associated with reinfarction following fibrinolytic administration in the Thrombolysis in Myocardial Infarction trials. *J Am Coll Cardiol* 2003; **42**: 7–16.

17 Keeley EC, Boura JA, Grines CL. Primary angioplasty versus intravenous thrombolytic therapy for acute myocardial infarction: a quantitative review of 23 randomised trials. *Lancet* 2003; **361**: 13–20.

18 Grines CL, Cox DA, Stone GW, *et al.* Coronary angioplasty with or without stent implantation for acute myocardial infarction. Stent Primary Angioplasty in Myocardial Infarction Study Group. *New Engl J Med* 1999; **341**: 1949–1956.

19 Stone GW, Grines CL, Cox DA, *et al.* Comparison of angioplasty with stenting, with or without abciximab, in acute myocardial infarction. *New Engl J Med* 2002; **346**: 957–966.

20 Zhu MM, Feit A, Chadow H, Alam M, Kwan T, Clark LT. Primary stent implantation compared with primary balloon angioplasty for acute myocardial infarction: a meta-analysis of randomized clinical trials. *Am J Cardiol* 2001; **88**: 297–301.

21 Leon MB, Baim DS, Popma JJ, *et al.* A clinical trial comparing three antithrombotic-drug regimens after coronary-artery stenting. *New Engl J Med* 1998; **339**: 1665–1671.

22 Antman EM, Anbe DT, Armstrong PW, *et al.* ACC/AHA Guidelines for the management of patients with ST-elevation myocardial infarction. *Circulation* 2004; **110**: e82–292.

23 Montalescot G, Sideris G, Meuleman C, *et al.* A randomized comparison of high clopidogrel loading doses in patients with non-ST-segment elevation acute coronary syndromes: the ALBION (Assessment of the Best Loading Dose of Clopidogrel to Blunt Platelet Activation, Inflammation and Ongoing Necrosis) trial. *J Am Coll Cardiol* 2006; **48**: 931–938.

24 Sabatine MS, Cannon CP, Gibson CM, *et al.* Effect of clopidogrel pretreatment before percutaneous coronary intervention in patients with ST-elevation myocardial infarction treated with fibrinolytics: the PCI-CLARITY study. *JAMA* 2005; **294**: 1224–1232.

25 Mehta SR, Yusuf S, Peters RJ, *et al.* Effects of pretreatment with clopidogrel and aspirin followed by long- term therapy in patients undergoing percutaneous coronary intervention: the PCI-CURE study. *Lancet* 2001; **358**: 527–533.

26 Steinhubl SR, Berger PB, Mann JT, 3rd, *et al.* Early and sustained dual oral antiplatelet therapy following percutaneous coronary intervention: a randomized controlled trial. *JAMA* 2002; **288**: 2411–2420.

27 Sabatine MS, Hamdalla H, Mehta S, Topol E, Steinhubl S, Cannon C. Benefit of clopidogrel pretreatment before PCI regardless of GP IIb/IIIa inhibitor use. *Eur Heart J* 2006; **27** (Abstract Suppl.): 862.

28 Fox KA, Mehta SR, Peters R, *et al.* Benefits and risks of the combination of clopidogrel and aspirin in patients undergoing surgical revascularization for non-ST-elevation acute coronary syndrome: the Clopidogrel in Unstable angina to prevent Recurrent ischemic Events (CURE) Trial. *Circulation* 2004; **110**: 1202–1208.

29 McLean DS, Sabatine MS, Guo W, McCabe CH, Cannon CP. Benefits and risks of clopidogrel pretreatment before coronary artery bypass grafting in patients with ST-elevation myocardial infarction treated with fibrinolytics in CLARITY-TIMI 28. *J Thromb Thrombolysis* 2007; **24**: 85–91.

30 Wiviott SD, Antman EM, Gibson CM, *et al.* Evaluation of prasugrel compared with clopidogrel in patients with acute coronary syndromes: design and rationale for the TRial to assess Improvement in Therapeutic Outcomes by optimizing platelet InhibitioN with prasugrel Thrombolysis In Myocardial Infarction 38 (TRITON-TIMI 38). *Am Heart J* 2006; **152**: 627–635.

31 Wiviott SD, Trenk D, Frelinger AL, *et al.* Prasugrel compared with high loading- and maintenance-dose clopidogrel in patients with planned percutaneous coronary intervention: the Prasugrel in Comparison to Clopidogrel for Inhibition of Platelet Activation and Aggregation-Thrombolysis in Myocardial Infarction 44 trial. *Circulation* 2007; **116**: 2923–2932.

32 Montalescot G, Wiviott SD, Braunwald E, et al. Prasugrel compared with clopidogrel in patients undergoing percutaneous coronary intervention for ST-elevation myocardial infarction in TRITON-TIMI 38. *Lancet*: in press.

33 Neumann FJ, Blasini R, Schmitt C, *et al.* Effect of glycoprotein IIb/IIIa receptor blockade on recovery of coronary flow and left ventricular function after the placement of coronary-artery stents in acute myocardial infarction. *Circulation* 1998; **98**: 2695–2701.

34 Montalescot G, Barragan P, Wittenberg O, *et al.* Platelet glycoprotein IIb/IIIa inhibition with coronary stenting for acute myocardial infarction. *New Engl J Med* 2001; **344**: 1895–1903.

35 Antoniucci D, Rodriguez A, Hempel A, *et al.* A randomized trial comparing primary infarct artery stenting with or without abciximab in acute myocardial infarction. *J Am Coll Cardiol* 2003; **42**: 1879–1885.

36 Brener SJ, Barr LA, Burchenal JEB, *et al.* Randomized, placebo-controlled trial of platelet glycoprotein IIb/IIIa blockade with primary angioplasty for acute myocardial infarction. *Circulation* 1998; **98**: 731–741.

37 Neumann F-J, Kastrati A, Schmitt C, *et al.* Effect of glycoprotein IIb/IIIa receptor blockade with abciximab on clinical and angiographic restenosis rate after the placement of coronary stents following acute myocardial infarction. *J Am Coll Cardiol* 2000; **35**: 915–921.

38 Montalescot G, Barragan P, Wittenberg O, *et al.* Platelet glycoprotein IIb/IIIa inhibition with coronary stenting for acute myocardial infarction. *New Engl J Med* 2001; **344**: 1895–1903.

39 EPISTENT Investigators. Randomised placebo-controlled and balloon-angioplasty-controlled trial to assess safety of coronary stenting with the use of platelet glycoprotein-IIb/IIIa blockade. *Lancet* 1998; **352**: 87–92.

40 De Luca G, Suryapranata H, Stone GW, *et al.* Abciximab as adjunctive therapy to reperfusion in acute ST-segment elevation myocardial infarction: a meta-analysis of randomized trials. *JAMA* 2005; **293**: 1759–1765.

41 Montalescot G, Antoniucci D, Kastrati A, *et al.* Abciximab in primary coronary stenting of ST-elevation myocardial infarction: a European meta-analysis on individual patients' data with long-term follow-up. *Eur Heart J* 2007; **28**: 443–449.

42 Zeymer U. Eptifibatide versus abciximab in primary PCI for acute ST-elevation myocardial infarction (EVA-AMI) trial. *American Heart Association Scientific Sessions*, Orlando, 2008.

43 Gurm HS, Smith DE, Collins JS, *et al.* The relative safety and efficacy of abciximab and eptifibatide in patients undergoing primary percutaneous coronary

intervention: insights from a large regional registry of contemporary percutaneous coronary intervention. *J Am Coll Cardiol* 2008; **51**: 529–535.

44 Lee DP, Herity NA, Hiatt BL, *et al*. Adjunctive platelet glycoprotein IIb/IIIa receptor inhibition with tirofiban before primary angioplasty improves angiographic outcomes: results of the TIrofiban Given in the Emergency Room before Primary Angioplasty (TIGER-PA) pilot trial. *Circulation* 2003; **107**: 1497–1501.

45 Zeymer U, Zahn R, Schiele R, *et al*. Early eptifibatide improves TIMI 3 patency before primary percutaneous coronary intervention for acute ST elevation myocardial infarction: results of the randomized integrilin in acute myocardial infarction (INTAMI) pilot trial. *Eur Heart J* 2005; **26**: 1971–1977.

46 van't Hof AW, Ernst N, de Boer MJ, *et al*. Facilitation of primary coronary angioplasty by early start of a glycoprotein 2b/3a inhibitor: results of the ongoing tirofiban in myocardial infarction evaluation (On-TIME) trial. *Eur Heart J* 2004; **25**: 837–846.

47 Stone GW, Cox D, Garcia E, *et al*. Normal flow (TIMI-3) before mechanical reperfusion therapy is an independent determinant of survival in acute myocardial infarction: analysis from the primary angioplasty in myocardial infarction trials. *Circulation* 2001; **104**: 636–641.

48 Gibson CM, Kirtane AJ, Murphy SA, *et al*. Early initiation of eptifibatide in the emergency department before primary percutaneous coronary intervention for ST-segment elevation myocardial infarction: results of the Time to Integrilin Therapy in Acute Myocardial Infarction (TITAN)-TIMI 34 trial. *Am Heart J* 2006; **152**: 668–675.

49 Maioli M, Bellandi F, Leoncini M, Toso A, Dabizzi RP. Randomized early versus late abciximab in acute myocardial infarction treated with primary coronary intervention (RELAx-AMI Trial). *J Am Coll Cardiol* 2007; **49**: 1517–1524.

50 Montalescot G, Borentain M, Payot L, Collet JP, Thomas D. Early vs late administration of glycoprotein IIb/IIIa inhibitors in primary percutaneous coronary intervention of acute ST-segment elevation myocardial infarction: a meta-analysis. *JAMA* 2004; **292**: 362–366.

51 Keeley EC, Boura JA, Grines CL. Comparison of primary and facilitated percutaneous coronary interventions for ST-elevation myocardial infarction: quantitative review of randomised trials. *Lancet* 2006; **367**: 579–588.

52 Ellis S. Facilitated Intervention with Enhanced Reperfusion Speed to Stop Events (FINESSE) Trial. *N Engl J Med* 2008; **358**: 2205–2217.

53 Smith SC, Jr, Feldman TE, Hirshfeld JW, Jr, *et al*. ACC/AHA/SCAI 2005 guideline update for percutaneous coronary intervention: a report of the American College of Cardiology/American Heart Association Task Force on Practice Guidelines (ACC/AHA/SCAI Writing Committee to Update 2001 Guidelines for Percutaneous Coronary Intervention). *Circulation* 2006; **113**: e166–286.

54 Silber S, Albertsson P, Aviles FF, *et al*. Guidelines for percutaneous coronary interventions. The Task Force for Percutaneous Coronary Interventions of the European Society of Cardiology. *Eur Heart J* 2005; **26**: 804–847.

Chapter 12

Antiplatelet therapy in chronic coronary artery disease

Kamran I. Muhammad and Deepak L. Bhatt

Chronic coronary artery disease (CAD) is an increasingly common condition, affecting an estimated 15.8 million Americans [1]. This condition confers an increased risk of myocardial infarction (MI) and death, resulting in considerable economic and social costs. Among several medical therapies that have been shown to mitigate the risks associated with chronic CAD, antiplatelet therapy plays a major role.

This chapter will focus on aspirin, clopidogrel and dual antiplatelet therapy in the medical management of chronic CAD and following percutaneous coronary intervention (PCI), and the potential use of antiplatelet agents in development.

Aspirin

A considerable body of evidence points to the role of aspirin in reducing vascular events and mortality in the setting of chronic CAD. Given its central role in chronic CAD, other antiplatelet agents are frequently compared to aspirin in trials to determine their effectiveness.

Aspirin after previous myocardial infarction

Early studies of aspirin therapy for secondary prevention after acute MI demonstrated a trend towards decreased mortality [2–5]. In 1994, the Antiplatelet Trialists' Collaboration group published a landmark meta-analysis of 145 trials, including a heterogeneous population of approximately 100,000 patients, which demonstrated a 25% relative risk reduction of vascular events

Antiplatelet Therapy in Ischemic Heart Disease, 1st edition. Edited by Stephen D. Wiviott.
© 2009 American Heart Association, ISBN: 9-781-4051-7626-2

(MI or stroke) and vascular death in patients treated with antiplatelet agents versus placebo (9.5% vs. 11.9%, p < 0.00001). Of these patients, 19,791 had a history of prior MI and within this group there was a similar 25% reduction of vascular events and vascular death (13.5% vs. 17.1%, p < 0.00001) [6]. While a variety of antiplatelet agents were employed in the various studies included in this meta-analysis, the most common agent used was aspirin.

In 2002, the newly renamed Antithrombotic Trialists' Collaboration (ATC) group published an updated meta-analysis including trials up to September 1997. A total of 287 studies were included with over 200,000 patients. The included trials focused on comparison of an antiplatelet regimen versus placebo or comparison of one antiplatelet regimen versus another in a heterogeneous population of patients deemed high risk for arterial vascular events. Focusing on the 12 trials that included 18,788 patients with previous MI, there was a 25% relative risk reduction of MI, stroke or vascular death (13.5% vs. 17.0%, p < 0.0001) with antiplatelet therapy for a mean duration of 27 months. Of these patients, 87% were participants in trials using aspirin. This overall reduction was driven by very significant reductions in non-fatal reinfarction (4.7% vs. 6.5%, p < 0.001) and vascular death (8.0% vs. 9.4%, p = 0.0006) as well as a smaller, but nevertheless significant, reduction in non-fatal stroke (0.9% vs. 1.4%, p = 0.002) (Figure 12.1) [7].

Given this extensive body of literature, it is clear that aspirin therapy in patients who have suffered prior MI is highly beneficial for preventing further vascular events and vascular death.

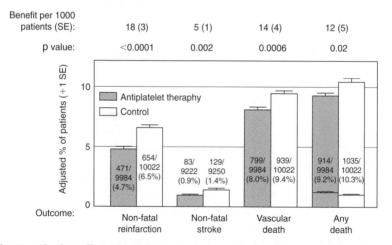

Fig. 12.1 Absolute effects of antiplatelet therapy on patients with previous MI (12 trials). Mean treatment duration was 2 years. SE = standard error. Reproduced with permission from: Antithrombotic Trialists' Collaboration. Collaborative meta-analysis of randomised trials of antiplatelet therapy for prevention of death, myocardial infarction, and stroke in high risk patients. *BMJ* 2002; **324** (7329): 71–86 [7].

Aspirin in chronic coronary artery disease without previous MI

Patients with chronic CAD, but without prior history of MI, have also been studied extensively. In the ATC meta-analysis, 2920 patients with stable angina were noted to have a 33% odds reduction in vascular events with anti-thrombotic treatment versus control (9.9% vs. 14.1%, p < 0.0001) [7]. Of these patients, 2739 (94%) were participants in trials using aspirin. The major trial that contributed to this group was the Swedish angina pectoris aspirin trial (SAPAT). SAPAT was a prospective, randomized, double-blinded study in which 2035 patients with stable angina were randomized to 75 mg of aspirin or placebo; patients with prior MI were excluded. In addition, all patients received sotalol. An impressive 34% reduction in the primary end-point of sudden death or MI was seen (8% vs. 12%, p = 0.003) [8].

Dosing considerations

The ATC meta-analysis also provides us with useful information regarding various dosing regimens of aspirin. Comparison of aspirin doses of ≥75 mg/day with <75 mg/day demonstrated no difference in the relative risk of vascular events. However, there are fewer data available for aspirin doses of <75 mg/day. In addition, comparison of high-dose aspirin, 500–1500 mg/day with doses of 75–325 mg/day also revealed no difference. When varying doses of aspirin, ranging from 500–1500 mg/day to <75 mg/day were compared to control, an expected significant reduction in the relative risk of vascular events was noted. However, there was no statistically increased benefit derived from higher daily aspirin doses as compared to lower daily doses [7].

For aspirin doses less than 325 mg/day there was no significant difference in the risk of major extracranial bleeding compared to placebo. In two trials comparing 75–325 mg/day with <75 mg/day, again no significant difference was noted in major extracranial bleeding [7]. However, a more recent analysis suggests that increasing doses of aspirin, particularly >100 mg/day, result in a higher risk of total bleeding complications with doses >200 mg/day resulting in a higher risk of major bleeding complications, especially gastrointestinal bleeding [9]. A recent, systematic review reaffirms that doses of aspirin greater than 75–81 mg/day do not afford added cardioprotection and are associated with a higher risk of gastrointestinal hemorrhage [10].

Therefore we conclude that lower doses of aspirin are probably as effective as higher doses for reducing the risk of vascular events with fewer bleeding complications. The optimal daily dose appears to be between 75 and 81 mg.

Interaction with non-steroidal anti-inflammatory medications

The ability of ibuprofen to antagonize the antiplatelet effect of aspirin has been demonstrated in patients taking these medications concurrently [11]. Studies to assess the clinical relevance of this observation have been conducted, yielding mixed results.

In a retrospective analysis of 7107 patients with known chronic CAD, the use of both aspirin and ibuprofen was associated with a greater hazard ratio of cardiovascular and all-cause mortality as compared to those taking aspirin alone (1.93, p = 0.001 and 1.73, p = 0.0305 respectively) [12]. This same study did not demonstrate an increased risk in patients using aspirin together with other non-steroidal anti-inflammatory medications (NSAIDs). It should be noted that this study had several limitations including small size, and lack of adjustment for tobacco use, body-mass index or severity of cardiovascular disease.

Other analyses have not demonstrated any significant diminution in the cardioprotective effect of aspirin in patients also taking NSAIDs, including ibuprofen [13]. Further study is needed to determine what interactions may occur between NSAIDs and aspirin [14,15].

Aspirin resistance

Given the central role of aspirin in the management of chronic CAD, aspirin resistance is a topic that has drawn considerable attention but remains to be fully characterized. Aspirin resistance results from a complex interplay of clinical, cellular and genetic factors [16]. Presently, aspirin resistance is a general term used to describe both clinical and laboratory-based observations in relation to aspirin therapy and is discussed in detail in Chapter 4.

ADP receptor antagonists

The agents in this class of antiplatelet medications exert their effect by inhibiting the binding of ADP to the G protein-coupled $P2Y_{12}$ receptor on the platelet, thereby reducing platelet aggregation and activation. Ticlopidine, and its successor clopidogrel, are the two major agents in this class that have been extensively studied. Novel agents, including prasugrel and AZD6140, are currently in Phase III clinical trials.

Ticlopidine

There are no significant data regarding the use of ticlopidine in the setting of chronic CAD. Ticlopidine has primarily been evaluated in the setting of unstable angina, acute MI and PCI, as well as other vascular disease states (peripheral arterial disease, cerebrovascular disease). Use of ticlopidine is limited by its adverse effects including neutropenia and thrombocytopenia.

Clopidogrel

The Clopidogrel versus Aspirin in Patients at Risk of Ischemic Events (CAPRIE) study was the first large randomized study to evaluate the effectiveness and safety of clopidogrel as an antiplatelet agent for secondary prevention of atherothrombotic disease [17].

CAPRIE enrolled 19,185 patients with recent MI (within 35 days), ischemic stroke or established peripheral arterial disease (PAD) and randomized them to aspirin 325 mg/day versus clopidogrel 75 mg/day with a mean follow-up duration of 1.91 years. Overall, there was a significant 8.7% relative risk reduction in the primary composite end-point of ischemic stroke, MI or vascular death in the clopidogrel treated group – a notable finding given that the control group was treated with aspirin which, as discussed, has been shown to have significant benefits on vascular outcomes compared to placebo (Figure 12.2). A further analysis of CAPRIE also demonstrated a statistically significant reduction in the rate of hospitalization for ischemic events or bleeding with clopidogrel as compared to aspirin [18].

However, focusing more specifically on the 6302 patients enrolled in CAPRIE based on recent MI, there was statistically non-significant trend towards benefit of aspirin over clopidogrel. This was in contrast to the groups with recent ischemic stroke or established PAD, in which clopidogrel appeared to reduce events compared to aspirin. The authors note that the study was designed to detect a treatment effect in the study population as a whole and not within each of the subgroups.

In an effort to understand this apparent discrepancy, a further analysis was performed combining patients with a history of remote MI from the ischemic

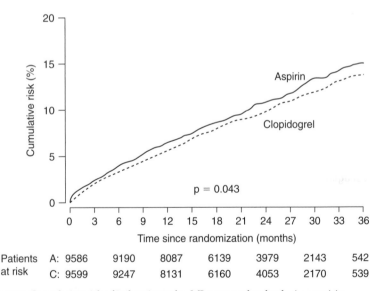

Patients	A: 9586	9190	8087	6139	3979	2143	542
at risk	C: 9599	9247	8131	6160	4053	2170	539

Fig. 12.2 Cumulative risk of ischemic stroke, MI, or vascular death. A = aspirin; C = clopidogrel. Reproduced with permission from: CAPRIE Steering Committee. A randomised, blinded, trial of clopidogrel versus aspirin in patients at risk of ischaemic events (CAPRIE). *Lancet* 1996; **348** (9038): 1329–1339 [17].

stroke and PAD subgroups (2144 patients) with those enrolled on the basis of recent MI, yielding a comprehensive cohort of patients with prior MI. Within this group, there was a 7.4% relative risk reduction (CI −5.2 to 18.6) associated with clopidogrel therapy versus aspirin. As this analysis was not prespecified in the protocol and its associated risk reduction had a large confidence interval spanning unity, it should be interpreted with caution. It must be stressed again that these data all compare clopidogrel to aspirin. It follows that, although not conclusively superior to aspirin in patients with prior MI, clopidogrel is certainly an effective antiplatelet agent for preventing vascular events when compared to placebo in this population.

Based on this, it appears that clopidogrel is an effective antiplatelet agent in chronic coronary disease for preventing vascular events. Clinically, aspirin remains the antiplatelet agent of choice given the considerations above, its cost and the overwhelming data behind its effectiveness. Situations where clopidogrel monotherapy for chronic CAD should be considered include aspirin intolerance/ allergy or high-risk secondary prevention for patients such as those enrolled in CAPRIE. In particular, subgroup analyses from CAPRIE suggest even greater benefit of clopidogrel over aspirin in patients with multiple, prior ischemic events [19]. These considerations also raise the question of whether dual antiplatelet therapy with aspirin plus clopidogrel may serve as an even more effective strategy for secondary prevention in chronic CAD. Recent studies have begun to shed light on this question and will be discussed in detail separately.

Clopidogrel resistance

As with aspirin resistance, clopidogrel resistance is an evolving area of study. Again, in the broad sense, the term has been used to refer to a spectrum of observations including clinical failure as well as variations in response to clopidogrel across individuals. Based on studies done primarily in the setting of PCI for acute MI, there is evidence that clopidogrel resistance leads to adverse cardiovascular outcomes [20,21], and is discussed in detail in Chapter 6.

Novel agents

Two oral ADP receptor antagonists, prasugrel and AZD6140, are currently in development. Prasugrel is a thienopyridine which, like ticlopidine and clopidogrel, requires conversion to an active metabolite that irreversibly binds to the $P2Y_{12}$ receptor. Studies have demonstrated that it is more potent than clopidogrel with a comparable safety profile [22,23]. AZD6140, a reversible inhibitor of the $P2Y_{12}$ receptor, has distinct pharmacologic properties allowing for more rapid, complete and sustained platelet inhibition as compared to clopidogrel [24]. These agents have yet to be fully studied in the setting of chronic CAD but it is anticipated that they will further expand the armamentarium of antiplatelet agents to treat this increasingly common disorder.

Dual antiplatelet therapy: clopidogrel plus aspirin

It has been established that dual antiplatelet therapy with clopidogrel plus aspirin is superior to therapy with aspirin alone in various cardiovascular settings including unstable angina, MI with and without ST-segment elevation, and in patients undergoing PCI [25–28]. The role of dual antiplatelet therapy in chronic CAD has recently become more fully defined.

The Clopidogrel for High Atherothrombotic Risk and Ischemic Stabilization, Management and Avoidance (CHARISMA) trial was a prospective, randomized study of 15,603 patients, with either established cardiovascular disease or those with multiple risk factors, assigned to receive either clopidogrel (75 mg/day) plus low-dose aspirin versus placebo plus low-dose aspirin with a median follow-up of 28 months [29]. There was a statistically non-significant 7.1% relative risk reduction in the primary end-point of MI, stroke or cardiovascular death and a statistically significant 7.7% relative risk reduction in the secondary end-point which included hospitalization for unstable angina, TIA or revascularization (Figure 12.3). There was a statistically significant increase in the risk of moderate bleeding (HR 1.62, $p < 0.001$) although no significant difference in fatal bleeding or intracranial hemorrhage was noted.

A prespecified analysis of the 12,153 patients with cardiovascular disease (documented CAD, cerebrovascular disease or symptomatic PAD) suggested a benefit in relation to the primary end-point with dual antiplatelet therapy. In contrast, the remaining 3284 patients enrolled on the basis of multiple risk factors, but without documented cardiovascular disease, derived no benefit from dual antiplatelet therapy.

Thus, CHARISMA provided the first evidence that dual antiplatelet therapy may be superior to aspirin therapy alone in patients with chronic CAD. This observation was further studied in an analysis of the CHARISMA trial which focused on the subset of 9478 patients with a history of prior MI (3846 patients), documented prior ischemic stroke (3245 patients) or symptomatic PAD (2838 patients), with 443 patients falling into multiple categories [30]. In this "CAPRIE-like" cohort from CHARISMA, there was a statistically significant 17% relative risk reduction in the primary end-point of cardiovascular death, MI or stroke (Figure 12.4) as well a 13% relative risk reduction in the secondary end-point, which included hospitalization for ischemic events in the patients treated with dual antiplatelet therapy. A comparable benefit was seen across subgroups, although the benefit in those with symptomatic PAD did not reach statistical significance. Again noted was a statistically significant increase in the risk of moderate bleeding. There was no increase in the risk of severe bleeding noted.

Patients originally enrolled in CHARISMA with chronic CAD but without a history of MI (including those with multivessel CAD, prior PCI and prior CABG) were excluded from this analysis. Comparison of this group to those

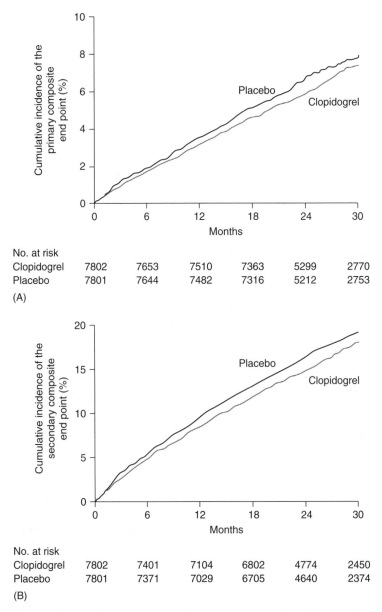

No. at risk
Clopidogrel	7802	7653	7510	7363	5299	2770
Placebo	7801	7644	7482	7316	5212	2753

(A)

No. at risk
Clopidogrel	7802	7401	7104	6802	4774	2450
Placebo	7801	7371	7029	6705	4640	2374

(B)

Fig. 12.3 (A) Cumulative incidence curves for the primary end point of MI, stroke or death from cardiovascular causes. (B) Cumulative incidence curves for the secondary endpoint, which included hospitalizations. Reproduced with permission from: Bhatt DL, Fox KA, Hacke W, Berger PB, Black HR, Boden WE, *et al*. Clopidogrel and aspirin versus aspirin alone for the prevention of atherothrombotic events. *New Engl J Med* 2006; **354** (16): 1706–1717 [29].

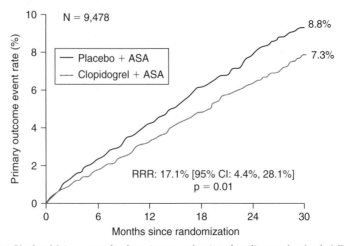

Fig. 12.4 Kaplan-Meier curves for the primary end point of cardiovascular death, MI, or stroke. ASA = aspirin; CI = confidence interval; RRR = relative risk reduction. Reproduced with permission from: Bhatt DL, Flather MD, Hacke W, Berger PB, Black HR, Boden WE, *et al.* Patients with prior myocardial infarction, stroke, or symptomatic peripheral arterial disease in the CHARISMA trial. *J Am Coll Cardiol* 2007; **49** (19): 1982–1988 [30].

with chronic CAD with history of prior MI, demonstrated that the latter benefited from dual antiplatelet therapy whereas the former did not (Figure 12.5). Thus, within the population of patients with chronic CAD, there appears to be a gradient of benefit with dual antiplatelet therapy favoring those with higher risk features, namely a history of prior, unstable plaque rupture with thrombosis.

In addition, although not reaching statistical significance, there was a suggestion that the benefit of dual antiplatelet therapy was greatest if given close to the incident ischemic event with reduction of benefit as time progressed (Figure 12.6A). In similar fashion there was a suggestion that the bleeding risk associated with dual antiplatelet over aspirin therapy alone appears to be greatest at the initiation of therapy with the excess risk becoming negligible in patients tolerating and continuing therapy after several months (Figure 12.6B).

As with other clinical settings in cardiovascular disease, there appears to be a benefit to be derived from intensification of antiplatelet therapy for patients with chronic CAD that have high risk characteristics, namely those with history of prior MI. CHARISMA, and the subsequent analysis of a "CAPRIE-like" cohort from CHARISMA, suggest that dual antiplatelet therapy with clopidogrel plus aspirin represents one effective strategy for intensification. Future studies will be needed to confirm, further refine and expand on this concept.

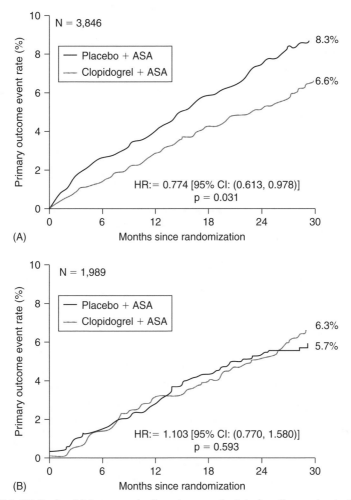

Fig. 12.5 (A) Kaplan–Meier curves for the primary endpoint of cardiovascular death, MI or stroke in patients enrolled with prior MI. (B) Kaplan–Meier curves for the primary end point in patients enrolled with CAD without prior MI. HR = hazard ratio. Other abbreviations as in Figure 12.4. Reproduced with permission from: Bhatt DL, Flather MD, Hacke W, Berger PB, Black HR, Boden WE, *et al.* Patients with prior myocardial infarction, stroke, or symptomatic peripheral arterial disease in the CHARISMA trial. *J Am Coll Cardiol* 2007; **49** (19): 1982–1988 [30].

Oral glycoprotein IIb/IIIa inhibitors

While there are numerous stimuli that serve to activate the platelet via binding to surface receptors and modification of intracellular signaling, a key common outcome of these interactions is activation of the platelet glycoprotein IIb/IIIa

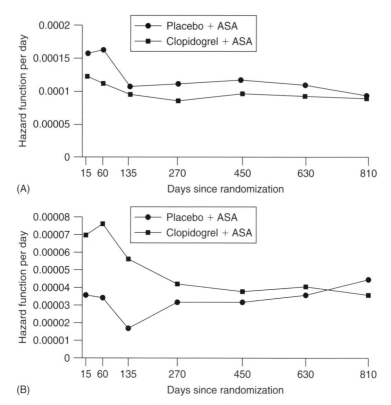

Fig. 12.6 (A) Instantaneous hazard for cardiovascular death, MI or stroke.
(B) Instantaneous hazard for severe or moderate bleeding. Abbreviations as in Figure
12.4. Reproduced with permission from: Bhatt DL, Flather MD, Hacke W, Berger
PB, Black HR, Boden WE, *et al*. Patients with prior myocardial infarction, stroke, or
symptomatic peripheral arterial disease in the CHARISMA trial. *J Am Coll Cardiol* 2007;
49 (19): 1982–1988 [30].

receptor (GP IIb/IIIa) with subsequent binding to fibrinogen, resulting in platelet aggregation and thrombus formation. The effectiveness of intravenous GP
IIb/IIIa inhibitors in the setting of the acute coronary syndromes (ACS) and
PCI has been well established [31]. Unfortunately the success seen with the
intravenous GP IIb/IIIa inhibitors has not been extended to their orally-
administered counterparts that, as a class, would have been well-suited for use
in chronic CAD.

Four large trials demonstrated excess mortality in patients receiving
oral GP IIb/IIIa inhibitors, primarily in the setting of ACS or elective PCI
[32–35]. A fifth trial, the most relevant to chronic CAD, randomized patients
with prior MI, angina, stroke or transient ischemic attack or PAD plus CAD

or cerebrovascular disease to receive the oral GP IIb/IIIa inhibitor lotrafiban versus placebo. Again noted was an increased risk of death in the lotrafiban group, driven primarily by excess vascular deaths, resulting in premature termination of this study [36]. Meta-analyses of oral GP IIb/IIIa trials confirm a highly significant 31% increase in mortality and suggest the risk is present whether these agents are substituted for, or added to, aspirin [37,38]. Furthermore, an increased risk of major bleeding was noted in each trial as well as in the pooled analyses but was not sufficient to account for the excess mortality.

Various mechanisms have been put forth to explain the increased mortality seen with oral GP IIb/IIIa inhibitors, including partial agonist activity of these agents resulting in platelet activation, genetic polymorphisms of the GP IIb/IIIa receptor influencing drug response, variability in plasma drug levels with oral dosing, and induction of cardiomyocyte apoptosis [39]. However, given the overwhelming evidence of harm with these agents, there is currently little interest in pursuing their development further.

Other antiplatelet agents

Dipyridamole

Dipyridamole achieves its antiplatelet effect by a variety of mechanisms, the most important of which may be enhancement of the NO/cyclic GMP signaling pathway via inhibition of the cyclic GMP phosphodiesterase type V enzyme [40]. While the majority of studies with this agent have been in the area of cerebrovascular disease, there is older literature evaluating its use in chronic CAD.

The Persantine-Asprin Reinfarction Study (PARIS) randomized over 2000 patients with history of MI to dipyridamole plus aspirin, aspirin alone or placebo and demonstrated no additive benefit with dipyridamole plus aspirin versus aspirin alone for reduction of death or MI [5]. The subsequent Persantine-Aspirin Reinfarction Study Part II (PARIS II) confirmed the superiority of dipyridamole plus aspirin over placebo for preventing the composite end-point of MI or cardiac death in patients with chronic CAD with history of prior MI [41].

Therefore, while combined dipyridamole and aspirin therapy is effective in reducing cardiac death and MI in patients with chronic CAD, there is no evidence that this approach is superior to aspirin therapy alone in this population. Further, there is no evidence available that suggests that dipyridamole can be substituted for aspirin in chronic CAD.

Cilostazol

Cilostazol exerts its antiplatelet effect by inhibition of the cyclic nucleotide phosphodiesterase type 3 enzyme [42]. While its ability to inhibit platelets *in vivo* is unclear, it has been shown to cause arterial vasodilatation and inhibit intimal hyperplasia and vascular smooth muscle proliferation. Studies have suggested that it may be more effective in preventing restenosis after PCI when compared to aspirin, clopidogrel or ticlopidine and, when added to clopidogrel and aspirin, may confer an even greater reduction in restenosis rates [43–47]. Its role in chronic CAD has not been studied and remains to be defined.

Antiplatelet therapy after percutaneous coronary intervention in chronic coronary artery disease

By virtue of their condition, patients with chronic CAD often require PCI with intracoronary stent placement. The appropriate use of antiplatelet therapy after coronary stenting is extensively covered in Chapter 17.

Among the studies addressing the use of antiplatelet therapy after PCI, the randomized, prospective CREDO trial is the most applicable to the setting of chronic CAD as it enrolled over 2000 patients referred for elective PCI and assigned them to receive 1 year of clopidogrel (75 mg/day) plus aspirin versus placebo plus aspirin. The patients in the clopidogrel arm also received a loading dose of clopidogrel (300 mg) prior to PCI and all patients received clopidogrel for 28 days after PCI. All patients received aspirin from the time of PCI through 1 year. Of the patients enrolled, 34% had a history of prior MI and 45% were undergoing PCI for stable angina or prior MI. At 1 year, there was a significant 27% risk reduction in the composite risk of death, MI or stroke in the patients who received long-term clopidogrel therapy [26].

Recent observational studies and meta-analyses have suggested that drug-eluting stents are associated with a higher incidence of late stent thrombosis as compared with bare metal stents, possibly translating into a small increased risk of late thrombotic events [48–52]. A variety of mechanisms for this phenomenon have been examined including hypersensitivity reactions, delayed endothelialization and possible long-term endothelial dysfunction due to drug-eluting stents [53–58]. Potential risk factors for late stent thrombosis include stenting at bifurcation lesions or across branch points, increasing length of the stented segment, left ventricular dysfunction and renal failure. Based on this, some have advocated longer dual antiplatelet therapy for those receiving drug-eluting stents: 12–24 months for typical patients and indefinitely for those at high risk [59].

Conclusion

As with other chronic diseases, there is no cure for chronic CAD. Therefore, effective therapies are needed to control disease progression and reduce disease-related complications. Antiplatelet therapy is among the most powerful and important therapies available for reducing complications related to chronic CAD, including recurrent ischemia, MI and cardiovascular death.

Aspirin is the best-studied and most effective of the antiplatelet agents for chronic CAD. Use of aspirin reduces the relative risk of vascular events, including MI, and cardiovascular death, by 25–30% in this population. Clopidogrel, an ADP receptor antagonist, is also an effective antiplatelet agent for the treatment of chronic CAD. Due to its cost, its use as monotherapy in this population is typically limited to those patients who are not candidates for aspirin therapy due to drug allergy or intolerance, although in high-risk secondary prevention it has modest superiority over aspirin.

Within chronic CAD, there is a spectrum of disease severity ranging from patients without prior MI to those with recurrent ischemia and MI. Recent data suggest that intensification of antiplatelet therapy, with the addition of clopidogrel to aspirin, in patients with high-severity chronic CAD provides added benefit as compared with aspirin therapy alone. It is expected that there will be ongoing research in this exciting area, with the goal of better defining the patients who will benefit from intensified therapies as well as determining the safest and most effective regimens of intensified antiplatelet therapies.

Two novel antiplatelet agents from the ADP receptor antagonist class, prasugrel and AZD6140, are currently under development. These agents have distinct pharmacologic properties that offer potential advantages over clopidogrel. Their role in the treatment of chronic CAD remains to be defined but if approved, may add to antiplatelet therapies available to treat this increasingly common disorder.

References

1 Rosamond W, Flegal K, Friday G, Furie K, Go A, Greenlund K, *et al*. Heart disease and stroke statistics – 2007 update: a report from the American Heart Association Statistics Committee and Stroke Statistics Subcommittee. *Circulation* 2007; **115**: e69–171.

2 Elwood PC, Cochrane AL, Burr ML, Sweetnam PM, Williams G, Welsby E, *et al*. A randomized controlled trial of acetyl salicylic acid in the secondary prevention of mortality from myocardial infarction. *BMJ* 1974; **1**: 436–440.

3 Coronary Drug Project Research Group. Aspirin in coronary heart disease. *J Chronic Dis* 1976; **2910**: 625–642.

4 Elwood PC, Sweetnam PM. Aspirin and secondary mortality after myocardial infarction. *Lancet* 1979; **2**: 1313–1315.

5 Persantine-Aspirin Reinfarction Study Research Group. Persantine and aspirin in coronary heart disease. *Circulation* 1980; **62**: 449–461.

6 Antiplatelet Trialists' Collaboration. Collaborative overview of randomised trials of antiplatelet therapy – I: Prevention of death, myocardial infarction, and stroke by prolonged antiplatelet therapy in various categories of patients. *BMJ* 1994; **308**: 81–106.

7 Antithrombotic Trialists' Collaboration. Collaborative meta-analysis of randomised trials of antiplatelet therapy for prevention of death, myocardial infarction, and stroke in high risk patients. *BMJ* 2002; **324**: 71–86.

8 Juul-Moller S, Edvardsson N, Jahnmatz B, Rosen A, Sorensen S, Omblus R. Double-blind trial of aspirin in primary prevention of myocardial infarction in patients with stable chronic angina pectoris. The Swedish Angina Pectoris Aspirin Trial (SAPAT) Group. *Lancet* 1992; **340**: 1421–1425.

9 Serebruany VL, Steinhubl SR, Berger PB, Malinin AI, Baggish JS, Bhatt DL, *et al*. Analysis of risk of bleeding complications after different doses of aspirin in 192,036 patients enrolled in 31 randomized controlled trials. *Am J Cardiol* 2005; **95**: 1218–1222.

10 Campbell CL, Smyth S, Montalescot G, Steinhubl SR. Aspirin dose for the prevention of cardiovascular disease: a systematic review. *JAMA* 2007; **297**: 2018–2024.

11 Catella-Lawson F, Reilly MP, Kapoor SC, Cucchiara AJ, DeMarco S, Tournier B, *et al*. Cyclooxygenase inhibitors and the antiplatelet effects of aspirin. *New Engl J Med* 2001; **345**: 1809–1817.

12 MacDonald TM, Wei L. Effect of ibuprofen on cardioprotective effect of aspirin. *Lancet* 2003; **361**: 573–574.

13 Garcia Rodriguez LA, Varas-Lorenzo C, Maguire A, Gonzalez-Perez A. Nonsteroidal antiinflammatory drugs and the risk of myocardial infarction in the general population. *Circulation* 2004; **109**: 3000–3006.

14 Helin-Salmivaara A, Virtanen A, Vesalainen R, Gronroos JM, Klaukka T, Idanpaan-Heikkila JE, *et al*. NSAID use and the risk of hospitalization for first myocardial infarction in the general population: a nationwide case-control study from Finland. *Eur Heart J* 2006; **27**: 1657–1663.

15 Bhatt DL. NSAIDS and the risk of myocardial infarction: do they help or harm? *Eur Heart J* 2006; **27**: 1635–1636.

16 Bhatt DL. Aspirin resistance: more than just a laboratory curiosity. *J Am Coll Cardiol* 2004; **43**: 1127–1129.

17 CAPRIE Steering Committee. A randomised, blinded, trial of clopidogrel versus aspirin in patients at risk of ischaemic events (CAPRIE). *Lancet* 1996; **348**: 1329–1339.

18 Bhatt DL, Hirsch AT, Ringleb PA, Hacke W, Topol EJ. Reduction in the need for hospitalization for recurrent ischemic events and bleeding with clopidogrel instead of aspirin. CAPRIE investigators. *Am Heart J* 2000; **140**: 67–73.

19 Ringleb PA, Bhatt DL, Hirsch AT, Topol EJ, Hacke W. Benefit of clopidogrel over aspirin is amplified in patients with a history of ischemic events. *Stroke* 2004; **35**: 528–532.

20 Matetzky S, Shenkman B, Guetta V, Shechter M, Bienart R, Goldenberg I, *et al*. Clopidogrel resistance is associated with increased risk of recurrent atherothrombotic events in patients with acute myocardial infarction. *Circulation* 2004; **109**: 3171–3175.

21 Gurbel PA, Bliden KP, Samara W, Yoho JA, Hayes K, Fissha MZ, *et al*. Clopidogrel effect on platelet reactivity in patients with stent thrombosis: results of the CREST Study. *J Am Coll Cardiol* 2005; **46**: 1827–1832.

22 Niitsu Y, Jakubowski JA, Sugidachi A, Asai F. Pharmacology of CS-747 (prasugrel, LY640315), a novel, potent antiplatelet agent with in vivo P2Y12 receptor antagonist activity. *Semin Thromb Hemost* 2005; **31**: 184–194.

23 Wiviott SD, Antman EM, Winters KJ, Weerakkody G, Murphy SA, Behounek BD, *et al*. Randomized comparison of prasugrel (CS-747, LY640315), a novel thienopyridine P2Y12 antagonist, with clopidogrel in percutaneous coronary intervention: results of

the Joint Utilization of Medications to Block Platelets Optimally (JUMBO)-TIMI 26 trial. *Circulation* 2005; **111**: 3366–3373.

24 Husted S, Emanuelsson H, Heptinstall S, Sandset PM, Wickens M, Peters G. Pharmacodynamics, pharmacokinetics, and safety of the oral reversible P2Y12 antagonist AZD6140 with aspirin in patients with atherosclerosis: a double-blind comparison to clopidogrel with aspirin. *Eur Heart J* 2006; **27**: 1038–1047.

25 Yusuf S, Zhao F, Mehta SR, Chrolavicius S, Tognoni G, Fox KK. Effects of clopidogrel in addition to aspirin in patients with acute coronary syndromes without ST-segment elevation. *New Engl J Med* 2001; **345**: 494–502.

26 Steinhubl SR, Berger PB, Mann JT, 3rd, Fry ET, DeLago A, Wilmer C, *et al.* Early and sustained dual oral antiplatelet therapy following percutaneous coronary intervention: a randomized controlled trial. *JAMA* 2002; **288**: 2411–2420.

27 Chen ZM, Jiang LX, Chen YP, Xie JX, Pan HC, Peto R, *et al.* Addition of clopidogrel to aspirin in 45,852 patients with acute myocardial infarction: randomised placebo-controlled trial. *Lancet* 2005; **366**: 1607–1621.

28 Sabatine MS, Cannon CP, Gibson CM, Lopez-Sendon JL, Montalescot G, Theroux P, *et al.* Addition of clopidogrel to aspirin and fibrinolytic therapy for myocardial infarction with ST-segment elevation. *New Engl J Med* 2005; **352**: 1179–1189.

29 Bhatt DL, Fox KA, Hacke W, Berger PB, Black HR, Boden WE, *et al.* Clopidogrel and aspirin versus aspirin alone for the prevention of atherothrombotic events. *New Engl J Med* 2006; **354**: 1706–1717.

30 Bhatt DL, Flather MD, Hacke W, Berger PB, Black HR, Boden WE, *et al.* Patients with prior myocardial infarction, stroke, or symptomatic peripheral arterial disease in the CHARISMA trial. *J Am Coll Cardiol* 2007; **49**: 1982–1988.

31 Kong DF, Califf RM, Miller DP, Moliterno DJ, White HD, Harrington RA, *et al.* Clinical outcomes of therapeutic agents that block the platelet glycoprotein IIb/IIIa integrin in ischemic heart disease. *Circulation* 1998; **98**: 2829–2835.

32 SYMPHONY Investigators. Comparison of sibrafiban with aspirin for prevention of cardiovascular events after acute coronary syndromes: a randomised trial. Sibrafiban versus aspirin to yield maximum protection from ischemic heart events post-acute coronary syndromes. *Lancet* 2000; **355**: 337–345.

33 Cannon CP, McCabe CH, Wilcox RG, Langer A, Caspi A, Berink P, *et al.* Oral glycoprotein IIb/IIIa inhibition with orbofiban in patients with unstable coronary syndromes (OPUS-TIMI 16) trial. *Circulation* 2000; **102**: 149–156.

34 O'Neill WW, Serruys P, Knudtson M, van Es GA, Timmis GC, van der Zwaan C, *et al.* Long-term treatment with a platelet glycoprotein-receptor antagonist after percutaneous coronary revascularization. EXCITE Trial Investigators. Evaluation of oral xemilofiban in controlling thrombotic events. *New Engl J Med* 2000; **342**: 1316–1324.

35 Second SYMPHONY Investigators. Randomized trial of aspirin, sibrafiban, or both for secondary prevention after acute coronary syndromes. *Circulation* 2001; **103**: 1727–1733.

36 Topol EJ, Easton D, Harrington RA, Amarenco P, Califf RM, Graffagnino C, *et al.* Randomized, double-blind, placebo-controlled, international trial of the oral IIb/IIIa antagonist lotrafiban in coronary and cerebrovascular disease. *Circulation* 2003; **108**: 399–406.

37 Chew DP, Bhatt DL, Sapp S, Topol EJ. Increased mortality with oral platelet glycoprotein IIb/IIIa antagonists: a meta-analysis of phase III multicenter randomized trials. *Circulation* 2001; **103**: 201–206.

38 Newby LK, Califf RM, White HD, Harrington RA, Van de Werf F, Granger CB, et al. The failure of orally administered glycoprotein IIb/IIIa inhibitors to prevent recurrent cardiac events. Am J Med 2002; 112: 647–658.

39 Chew DP, Bhatt DL, Topol EJ. Oral glycoprotein IIb/IIIa inhibitors: why don't they work? Am J Cardiovasc Drugs 2001; 1: 421–428.

40 Aktas B, Utz A, Hoenig-Liedl P, Walter U, Geiger J. Dipyridamole enhances NO/cGMP-mediated vasodilator-stimulated phosphoprotein phosphorylation and signaling in human platelets: in vitro and in vivo/ex vivo studies. Stroke 2003; 34: 764–769.

41 Klimt CR, Knatterud GL, Stamler J, Meier P. Persantine-Aspirin Reinfarction Study. Part II. Secondary coronary prevention with persantine and aspirin. J Am Coll Cardiol 1986; 7: 251–269.

42 Schror K. The pharmacology of cilostazol. Diabetes Obes Metab 2002; 4 (Suppl. 2): S14–19.

43 Kunishima T, Musha H, Eto F, Iwasaki T, Nagashima J, Masui Y, et al. A randomized trial of aspirin versus cilostazol therapy after successful coronary stent implantation. Clin Ther 1997; 19: 1058–1066.

44 Tsuchikane E, Fukuhara A, Kobayashi T, Kirino M, Yamasaki K, Kobayashi T, et al. Impact of cilostazol on restenosis after percutaneous coronary balloon angioplasty. Circulation 1999; 100: 21–26.

45 Kamishirado H, Inoue T, Mizoguchi K, Uchida T, Nakata T, Sakuma M, et al. Randomized comparison of cilostazol versus ticlopidine hydrochloride for antiplatelet therapy after coronary stent implantation for prevention of late restenosis. Am Heart J 2002; 144: 303–308.

46 Lee SW, Park SW, Hong MK, Lee CW, Kim YH, Park JH, et al. Comparison of cilostazol and clopidogrel after successful coronary stenting. Am J Cardiol 2005; 95: 859–862.

47 Douglas JS, Jr, Holmes DR, Jr, Kereiakes DJ, Grines CL, Block E, Ghazzal ZM, et al. Coronary stent restenosis in patients treated with cilostazol. Circulation 2005; 112: 2826–2832.

48 Moreno R, Fernandez C, Hernandez R, Alfonso F, Angiolillo DJ, Sabate M, et al. Drug-eluting stent thrombosis: results from a pooled analysis including 10 randomized studies. J Am Coll Cardiol 2005; 45: 954–959.

49 Bavry AA, Kumbhani DJ, Helton TJ, Borek PP, Mood GR, Bhatt DL. Late thrombosis of drug-eluting stents: a meta-analysis of randomized clinical trials. Am J Med 2006; 119: 1056–1061.

50 Kuchulakanti PK, Chu WW, Torguson R, Ohlmann P, Rha SW, Clavijo LC, et al. Correlates and long-term outcomes of angiographically proven stent thrombosis with sirolimus- and paclitaxel-eluting stents. Circulation 2006; 113: 1108–1113.

51 Rodriguez AE, Mieres J, Fernandez-Pereira C, Vigo CF, Rodriguez-Alemparte M, Berrocal D, et al. Coronary stent thrombosis in the current drug-eluting stent era: insights from the ERACI III trial. J Am Coll Cardiol 2006; 47: 205–207.

52 Ellis SG, Colombo A, Grube E, Popma J, Koglin J, Dawkins KD, et al. Incidence, timing, and correlates of stent thrombosis with the polymeric paclitaxel drug-eluting stent: a TAXUS II, IV, V, and VI meta-analysis of 3,445 patients followed for up to 3 years. J Am Coll Cardiol 2007; 49: 1043–1051.

53 Grewe PH, Deneke T, Machraoui A, Barmeyer J, Muller KM. Acute and chronic tissue response to coronary stent implantation: pathologic findings in human specimen. *J Am Coll Cardiol* 2000; **35**: 157–163.

54 Farb A, Burke AP, Kolodgie FD, Virmani R. Pathological mechanisms of fatal late coronary stent thrombosis in humans. *Circulation* 2003; **108**: 1701–1706.

55 Nebeker JR, Virmani R, Bennett CL, Hoffman JM, Samore MH, Alvarez J, *et al.* Hypersensitivity cases associated with drug-eluting coronary stents: a review of available cases from the Research on Adverse Drug Events and Reports (RADAR) project. *J Am Coll Cardiol* 2006; **47**: 175–181.

56 Joner M, Finn AV, Farb A, Mont EK, Kolodgie FD, Ladich E, *et al.* Pathology of drug-eluting stents in humans: delayed healing and late thrombotic risk. *J Am Coll Cardiol* 2006; **48**: 193–202.

57 Kotani J, Awata M, Nanto S, Uematsu M, Oshima F, Minamiguchi H, *et al.* Incomplete neointimal coverage of sirolimus-eluting stents: angioscopic findings. *J Am Coll Cardiol* 2006; **47**: 2108–2111.

58 Hofma SH, van der Giessen WJ, van Dalen BM, Lemos PA, McFadden EP, Sianos G, *et al.* Indication of long-term endothelial dysfunction after sirolimus-eluting stent implantation. *Eur Heart J* 2006; **27**: 166–170.

59 Rabbat MG, Bavry AA, Bhatt DL, Ellis SG. Understanding and minimizing late thrombosis of drug-eluting stents. *Cleve Clin J Med* 2007; **74**: 129–136.

Chapter 13

Antiplatelet therapy in peripheral arterial disease

Esther S. Kim and Heather L. Gornik

Introduction

Peripheral arterial disease (PAD), or atherosclerosis of the lower extremities, is a common disorder which increases in prevalence with age and other well-established cardiovascular risk factors such as smoking and diabetes [1,2]. The prevalence of PAD is estimated to be as high as 15% of the United States population above the age of 70 years [2]. The presence of PAD is a marker of extensive systemic atherosclerosis [3]. In addition to functional impairment, patients with PAD are at an increased risk of a major cardiovascular event, including stroke and myocardial infarction (MI) [4–6], a two-to-three-fold increased risk of all-cause mortality, and three-to-sixfold increased risk of cardiovascular mortality compared to patients without PAD [6–9]. While the risk of worsening claudication and amputation are often the primary concern of the patient suffering from PAD, the likelihood of a life-threatening cardiovascular event or death is a much more immediate threat. Previous epidemiologic studies reported a 5-year likelihood of stroke, myocardial infarction or death between 20 and 30% among patients with claudication compared to an estimated likelihood of limb loss at 5 years of less than 4% [10]. Recently, in a multinational registry of more than 68,000 patients with atherosclerotic vascular disease, there was a 21% 1-year incidence of cardiovascular death, MI, stroke or hospitalization for other cardiovascular events among patients followed with PAD, compared to a 15% event rate among patients with coronary artery disease alone [11].

Antiplatelet Therapy in Ischemic Heart Disease, 1st edition. Edited by Stephen D. Wiviott.
© 2009 American Heart Association, ISBN: 9-781-4051-7626-2

Given these data, it is not surprising that aggressive cardiovascular risk factor modification is recommended for all patients with PAD to prevent limb-related morbidity and cardiovascular morbidity and mortality [12,13]. Antiplatelet therapy is the cornerstone of these recommended cardiovascular risk-modifying therapies. In this chapter we review the role of specific antiplatelet agents in the management of PAD, focusing on the commonly prescribed agents: aspirin, thienopyridines and phosphodiesterase inhibitors. We emphasize both the cardiovascular risk reduction associated with antiplatelet therapy and the potential for these agents to improve leg symptoms and limb-related outcomes, such as claudication and bypass graft patency. Less commonly encountered antiplatelet agents which may be used in the treatment of PAD will also be discussed.

Aspirin

Cardiovascular risk reduction

The strongest evidence to support the use of aspirin in the management of PAD is derived from large meta-analyses of randomized controlled trials (RCTs) of antiplatelet therapy in the treatment of coronary and noncoronary atherosclerosis [14,15]. The majority of trials in these meta-analyses randomized patients to aspirin, although trials of other antiplatelet agents (discussed later in this chapter) were also included. The first Antiplatelet Trialists' Collaboration, a meta-analysis of 145 RCTs comparing antiplatelet agents to control in approximately 70,000 patients with vascular disease, demonstrated a 25% reduction in the risk of MI, stroke or vascular death with antiplatelet therapy [14]. In the second Antiplatelet Trialists' Collaboration meta-analysis, which reported data from 9,214 patients with PAD separately, there was an overall 23% odds reduction in MI, stroke or vascular death associated with randomization to antiplatelet therapy. Patients with intermittent claudication, those undergoing lower extremity bypass surgery and those undergoing percutaneous peripheral intervention obtained similar benefits from antiplatelet therapy (Figure 13.1) [16].

Few of the PAD-specific trials in the Antiplatelet Trialists'Collaboration meta-analysis randomized patients to aspirin versus placebo [16]. Indeed, while aspirin may prevent major vascular events when grouped with other antiplatelet therapies in meta-analyses, there have been few RCTs investigating the effect of aspirin alone on stroke, MI or death among patients with PAD. For this reason, professional labeling of aspirin for the specific indication of PAD was not approved by the Food and Drug Administration (FDA) [17]. Since the publication of the second Antithrombotic Trialists' Collaboration meta-analysis in 2002, one additional RCT has demonstrated a cardiovascular morbidity and mortality benefit of aspirin among patients with PAD. The Critical Leg Ischaemia Prevention Study (CLIPS) [18] randomized 366 patients

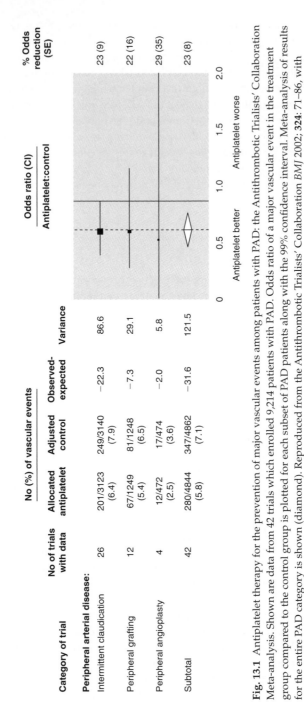

Fig. 13.1 Antiplatelet therapy for the prevention of major vascular events among patients with PAD: the Antithrombotic Trialists' Collaboration Meta-analysis. Shown are data from 42 trials which enrolled 9,214 patients with PAD. Odds ratio of a major vascular event in the treatment group compared to the control group is plotted for each subset of PAD patients along with the 99% confidence interval. Meta-analysis of results for the entire PAD category is shown (diamond). Reproduced from the Antithrombotic Trialists' Collaboration *BMJ* 2002; **324**: 71–86, with permission.

with symptomatic or asymptomatic PAD to receive aspirin (100 mg daily), antioxidant vitamins, both or neither treatment in a 2 × 2 placebo-controlled factorial design. Patients were followed for a period of 2 years for the development of MI, stroke, pulmonary embolism, vascular death and critical limb ischemia. Compared with placebo, randomization to aspirin was associated with a 64% reduction in the risk of a major vascular event.

Claudication and limb-related outcomes

The use of aspirin to delay the development or progression of PAD or symptoms of claudication has been investigated in a handful of clinical trials. Among the more than 22,000 healthy male participants in the Physicians Health Study, those randomized to aspirin (325 mg every other day) had a 46% reduction in the relative risk of needing peripheral arterial surgery during the 5-year follow-up period compared to placebo [19]. There was no significant difference in the risk of developing intermittent claudication between the two groups. A small study of 54 patients reported improved walking distance and resting limb blood flow among patients treated with a combination of aspirin and dipyridamole [20]. Hess and colleagues randomized 240 patients with PAD to receive aspirin, aspirin plus dipyridamole or placebo for a period of 2 years. Patients randomized to either aspirin or aspirin plus dipyridamole had slower angiographic progression of lower extremity PAD when compared to placebo [21].

Improved patency following revascularization

There have been few RCTs investigating the efficacy of aspirin alone in preventing graft occlusion after lower extremity bypass surgery. A meta-analysis of 11 trials of prevention of peripheral arterial graft occlusion by the Antiplatelet Trialists' Collaboration demonstrated a 38% reduction in the odds of graft occlusion among patients randomized to antiplatelet therapy compared to compared to those randomized to control (15.8% versus 23.6%, p = 0.0001) [15]. Based on the trials included in this meta-analysis (all published prior to March, 1990), there was no evidence that any antiplatelet regimen was better than medium-dose aspirin (75–325 mg daily) alone in preventing graft occlusion. A subsequent meta-analysis of five clinical trials enrolling 816 patients undergoing infrainguinal bypass surgery found a relative risk reduction of 22% (RR 0.78, 95% CI 0.64–0.95) for graft occlusion among patients randomized to aspirin with or without dipyridamole compared to placebo [22]. A separate meta-analysis investigating the effect of aspirin on the risk of vein graft occlusion for venous versus prosthetic conduits found that while aspirin, with or without dipyridamole, improves graft patency of prosthetic grafts, this finding may not be true in vein grafts [23]. In a retrospective study of 125 infrainguinal bypass procedures performed for critical limb ischemia, there was no difference in 2-year patency rates among patients treated with or without aspirin [24]. Of note, however, the majority of bypass grafts in this study were performed using autologous vein conduit (104 of 125 bypasses).

The role of aspirin for prevention of reocclusion after peripheral transluminal angioplasty (PTA) of the lower extremities has been studied in few clinical trials with conflicting results. In one study of 199 patients who underwent femoropopliteal PTA and were randomized to placebo or dipyridamole with one of two doses of aspirin (330 mg t.i.d. or 100 mg t.i.d.), there was improvement or no deterioration of angiographic or clinical measures with antiplatelet therapy compared to placebo (61% with high dose aspirin plus dipyridamole versus 37% with placebo, p = 0.01) [25]. In contrast, another study of 233 patients who underwent PTA and were randomized to either placebo or aspirin (50 mg daily) plus dipyridamole (400 mg daily) found no difference in patency between the two groups after 1 year [26].

Guidelines and recommendations

Major professional organizations have recommended the use of aspirin in the management of patients with PAD, with emphasis upon the potential for prevention of major cardiovascular events [12,13,27]. The American College of Cardiology/American Heart Association (ACC/AHA) give aspirin therapy (75–325 mg daily) its highest recommendation (Class IA) to reduce the risk of MI, stroke or vascular death in all patients with PAD, regardless of the presence of claudication [12] (Table 13.1). The American College of

Table 13.1 2005 American College of Cardiology/American Heart Association PAD guidelines: antiplatelet and anticoagulant therapy

Class I

1. Antiplatelet therapy is indicated to reduce the risk of MI, stroke or vascular death in individuals with atherosclerotic lower extremity peripheral arterial disease. *(Level of Evidence: A)*
2. Aspirin, in daily doses of 75 to 325 mg, is recommended as safe and effective antiplatelet therapy to reduce the risk of MI, stroke or vascular death in individuals with atherosclerotic lower extremity peripheral arterial disease. *(Level of Evidence: A)*
3. Clopidogrel (75 mg per day) is recommended as an effective alternative antiplatelet therapy to aspirin to reduce the risk of MI, stroke, or vascular death in individuals with atherosclerotic lower extremity peripheral arterial disease. *(Level of Evidence: B)*

Class III

Oral anticoagulation therapy with warfarin is not indicated to reduce the risk of adverse cardiovascular ischemic events in individuals with atherosclerotic lower extremity peripheral arterial disease. *(Level of Evidence: C)*

Chest Physicians (ACCP) recommends lifelong aspirin (75 to 325 mg daily) in patients with PAD who have clinically manifest coronary or cerebrovascular disease (Grade 1A) [27]. Lifelong aspirin therapy is also recommended for patients with PAD who do not have clinically manifest coronary or cerebrovascular disease (Grade 1C+). The Trans-Atlantic Inter-Society Consensus Document on Management of Peripheral Arterial Disease (TASC II) recommends that all symptomatic patients with PAD should be prescribed long-term antiplatelet therapy, regardless of concomitant coronary or cerebrovascular disease (Grade A) [13].

For patients with PAD who have undergone revascularization with prosthetic infrainguinal bypass surgery, the ACCP recommends aspirin therapy (Grade 1A). The ACCP also recommends aspirin (75 to 162 mg daily) for all patients who have undergone lower extremity PTA, with or without stenting (Grade 1C+) [27]. The ACC/AHA recommends that all patients undergoing lower extremity revascularization procedures should be treated with antiplatelet therapy (usually aspirin or clopidogrel) indefinitely for purposes of cardiovascular event prevention (Class IA) [12].

Thienopyridines

Cardiovascular risk reduction

The thienopyridines, ticlopidine and clopidogrel, have been shown to benefit patients with PAD, with benefit in cardiovascular risk reduction and improved outcomes following lower extremity revascularization procedures.

Ticlopidine has been shown to decrease cardiovascular mortality in a number of small clinical trials and meta-analyses [28–32]. A meta-analysis of RCTs which investigated the ability of ticlodipine to reduce cardiovascular events in patients with intermittent claudication found a significant reduction in both fatal and non-fatal cardiovascular events among patients randomized to ticlopidine versus placebo, but only four studies randomizing a total of 618 patients were include in the meta-analysis [31]. More recently, multicenter studies have investigated the use of ticlopidine among patients with PAD. The Argentinian EMATAP trial (Estudio Multicentrico Argentino de la Ticlopidine en las Arteriopatias Perifericas) randomized 615 patients with intermittent claudication to ticlopidine or placebo [28]. Randomization to ticlodipine (500 mg twice daily) for 24 weeks resulted in a statistically significant reduction in mortality and non-fatal thrombotic events compared to placebo during a 6-month follow-up period (3.0% ticlopidine vs. 6.8% placebo, RR = 0.44, p = 0.027). In the Swedish Ticlpidine Multicentre (STIMS) Study, 687 patients with intermittent claudication were randomized to ticlopidine (250 mg twice daily) or placebo and followed for a 5-year period for the incidence of death, MI, stroke or TIA [29]. Patients randomized to ticlopidine experienced a 29.1% reduction in all-cause mortality (18.5% ticlopidine vs. 26.1% placebo, p = 0.015) due primarily to a reduction in coronary-artery-related deaths. Surprisingly, there was no significant benefit of ticlopidine on the incidence of the primary end-point of fatal or non-fatal MI, stroke or TIA. In a more recent meta-analysis of antiplatelet therapy for PAD, the use of ticlopidine was associated with a 32% reduction in mortality compared to placebo [32].

In contrast to the modest size of trials demonstrating evidence in support of the use of ticlopidine for cardiovascular risk reduction among patients with PAD, the evidence base to support the use of clopidogrel for this purpose includes thousands of patients, though only from two mega trials. The CAPRIE trial [33] (Clopidogrel versus Aspirin in Patients at Risk of Ischaemic Events) randomized 19,185 patients with atherosclerotic vascular disease, including PAD, to clopidogrel (75 mg daily) or aspirin (325 mg daily) and followed them over a mean of 1.9 years for the occurrence of stroke, MI or vascular death. The primary finding of this study was an 8.7% reduction in the relative risk of the composite end-point among patients randomized to clopidogrel (annual event rates 5.32% clopidogrel vs. 5.83% aspirin, p = 0.043). Among the subgroup of patients enrolled with a diagnosis of PAD, including those with claudication and abnormal ABI or those with a prior history of lower extremity revascularization or amputation, there was a 23.8% reduction in the relative risk of the combined outcome of stroke, MI or vascular death attributed to clopidogrel (annual event rate 3.71% clopidogrel vs. 4.85% aspirin, p = 0.0028). The relative risk reduction in the PAD subgroup was of greater magnitude in comparison to the subgroup of patients enrolled with prior stroke or MI (Figure 13.2).

Building upon the findings of the CAPRIE study, the Clopidogrel for High Atherothrombotic Risk and Ischemic Stabilization Trial (CHARISMA) explored the relative benefits of dual antiplatelet therapy with aspirin plus clopidogrel versus aspirin alone in the prevention of recurrent events among patients with atherosclerotic vascular disease or multiple risk factors [34]. In CHARISMA, a total of 15,603 patients with clinically evident cardiovascular disease (CVD) or multiple risk factors for CVD were randomized to clopidogrel (75 mg daily) in combination with aspirin therapy (75 to 162 mg daily) or aspirin (75 to 162 mg daily) plus placebo. Patients were followed for the composite outcome of MI, stroke or vascular death over a median of 28 months. Overall, there was a no significant difference in the rate of the composite outcome between the two groups (relative risk = 0.93, p = 0.22). However, in a subsequent subgroup analysis of the 9478 patients enrolled with prior MI, ischemic stroke or symptomatic PAD [35], dual antiplatelet therapy as associated with a 17% reduction in the primary end-point (relative risk = 0.83, p = 0.01) (Figure 13.3). In contrast to the findings of the CAPRIE trial, a separate analysis of the 2838 patients in CHARISMA with symptomatic PAD found no significant difference in the occurrence of the composite end-point with clopidogrel plus aspirin versus aspirin alone. There was a statistically significant benefit associated

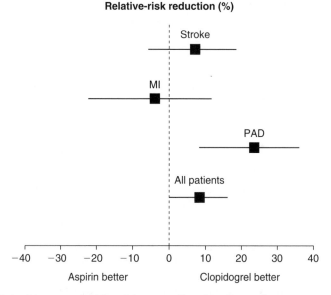

Relative-risk reduction (%)

Aspirin better   Clopidogrel better

Fig. 13.2 Aspirin versus clopidogrel for prevention of cardiovascular events among patients with atherosclerotic vascular disease: the CAPRIE trial. Shown are the relative risk reduction and 95% confidence interval for the combined outcome of stroke, MI, or vascular death for each subgroup of patients enrolled. MI = myocardial infarction, PAD = peripheral arterial disease. Among patients enrolled in CAPRIE with symptomatic PAD, there was a 23.8% relative risk reduction in the clopidogrel group. Reproduced with permission from *Lancet* 1996; **348**: 1329–1339.

with dual antiplatelet therapy among the patients randomized with prior MI or ischemic stroke.

Claudication and limb-related outcomes

There is scant evidence in support of a benefit of thienopyridines on the symptoms of PAD. In a subgroup of the STIMS trial of ticlopidine versus placebo for PAD, 101 patients with intermittent claudication were followed for symptoms and limb-related outcomes over a period of 5 years [37]. Among the patients randomized to ticlopidine, there was marginal improvement in blood flow parameters (venous occlusion plethysmography), ankle-brachial index (ABI) and walking distance. Other small clinical trials have reported more significant increases in walking distance [30,38] and ABI [30] for patients with intermittent claudication randomized to ticlopidine. Further, a separate analysis of the STIM trial found that ticlopidine prevented the need for future vascular surgery with an odds ratio of 0.49 (p < 0.001) when compared with placebo [39]. There have been no randomized clinical trials investigating the effect of

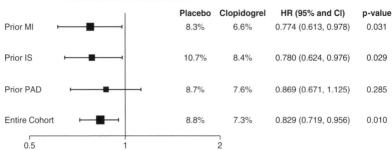

Fig. 13.3 Dual antiplatelet therapy versus aspirin alone for prevention of cardiovascular events among patients with atherosclerotic vascular disease: the CHARISMA trial. Shown are hazard ratios with 95% confidence intervals for the composite end-point of cardiovascular death, MI or stroke for patients randomized to clopidogrel plus aspirin versus aspirin alone (aspirin + placebo). Data are presented according to subset of disease on enrollment. In comparison to CAPRIE [33], there was no significant difference in the rate of the composite end-point among the patients with PAD randomized to dual antiplatelet therapy, although there was a benefit among the subset of patients with prior MI or prior ischemic stroke. Reproduced with permission from *J Am Coll Cardiol* 2007; **49**: 1982–1988.

clopidogrel on claudication symptoms or functional outcomes among patients with PAD.

Improved patency following revascularization

Despite widespread clinical use following lower extremity revascularization procedures, particularly endovascular intervention, there is little data to support the use of either ticlopidine or clopidogrel for improved patency outcomes in patients with PAD. One RCT investigated the ability of ticlopidine to maintain patency of lower extremity saphenous-vein bypass grafts [40]. In this study of 243 patients with femoropopliteal or femorotibial grafts randomized to ticlopidine or placebo, the 2-year patency rate in the ticlopidine group was 82% compared to 63% in the placebo group (p = 0.002). There are currently no clinical trial data to support the use of clopidogrel alone to improve patency after bypass grafting or PTA [27]. While there have been two randomized placebo-controlled clinical trials with laboratory end-points measuring the antiplatelet effect of clopidogrel added to aspirin therapy versus placebo and aspirin in patients undergoing angioplasty [41] and after bypass grafting [42], there have been no trials performed in these patients which assess for clinical outcomes with dual antiplatelet therapy. While clopidogrel and aspirin are commonly prescribed following percutaneous revascularization of the lower extremities, it is clear that this practice is based upon extrapolation of data from percutaneous coronary intervention trials, rather than trials specific to patients with PAD.

Guidelines and recommendations

The ACC/AHA Guidelines recommend clopidogrel 75 mg daily as an alternative to aspirin (Class IB) for the prevention of major vascular events in patients with PAD (Table 13.1) [12]. This recommendation is echoed by the ACCP which recommends the use of clopidogrel for patients with PAD over no antiplatelet therapy (Grade 1C+), but suggests the use of aspirin over clopidogrel if possible (Grade 2A), citing cost-effectiveness [27]. While ticlopidine has been shown to reduce cardiovascular events and improve symptoms in patients with intermittent claudication, its use is associated with a significant risk of hematological disturbances and requires close laboratory monitoring. Because of these potential severe side effects, the ACCP recommends the use of clopidogrel over ticlopidine (Grade 1C+) for patients who are not able to take aspirin [27]. Dual antiplatelet therapy with aspirin plus a thienopyridine for patients with PAD is not generally recommended.

Cilostazol

Cilostazol is a type 3 phosphodiesterase inhibitor which inhibits platelets both *in vitro* and *in vivo* [43]. Cilostazol is prescribed for the treatment of claudication, and along with pentoxyifylline, is one of two FDA approved agents for this indication. There have been no clinical trials showing any improvement in cardiovascular morbidity or mortality among patients with PAD treated with this drug.

Cilostazol (100 mg twice daily) has been shown to improve walking distance in patients with intermittent claudication in numerous RCTs with a demonstrated improvement in maximal walking distance between 21 and 47% and an improvement in pain-free walking distance between 22 and 59% [44–47] (Figure 13.4). The improvement in walking distances with cilostazol was statistically significant when compared to placebo. Cilostazol improved ABI slightly in one trial [44] but failed to do better than placebo in improving ABIs in another [46]. A Cochrane Collaboration Review of cilostazol for claudication, which included eight randomized clinical trials, found an improvement in the weighted mean difference for maximal walking distance with both cilostazol 50 mg twice daily and 100 mg twice daily compared with placeb [48]. In another meta-analysis of six randomized trials of 1,751 patients, randomization to cilostazol was not only associated with improvements in walking distance, but significant improvements in health-related quality of life compared to placebo [49].

A retrospective study of 141 patients undergoing femoropopliteal revacularization demonstrated that cilostazol use was associated with a significantly

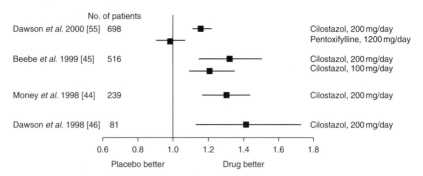

Fig. 13.4 Results of four randomized, placebo-controlled trials of cilostazol (and pentoxifylline) for the treatment of claudication. The data shown are as the geometric mean ratios of the maximal treadmill walking distance (on the horizontal axis) and 95% confidence intervals for cilostazol as compared with placebo [44–46,54]. Adapted with permission from *NEJM* 2001; **344**: 1608–1621 [56]. *Copyright©2001 Massachusetts Medical Society. All rights reserved.*

reduced need for repeat PTA (12% cilostazol vs. 32% no cilostazol, $p < 0.01$) [50]. Similar findings have been reported in a randomized clinical trial of prevention of coronary restenosis with cilostazol [51].

Guidelines and recommendations

The use of cilostazol for the treatment of claudication is given a Class IA recommendation by the ACC/AHA (Table 13.2) [12]. The Trans-Atlantic Inter-Society Consensus recommends a trial of cilostazol as first-line pharmacotherapy for symptomatic relief of claudication [13]. In striking contrast, the ACCP recommends the use of cilostazol only in patients with disabling intermittent claudication who are not candidates for percutaneous or surgical intervention and who have failed conservative therapy (Grade 2A). They specifically suggest not using cilostazol in patients with less than disabling claudication (Grade 2A) based on its cost and what the ACCP considers to be a modest improvement in functional outcomes and health-related quality of life [27].

Contraindications and potential side effects

Cilostazol, like milrinone, is a type 3 phosphodiesterase inhibitor. Milrinone has been found to increase mortality in patients with chronic heart failure [52], and concerns regarding excess death associated with this class of drugs has resulted in a black box warning that cilostazol should not be used in patients with heart failure of any severity [43]. Cilostazol is also contraindicated in patients with moderate-to-severe renal or hepatic impairment, hemostatic disorders or active pathological bleeding. The most common side effects of cilostazol include headache, diarrhea, palpitations, peripheral edema and dizziness.

Table 13.2 2005 American College of Cardiology/American Heart Association PAD guidelines: cilostazol and pentoxifylline for claudication

Class I

1. Cilostazol (100 mg orally 2 times per day) is indicated as an effective therapy to improve symptoms and increase walking distance in patients with lower extremity PAD and intermittent claudication (in the absence of heart failure). *(Level of Evidence: A)*
2. A therapeutic trial of cilostazol should be considered in all patients with lifestyle-limiting claudication (in the absence of heart failure). *(Level of Evidence: A)*

Class II-B

1. Pentoxifylline (400 mg 3 times per day) may be considered as second-line alternative therapy to cilostazol to improve walking distance in patients with intermittent claudication. *(Level of Evidence: A)*.
2. The clinical effectiveness of pentoxifylline as therapy for claudication is marginal and not well established. *(Level of Evidence: C)*.

Pentoxifylline

Pentoxifylline is a methylxanthine derivative with weak antiplatelet properties. While there have been many small clinical trials showing improvement in walking distance in patients with claudication treated with pentoxifylline versus placebo, there have been no studies demonstrating a reduction in major cardiovascular events or mortality.

A meta-analysis of clinical trials of pentoxifylline between 1976 and 1994 showed an improvement in pain-free walking distance in a total of 612 patients of 29.4 meters compared to placebo (95% CI 13.0 to 45.9 meters) and an improvement in maximal walking distance of 48.4 meters (95% CI 18.3 to 78.6 meters) compared to placebo [53]. The clinical significance of the improvement associated with pentoxifylline is questionable – less than an improvement of one city block of walking distance. Since the publication of the meta-analysis, there have been a few additional RCTs of pentoxifylline for claudication. The largest of these studies included 200 patients who were randomized to pentoxifylline (400 mg four times daily) or placebo. A the end of 40 weeks, there was a 386% increase in pain-free walking distance compared to a 369% increase in the placebo group (p < 0.02), representing a 38% excess increase in total walking distance in the pentoxifylline group over placebo. Similarly, there were large increases in maximal walking distance in both the pentoxifylline (329%) and placebo (183%) groups (p < 0.02) [54]. Of note, these were unusually large improvements in walking distances in both the pentoxifylline and placebo groups, which have not been reproduced in other studies.

One multicenter RCT compared cilostazol (100 mg twice daily) to pentoxifylline (400 mg three times daily) or placebo among 698 patients with intermittent claudication [55]. After 24 weeks of treatment, increase in maximal walking distance among patients randomized to cilostazol was significantly greater than that of patients randomized to either pentoxifylline or placebo (107 m versus 64 m versus 65 m in the cilostazol, pentoxifylline and placebo groups respectively, p < 0.001). Indeed, the treatment effect of pentoxifylline was similar to that of placebo. A figure of the comparative effects of cilostazol and pentoxifylline on walking distance in the four major RCT is shown in Figure 13.4 [56]. As the largest and most rigorously designed of the pentoxifylline trials, the study by Dawson and colleagues provide data that call into question the role of pentoxifylline as a medical therapy for claudication. In most recent treatment guidelines for PAD, pentoxifylline has been relegated to second line therapy for claudication (Table 13.2).

One trial investigated the potential role of pentoxifylline for maintaining graft patency among patients who have undergone peripheral artery bypass surgery [57]. This small study followed 110 patients with peripheral arterial bypass grafts over a period of 2 years and found that those treated with pentoxifylline (400 mg daily) had higher patency rates compared to those treated with placebo. In a second arm of the study, randomization to pentoxifylline was also associated with improved patency of aortocoronary bypass grafts at 2 years follow-up.

Guidelines and recommendations

The ACCP recommends against the use of pentoxifylline for claudication citing a lack of convincing evidence of the efficacy of pentoxifylline over placebo (Grade 1B) [27]. In contrast, the ACC/AHA recommends that pentoxifylline (400 mg three times a day) be considered as a second-line alternative agent to cilostazol for patients with intermittent claudication to improve walking distance [12]. It may be considered for patients in whom cilostazol is contraindicated, such as those with congestive heart failure.

Contraindications and potential side effects

Pentoxifylline is generally well-tolerated, although reported adverse effects include sore throat, dyspepsia, nausea and diarrhea [58]. Its use is not recommended in patients with hypersensitivity to pentoxifylline, xanthines (e.g. caffeine, theophylline), any component of the formulation or history of recent cerebral and/or retinal hemorrhage. Pentoxifylline should be prescribed with caution among patients taking theophylline, and drug levels of the later must be carefully followed as they can increase significantly with coadministration of the two medications [58].

Other antiplatelet agents

A handful of alternative antiplatelet agents have been investigated for use in the management of PAD. In general, these drugs have limited evidence in support of efficacy, although they may be available for clinical use in certain parts of the world.

Triflusal is an antiplatelet agent structurally related to the salicylates, which inhibits platelet aggregation primarily by inhibition of platelet arachidonic acid metabolism. In a single clinical trial, treatment with triflusal (300 mg twice daily) for 24 weeks improved both maximal and pain-free walking distances compared to placebo in patients with intermittent claudication [59]. Though available in some European countries, triflusal is not been approved for use by the United States FDA.

Picotamide is an inhibitor of thromboxane A2 and is also an antagonist of the thomboxane A2 receptor. Picotamide has been shown to reduce cardiovascular morbidity and mortality compared to placebo among 2304 patients with symptomatic PAD over a period 18 months (23% relative risk reduction, p = 0.029) [60]. In a trial of 1,209 patients with type 2 diabetes mellitus and PAD, picotamide reduced overall mortality by 45% versus aspirin (320 mg once daily, p = 0.047) [61], although there was no difference between the two groups for the combined end-point of mortality and major cardiovascular morbidity. Treatment with picotamide increased pain-free walking distance compared to placebo in two small randomized trials, each enrolling fewer than 50 patients [62,63]. Picotamide is not approved for use in the United States, but is used in some European countries.

Naftidrofuryl is an antagonist of the 5-hydroxytryptamine-2 receptor with demonstrated *in vivo* and *in vitro* antiplatelet activity [64]. Treatment with naftidrofuryl has been shown to increase pain-free walking distance compared to placebo in a meta-analysis of five randomized trials [65]. More recent trials have confirmed these findings and also found a significant improvement in maximal walking distance compared to placebo [66,67]. While available in Europe for many years and an alternative to cilostazol for medical management of claudication in the TASC II guidelines, naftidrofuryl is not approved for use in the United States [13]. Serotonin receptor antagonism for the medical treatment of claudication is an active area of clinical investigation, and RCTs of new agents are ongoing.

Conclusion

Antiplatelet therapy is the cornerstone of management of PAD, both for prevention of cardiovascular events and death and for the treatment of claudication symptoms. All patients with PAD and without contraindications, regardless of the presence or severity of claudication, should be treated with an antiplatelet agent (aspirin or clopidogrel) to prevent stroke, MI and cardiovascular death. Medical treatment with cilostazol should be considered as an option for improving function and quality of life among patients with claudication. All patients with PAD and without contraindications who undergo lower extremity revascularization procedures should be treated with antiplatelet therapy long term, the nature of which (aspirin or clopidogrel alone versus a defined course of dual antiplatelet therapy) depends upon the specifics of the procedure performed.

References

1 Pasternak RC, Criqui MH, Benjamin EJ, Fowkes FG, Isselbacher EM, McCullough PA, *et al.* Atherosclerotic Vascular Disease Conference: Writing Group I: epidemiology. *Circulation* 2004; **109**: 2605–2612.

2 Selvin E, Erlinger TP. Prevalence of and risk factors for peripheral arterial disease in the United States: results from the National Health and Nutrition Examination Survey, 1999–2000. *Circulation* 2004; **110**: 738–743.

3 Criqui MH, Denenberg JO, Langer RD, Fronek A. The epidemiology of peripheral arterial disease: importance of identifying the population at risk. *Vasc Med* 1997; **2**: 221–226.

4 Dormandy J, Mahir M, Ascady G, Balsano F, De Leeuw P, Blombery P, *et al.* Fate of the patient with chronic leg ischaemia. A review article. *J Cardiovasc Surg* (Torino) 1989; **30**: 50–57.

5 Criqui MH, Langer RD, Fronek A, Feigelson HS, Klauber MR, McCann TJ, *et al.* Mortality over a period of 10 years in patients with peripheral arterial disease. *New Engl J Med* 1992; **326**: 381–386.

6 Leng GC, Fowkes FG, Lee AJ, Dunbar J, Housley E, Ruckley CV. Use of ankle brachial pressure index to predict cardiovascular events and death: a cohort study. *BMJ* 1996; **313**: 1440–1444.

7 Kannel WB, McGee DL. Update on some epidemiologic features of intermittent claudication: the Framingham Study. *J Am Geriatr Soc* 1985; **33**: 13–18.

8 Newman AB, Sutton-Tyrrell K, Vogt MT, Kuller LH. Morbidity and mortality in hypertensive adults with a low ankle/arm blood pressure index. *JAMA* 1993; **270**: 487–489.

9 McKenna M, Wolfson S, Kuller L. The ratio of ankle and arm arterial pressure as an independent predictor of mortality. *Atherosclerosis* 1991; **87**: 119–128.

10 Weitz JI, Byrne J, Clagett GP, Farkouh ME, Porter JM, Sackett DL, *et al.* Diagnosis and treatment of chronic arterial insufficiency of the lower extremities: a critical review. *Circulation* 1996; **94**: 3026–3049.

11 Steg PG, Bhatt DL, Wilson PW, D'Agostino R, Sr, Ohman EM, Rother J, *et al.* One-year cardiovascular event rates in outpatients with atherothrombosis. *JAMA* 2007; **297**: 1197–1206.

12 Hirsch AT, Haskal ZJ, Hertzer NR, Bakal CW, Creager MA, Halperin JL, *et al.* ACC/AHA 2005 guidelines for the management of patients with peripheral arterial disease (lower extremity, renal, mesenteric, and abdominal aortic): executive summary a collaborative report from the American Association for Vascular Surgery/Society for

Vascular Surgery, Society for Cardiovascular Angiography and Interventions, Society for Vascular Medicine and Biology, Society of Interventional Radiology, and the ACC/AHA Task Force on Practice Guidelines (Writing Committee to Develop Guidelines for the Management of Patients With Peripheral Arterial Disease) endorsed by the American Association of Cardiovascular and Pulmonary Rehabilitation; National Heart, Lung, and Blood Institute; Society for Vascular Nursing; TransAtlantic Inter-Society Consensus; and Vascular Disease Foundation. *J Am Coll Cardiol* 2006; **47**: 1239–1312.

13 Norgren L, Hiatt WR, Dormandy JA, Nehler MR, Harris KA, Fowkes FG, *et al.* Inter-Society Consensus for the Management of Peripheral Arterial Disease (TASC II). *Eur J Vasc Endovasc Surg* 2007; **33** (Suppl. 1): S1–75.

14 Antiplatelet Trialists' Collaboration. Collaborative overview of randomised trials of antiplatelet therapy – I: Prevention of death, myocardial infarction, and stroke by prolonged antiplatelet therapy in various categories of patients. *BMJ* 1994; **308**: 81–106.

15 Antiplatelet Trialists' Collaboration. Collaborative overview of randomised trials of antiplatelet therapy – II: Maintenance of vascular graft or arterial patency by antiplatelet therapy. *BMJ* 1994; **308**: 159–168.

16 Antithrombotic Trialists' Collaboration. Collaborative meta-analysis of randomised trials of antiplatelet therapy for prevention of death, myocardial infarction, and stroke in high risk patients. *BMJ* 2002; **324**: 71–86.

17 Food and Drug Administration. Internal analgesic, antipyretic and antirheumatic drug products for over-the-counter human use: final rule for professional labeling of aspirin, buffered aspirin and aspirin in combination with antacid drug products. *Federal Register* 2005; **63**: 56802–56819.

18 Catalano M, Born G, Peto R. Prevention of serious vascular events by aspirin amongst patients with peripheral arterial disease: randomized, double-blind trial. *J Intern Med* 2007; **261**: 276–284.

19 Goldhaber SZ, Manson JE, Stampfer MJ, LaMotte F, Rosner B, Buring JE, *et al.* Low-dose aspirin and subsequent peripheral arterial surgery in the Physicians' Health Study. *Lancet* 1992; **340**: 143–145.

20 Libretti A, Catalano M. Treatment of claudication with dipyridamole and aspirin. *Int J Clin Pharmacol Res* 1986; **6**: 59–60.

21 Hess H, Mietaschk A, Deichsel G. Drug-induced inhibition of platelet function delays progression of peripheral occlusive arterial disease. A prospective double-blind arteriographically controlled trial. *Lancet* 1985; **1**: 415–419.

22 Tangelder MJ, Lawson JA, Algra A, Eikelboom BC. Systematic review of randomized controlled trials of aspirin and oral anticoagulants in the prevention of graft occlusion and ischemic events after infrainguinal bypass surgery. *J Vasc Surg* 1999; **30**: 701–709.

23 Watson HR, Skene AM, Belcher G. Graft material and results of platelet inhibitor trials in peripheral arterial reconstructions: reappraisal of results from a meta-analysis. *Br J Clin Pharmacol* 2000; **49**: 479–483.

24 Mahmood A, Sintler M, Edwards AT, Smith SR, Simms MH, Vohra RK. The efficacy of aspirin in patients undergoing infra-inguinal bypass and identification of high risk patients. *Int Angiol* 2003; **22**: 302–307.

25 Heiss HW, Just H, Middleton D, Deichsel G. Reocclusion prophylaxis with dipyridamole combined with acetylsalicylic acid following PTA. *Angiology* 1990; **41**: 263–269.

26 Study Group on Pharmacological Treatment after PTA. Platelet inhibition with ASA/ dipyridamole after percutaneous balloon angioplasty in patients with symptomatic lower limb arterial disease. A prospective double-blind trial. *Eur J Vasc Surg* 1994; **8**: 83–88.

27 Clagett GP, Sobel M, Jackson MR, Lip GY, Tangelder M, Verhaeghe R. Antithrombotic therapy in peripheral arterial occlusive disease: the Seventh ACCP Conference on Antithrombotic and Thrombolytic Therapy. *Chest* 2004; **126** (3 Suppl.): 609S–626S.

28 Blanchard J, Carreras LO, Kindermans M. Results of EMATAP: a double-blind placebo-controlled multicentre trial of ticlopidine in patients with peripheral arterial disease. *Nouv Rev Fr Hematol* 1994; **35**: 523–528.

29 Janzon L, Bergqvist D, Boberg J, Boberg M, Eriksson I, Lindgarde F, *et al.* Prevention of myocardial infarction and stroke in patients with intermittent claudication; effects of ticlopidine. Results from STIMS, the Swedish Ticlopidine Multicentre Study. *J Intern Med* 1990; **227**: 301–308.

30 Balsano F, Coccheri S, Libretti A, Nenci GG, Catalano M, Fortunato G, *et al.* Ticlopidine in the treatment of intermittent claudication: a 21-month double-blind trial. *J Lab Clin Med* 1989; **114**: 84–91.

31 Boissel JP, Peyrieux JC, Destors JM. Is it possible to reduce the risk of cardiovascular events in subjects suffering from intermittent claudication of the lower limbs? *Thromb Haemost* 1989; **62**: 681–685.

32 Girolami B, Bernardi E, Prins MH, ten Cate JW, Prandoni P, Hettiarachchi R, *et al.* Antithrombotic drugs in the primary medical management of intermittent claudication: a meta-analysis. *Thromb Haemost* 1999; **81**: 715–722.

33 CAPRIE Steering Committee. A randomised, blinded, trial of clopidogrel versus aspirin in patients at risk of ischaemic events (CAPRIE). *Lancet* 1996; **348**: 1329–1339.

34 Bhatt DL, Fox KA, Hacke W, Berger PB, Black HR, Boden WE, *et al.* Clopidogrel and aspirin versus aspirin alone for the prevention of atherothrombotic events. *New Engl J Med* 2006; **354**: 1706–1717.

35 Bhatt DL, Flather MD, Hacke W, Berger PB, Black HR, Boden WE, *et al.* Patients with prior myocardial infarction, stroke, or symptomatic peripheral arterial disease in the CHARISMA trial. *J Am Coll Cardiol* 2007; **49**: 1982–1988.

36 Wiviott SD, Antman EM, Gibson CM, Montalescot G, Riesmeyer J, Weerakkody G, *et al.* Evaluation of prasugrel compared with clopidogrel in patients with acute coronary syndromes: design and rationale for the TRial to assess Improvement in Therapeutic Outcomes by optimizing platelet InhibitioN with prasugrel Thrombolysis In Myocardial Infarction 38 (TRITON-TIMI 38). *Am Heart J* 2006; **152**: 627–635.

37 Fagher B. Long-term effects of ticlopidine on lower limb blood flow, ankle/ brachial index and symptoms in peripheral arteriosclerosis. A double-blind study. The STIMS Group in Lund. Swedish Ticlopidine Multicenter Study. *Angiology* 1994; **45**: 777–788.

38 Arcan JC, Blanchard J, Boissel JP, Destors JM, Panak E. Multicenter double-blind study of ticlopidine in the treatment of intermittent claudication and the prevention of its complications. *Angiology* 1988; **39**: 802–811.

39 Bergqvist D, Almgren B, Dickinson JP. Reduction of requirement for leg vascular surgery during long-term treatment of claudicant patients with ticlopidine: results from the Swedish Ticlopidine Multicentre Study (STIMS). *Eur J Vasc Endovasc Surg* 1995; **10**: 69–76.

40 Becquemin JP. Effect of ticlopidine on the long-term patency of saphenous-vein bypass grafts in the legs. Etude de la Ticlopidine apres Pontage Femoro-Poplite and the Association Universitaire de Recherche en Chirurgie. *New Engl J Med* 1997; **337**: 1726–1731.

41 Cassar K, Ford I, Greaves M, Bachoo P, Brittenden J. Randomized clinical trial of the antiplatelet effects of aspirin-clopidogrel combination versus aspirin alone after lower limb angioplasty. *Br J Surg* 2005; **92**: 159–165.

42 Smout JD, Mikhailidis DP, Shenton BK, Stansby G. Combination antiplatelet therapy in patients with peripheral vascular bypass grafts. *Clin Appl Thromb Hemost* 2004; **10**: 9–18.

43 US Food and Drug Administration. *Cilostazol Package Insert*. http://www.fda.gov/cder/news/cilostazol/cilo_label.htm.

44 Money SR, Herd JA, Isaacsohn JL, Davidson M, Cutler B, Heckman J, *et al.* Effect of cilostazol on walking distances in patients with intermittent claudication caused by peripheral vascular disease. *J Vasc Surg* 1998; **27**: 267–274; discussion 274–275.

45 Beebe HG, Dawson DL, Cutler BS, Herd JA, Strandness DE, Jr., Bortey EB, *et al.* A new pharmacological treatment for intermittent claudication: results of a randomized, multicenter trial. *Arch Intern Med* 1999; **159**: 2041–2050.

46 Dawson DL, Cutler BS, Meissner MH, Strandness DE, Jr. Cilostazol has beneficial effects in treatment of intermittent claudication: results from a multicenter, randomized, prospective, double-blind trial. *Circulation* 1998; **98**: 678–686.

47 Strandness DE, Jr., Dalman RL, Panian S, Rendell MS, Comp PC, Zhang P, *et al.* Effect of cilostazol in patients with intermittent claudication: a randomized, double-blind, placebo-controlled study. *Vasc Endovascular Surg* 2002; **36**: 83–91.

48 Robless P, Mikhailidis DP, Stansby GP. Cilostazol for peripheral arterial disease. *Cochrane Database Syst Rev* 2007: CD003748.

49 Regensteiner JG, Ware JE, Jr., McCarthy WJ, Zhang P, Forbes WP, Heckman J, *et al.* Effect of cilostazol on treadmill walking, community-based walking ability, and health-related quality of life in patients with intermittent claudication due to peripheral arterial disease: meta-analysis of six randomized controlled trials. *J Am Geriatr Soc* 2002; **50**: 1939–1946.

50 Iida O, Nanto S, Uematsu M, Morozumi T, Kotani J, Awata M, *et al.* Cilostazol reduces target lesion revascularization after percutaneous transluminal angioplasty in the femoropopliteal artery. *Circ J* 2005; **69**: 1256–1259.

51 Douglas JS, Jr., Holmes DR, Jr., Kereiakes DJ, Grines CL, Block E, Ghazzal ZM, *et al.* Coronary stent restenosis in patients treated with cilostazol. *Circulation* 2005; **112**: 2826–2832.

52 Packer M, Carver JR, Rodeheffer RJ, Ivanhoe RJ, DiBianco R, Zeldis SM, *et al.* Effect of oral milrinone on mortality in severe chronic heart failure. The PROMISE Study Research Group.*New Engl J Med* 1991; **325**: 1468–1475.

53 Hood SC, Moher D, Barber GG. Management of intermittent claudication with pentoxifylline: meta-analysis of randomized controlled trials. CMAJ. 1996 Oct 15;**155**(8):1053-1059.

54 Cesarone MR, Belcaro G, Nicolaides AN, Griffin M, De Sanctis MT, Incandela L, *et al.* Treatment of severe intermittent claudication with pentoxifylline: a 40-week, controlled, randomized trial. *Angiology* 2002; **53** (Suppl. 1): S1–5.

55 Dawson DL, Cutler BS, Hiatt WR, Hobson RW, 2nd, Martin JD, Bortey EB, *et al.* A comparison of cilostazol and pentoxifylline for treating intermittent claudication. *Am J Med* 2000; **109**: 523–530.

56 Hiatt WR. Medical treatment of peripheral arterial disease and claudication. *New Engl J Med* 2001; **344**: 1608–1621.

57 Angelides NS, Minas C. Can aortocoronary and peripheral venous bypass graft patency be improved by the administration of pentoxifylline on a long-term basis? *Cardiologia* 1999; **44**: 1059–1064.

58 US Food and Drug Administration. *Pentoxifylline Package Insert.* http://www.fda.gov/cder/foi/nda/97/018631_s030ap.pdf.

59 Auteri A, Angaroni A, Borgatti E, Catalano M, De Vizzi GB, Forconi S, *et al.* Triflusal in the treatment of patients with chronic peripheral arteriopathy: multicentre double-blind clinical study vs placebo. *Int J Clin Pharmacol Res* 1995; **15**: 57–63.

60 Balsano F, Violi F. Effect of picotamide on the clinical progression of peripheral vascular disease. A double-blind placebo-controlled study. The ADEP Group. *Circulation* 1993; **87**: 1563–1569.

61 Neri Serneri GG, Coccheri S, Marubini E, Violi F. Picotamide, a combined inhibitor of thromboxane A2 synthase and receptor, reduces 2-year mortality in diabetics with peripheral arterial disease: the DAVID study. *Eur Heart J* 2004; **25**: 1845–1852.

62 Coto V, Cocozza M, Oliviero U, Lucariello A, Picano T, Coto F, *et al.* Clinical efficacy of picotamide in long-term treatment of intermittent claudication. *Angiology* 1989; **40**: 880–885.

63 Canonico V, Ammaturo V, Guarini P, Tedeschi C, Nunziata G, Nappi A, *et al.* [The clinico-instrumental evaluation of the efficacy of picotamide in treating chronic obstructive arteriopathies of the lower extremities]. *Minerva Cardioangiol* 1991; **39**: 75–80.

64 Kirsten R, Erdeg B, Moxter D, Hesse K, Breidert M, Nelson K. Platelet aggregation after naftidrofuryl application in vitro and ex vivo. *Int J Clin Pharmacol Ther* 1995; **33**: 81–84.

65 Lehert P, Comte S, Gamand S, Brown TM. Naftidrofuryl in intermittent claudication: a retrospective analysis. *J Cardiovasc Pharmacol* 1994; **23** Suppl 3: S48–52.

66 Kieffer E, Bahnini A, Mouren X, Gamand S. A new study demonstrates the efficacy of naftidrofuryl in the treatment of intermittent claudication. Findings of the Naftidrofuryl Clinical Ischemia Study (NCIS). *Int Angiol* 2001; **20**: 58–65.

67 Boccalon H, Lehert P, Mosnier M. [Effect of naftidrofuryl on physiological walking distance in patients with intermittent claudication]. *Ann Cardiol Angeiol* (Paris) 2001; **50**: 175–182.

Chapter 14

Clinical use of antiplatelet agents in cardiovascular disease: cerebrovascular diseases

Larry B. Goldstein

The efficacies of several platelet antiaggregant drugs have been evaluated in randomized trials of both primary and secondary ischemic stroke prevention as well as for the treatment of patients with acute ischemic stroke. These trial results help to inform therapeutic decisions for individual patients; however, gaps in the available data still provide a challenge for physicians.

Antiplatelet agents for the primary prevention of ischemic stroke

The clinical usefulness of platelet antiaggregants for prevention of a first stroke is dependent on the patient's risk of ischemic vascular events. The effects on stroke need to be considered in the context of overall cardiovascular protection as risk factors for stroke overlap with those for coronary heart and peripheral vascular disease. These risks are important to consider because even low doses of platelet antiaggregants can be associated with increased chances of central and systemic bleeding complications that exceed stroke reduction in persons at low stroke risk. The Antiplatelet Trialists' Collaborators evaluated studies of the effects of five different platelet antiaggregants including aspirin, ticlopidine, dipyridamole, suloctidil and sulfinpyrazone, alone or in combination, on non-fatal stroke, non-fatal MI and vascular death in 30,000 "low risk" patients randomized in three clinical trials [1]. Subjects in these studies had no prior history of cardiac, cerebrovascular or peripheral vascular disease. There was an overall non-significant 10% reduction in the listed outcome events with platelet antiaggregants, mainly due to a 29% reduction in non-fatal myocardial infarction. There was a non-significant increase in the risk of non-fatal

Antiplatelet Therapy in Ischemic Heart Disease, 1st edition. Edited by Stephen D. Wiviott.
© 2009 American Heart Association, ISBN: 9-781-4051-7626-2

stroke in platelet antiaggregant-treated patients, primarily due to a greater risk of intracranial hemorrhage. Therefore, there is no evidence of a reduction in stroke risk with platelet antiaggregants in persons at low risk. The US Preventive Services Task Force recommends aspirin (75 mg/d) for cardiac prophylaxis for persons whose 5-year coronary heart disease risk is ≥3% [2]. The 2002 update of the AHA Guidelines for the primary prevention of cardiovascular disease and stroke recommends a ≥10% risk over 10 years rather than a >3% risk over 5 years to maximize the benefits of aspirin as compared to its associated increased risk of brain and systemic bleeding [3].

The studies reviewed by the Antiplatelet Trialists' Collaborators included few women. More recently, the Women's Health Study (WHS) randomized 39,876 initially asymptomatic women 45 years of age or older to receive 100 mg of aspirin or placebo on alternate days [4]. These women were followed for 10 years for the occurrence of the study's primary end-point (non-fatal MI, non-fatal stroke or cardiovascular death). As was the case for men, there was no overall benefit as reflected in the study's primary end-point (RR = 0.91, 95% CI 0.80 to 1.03; p = 0.13). There was, however, a 17% reduction in the risk of stroke (RR = 0.83, 95% CI 0.69 to 0.99; p = 0.04). This reflected a 24% reduction in the risk of ischemic stroke (RR = 0.76, 95% CI 0.63 to 0.93; p = 0.009), an effect that was partially attenuated by a non-significant increase in the risk of hemorrhagic stroke (RR = 1.24, 95% CI 0.82 to 1.87; p = 0.31). The overall average stroke rates were 0.11% per year in aspirin-treated women and 0.13% per year in those treated with placebo (absolute risk reduction = 0.02% per year, Numbers needed to treat (NNT) = 5000). Gastrointestinal (GI) hemorrhage requiring transfusion was more frequent in the aspirin group (RR = 1.40, 95% CI 1.07 to 1.83; p = 0.02). The average GI hemorrhage rates were 0.06% per year for aspirin and 0.05% per year for placebo (absolute risk increase = 0.01% per year, Numbers needed to harm (NNH) = 10,000). The most consistent benefit for aspirin was in women 65 years of age or older at study entry, among whom the risk of major cardiovascular events was reduced by 26% (RR = 0.74, 95% CI 0.59 to 0.92; p = 0.008), but in whom there was not a significant reduction in stroke (RR = 0.78; 95% CI 0.57 to 1.08; p = 0.13). *Post hoc* subgroup analyses found reductions in stroke for those women with a history of hypertension (RR = 0.76; 95% CI 0.59 to 0.98; p = 0.04), hyperlipidemia (RR = 0.62; 95% CI 0.47 to 0.83; p = 0.001), diabetes (RR = 0.46; 95% CI 0.25 to 0.85; p = 0.01), or having a 10-year cardiovascular risk ≥10% (RR = 0.54; 95% CI 0.30 to 0.98; p = 0.04).

The definition of "primary stroke prevention" becomes somewhat clouded in populations with established cardiovascular disease who have never had a stroke or Transient Ischemic Attack (TIA). Although a primary prevention population from the standpoint of stroke, this represents a secondary (i.e. high-risk) prevention population based on the presence of disease affecting other vascular beds. Having coronary heart or peripheral (i.e. non-cerebrovascular) disease is also associated with an increased risk of stroke. As with overall primary prevention populations at high stroke risk because of the presence of other conditions, the benefit of treatment in these patients generally outweighs the risk of bleeding complications. For example, the Second International Study of Infarct Survival Study evaluated 160 mg/day of aspirin beginning within 24 hours of MI and continued for 5 weeks [5]. Treatment was associated with a 21% reduction in vascular mortality (RR = 0.21, 95% CI 0.14 to 0.27; p < 0.001), a 49% reduction in myocardial reinfarction rates (RR = 0.45, 95% CI 0.33 to 0.55; p < 0.0001), and a 42% reduction in stroke (RR = 0.42, 95% CI 0.17 to 0.59; p = 0.004).

Two studies have compared the combination of aspirin and clopidogrel in patients with acute coronary syndromes. In the Clopidogrel in Unstable Angina to Prevent Recurrent Events (CURE) trial, treatment was begun within 24 hours of symptom onset in patients with non-ST-segment elevation acute coronary syndromes with patients subsequently followed for 3–12 months [6]. There was a 20% relative reduction in the proportion of patients having a primary end-point (death from cardiovascular causes, non-fatal myocardial infarction or stroke) with the combination (9.3% vs. 11.4%; RR = 0.80, 95% CI 0.72 to 0.90, p < 0.001). The risk of stroke was similar in the two treatment groups (1.2% vs. 1.4% for the combination vs. aspirin alone; RR = 0.86, 95% CI 0.63 to 1.18). The combination was associated with a higher risk of major bleeding complications (3.7% vs. 2.7%; RR = 1.38, 95% CI 1.13 to 1.67, p = 0.001). The Clopidogrel and Metoprolol in Myocardial Infarction Trial (COMMIT) included subjects who presented within 24 hours of suspected acute MI with ST-elevation, ST depression or left-bundle branch block and who were not scheduled for a primary percutaneous coronary intervention [7]. Co-primary outcomes were the composite of death, reinfarction or stroke, and death from any cause during the scheduled treatment period (i.e. until hospital discharge or day 28). There were reductions in both primary outcomes with combination treatment with clopidogrel plus aspirin as compared with aspirin alone (9.2% vs. 10.1%, OR = 0.91, 95% CI 0.86 to 0.97, p = 0.002 for death, reinfarction or stroke and 7.5% vs. 8.1%, OR = 0.93, 95% CI 0.87 to 0.99, p = 0.03 death from any cause). The risk of stroke was again similar in the two treatment groups (0.9% vs. 1.1%, OR = 0.86, 95% CI 0.72 to 1.03, p = 0.11) with identical proportions of subjects having non-fatal strokes (0.6% in each treatment group). There was no increase in the risk of bleeding complications. Although the two studies were not powered to detect a difference in stroke outcomes, the point estimates in each favored a reduction in stroke with the combination of aspirin and clopidogrel. However, because the 95% CIs for stroke end-points cross unity in each study, neither proves a benefit in reducing stroke.

Antiplatelet therapy (90% aspirin) is associated with an approximate 22% (95% CI 2 to 38%) reduction in the risk of stroke in patients with non-valvular atrial fibrillation compared to placebo [8]. Treatment with adjusted-dose warfarin is associated with a 36% (95% CI 14 to 52%) reduction in stroke risk compared with aspirin [8]. Anticoagulation with warfarin is recommended for prevention of a first stroke in patients with non-valvular atrial fibrillation in whom the risk of ischemic stroke is more than 2.5% per year (based on risk factors such as the presence of congestive heart failure, hypertension, age over 75 years and diabetes mellitus) in whom the reduction in stroke outweighs the risk of warfarin-related bleeding complications [9]. Those at low risk (1% per year or less) can be treated with aspirin whereas either aspirin or warfarin are reasonable alternatives for those at low to moderate risk (i.e. ~1.5% per year).

Patients in each of the major randomized trials of endarterectomy for asymptomatic stenosis were treated with aspirin because of their high risk of atheroembolic events [10–12]. Surgically treated patients were not given aspirin in one smaller trial [13]. There were no major strokes or deaths in either the aspirin or surgically treated groups. The study was stopped early because 26% of those in the surgical arm (no aspirin) had myocardial infarctions as compared with 9% of those in the medical (aspirin-treated) arm ($p = 0.002$).

Taken together, the available data show no benefit of platelet antiaggregants in reducing the chances of a first stroke in low risk populations in which bleeding complications with even low doses of aspirin negate any benefit. Platelet antiaggregant therapy is likely of value for reducing the risk of cardiovascular events in higher risk primary prevention populations. Treatment with aspirin is associated with a reduction in stroke as well as other cardiovascular events in patients with acute MI. In high-risk cardiac populations with non-ST elevation acute coronary syndromes or acute MI with ST segment changes or left-bundle branch block, there is no proven reduction in stroke outcomes with combination treatment with aspirin and clopidogrel as compared to aspirin alone, with treatment decisions guided by the effect on each study's combined end-points. Table 14.1 gives relevant treatment recommendations as reflected in the current American Heart Association/American Stroke Association guidelines for the use of antiplatelet drugs for the primary prevention of ischemic stroke [9].

Antiplatelet agents for prevention of recurrent ischemic stroke

The Antiplatelet Trialists' Collaborators meta-analysis evaluated the effects of platelet antiaggregants in 23,020 patients with prior stroke or TIA who had been randomized in 21 trials [14]. Antiplatelet treatment was associated with a 22% reduction in the combined risk of myocardial infarction, stroke or vascular death (17.8% vs. 21.4%, $p < 0.05$). This was based on reductions of 25 ± 5 recurrent non-fatal strokes ($p < 0.0001$), 7 ± 4 vascular deaths ($p = 0.04$), and 6 ± 2 non-fatal myocardial infarctions for every 1000 treated patients. These benefits exceeded the risk of bleeding (about 1 to 2 additional major extracranial hemorrhages per 1000 treated patients per year).

Two controlled trials with direct comparative data showed no differential effect of different doses of aspirin in non-surgical patients with prior stroke or

Table 14.1 AHA/ASA guidelines for the use of antiplatelet agents for the primary prevention of ischemic stroke [9]

1. Aspirin is not recommended for the prevention of a first stroke in men.

2. The use of aspirin is recommended for cardiovascular (including but not specific to stroke) prophylaxis among persons whose risk is sufficiently high for the benefits to outweigh the risks associated with treatment (a 10-year risk of cardiovascular events of 6% to 10%).

3. Aspirin can be useful for prevention of a first stroke among women whose risk is sufficiently high for the benefits to outweigh the risks associated with treatment.

4. Aspirin is recommended for patients with non-valvular atrial fibrillation who are at low risk (1% per year or less) for ischemic stroke whereas either aspirin or warfarin are reasonable alternatives for those at low to moderate (i.e. ~1.5% per year). Anticoagulation with warfarin is recommended for those without contraindications at high risk of ischemic stroke.

5. The use of aspirin is recommended in patients having endarterectomy for asymptomatic stenosis unless contraindicated because aspirin was used in all of the cited trials as an antiplatelet drug except in the surgical arm of one study, in which there was a higher rate of MI in those who were not given aspirin.

TIA (1200 vs. 300 mg/day and 283 vs. 30 mg/day) [15,16]. In contrast, a double-blind, controlled trial of 2849 endarterectomy patients compared the efficacy of aspirin at doses of 81 mg (n = 709), 325 mg (n = 708), 650 mg (n = 715) or 1300 mg (n = 717) daily that was started before surgery and continued for 3 months [17]. As compared to patients given the two higher doses of aspirin, those given the two lower doses had lower combined rates of stroke, myocardial infarction and death at 30 days (5.4 vs. 7.0%, p = 0.07) and at 3 months (6.2 vs. 8.4%, p = 0.03). Although lower doses of aspirin are generally thought to be associated with a lower risk of gastrointestinal hemorrhage as compared to higher doses, a meta-analysis of 24 randomized controlled trials (including about 66,000 participants) found no relationship between dose (50 to 1500 mg/day) and risk [18].

Treatment with aspirin is the standard comparator drug in randomized trials of other platelet antiaggregants for secondary stroke prevention. The Ticlopidine Aspirin Stroke Study (TASS) compared ticlopidine with aspirin (1300 mg/day) in patients with TIA or minor stroke [19]. The 3-year rate of non-fatal stroke or death was 17% for ticlopidine and 19% for aspirin (RR = 12%, 95% CI –2 to 26%, p = 0.048); the rates of fatal and non-fatal stroke at 3 years were 10% for ticlopidine and 13% for aspirin (RR = 21%, 95% CI 4 to 38%, p = 0.024). Although ticlopidine was somewhat more efficacious than aspirin, its use is limited because of the risk of side effects, including leukopenia, diarrhea and thrombotic thrombocytopenic purpura [20,21].

A subgroup analysis of the TASS trial found a 24% relative risk reduction for stroke or death at 2 years favoring ticlopidine over aspirin among black patients [22]. The African American Antiplatelet Stroke Prevention Study (AAASPS) randomized 1809 African American patients with non-cardioembolic ischemic stroke to ticlopidine or aspirin [23]. There was no statistically significant difference between ticlopidine and aspirin in the prevention of recurrent stroke, myocardial infarction or vascular death, further limiting ticlopidine's use.

The Clopidogrel versus Aspirin in Patients at Risk of Ischemic Events (CAPRIE) trial randomized 15,000 patients with prior myocardial infarction, symptomatic peripheral arterial disease or atherothrombotic stroke within 6 months to clopidogrel 75 mg or aspirin 325 mg per day [24]. Overall, clopidogrel treatment was associated with an 8.7% (95% CI 0.3% to 16.5%, p = 0.043) relative reduction in the combined risk of non-fatal stroke, non-fatal myocardial infarction or vascular death (0.51% annual reduction) [24]. Although not powered for subgroup analyses, there was not a reduction in these combined end-points in the strata of patients who entered the trial with stroke (RR = 7.3%, 95% CI –5.7 to 18.7%, p = 0.26).

Combination antiplatelet therapy offers the potential for greater reductions in ischemic events as compared to single drugs in patients at particularly high risk. The Clopidogrel for High Atherothrombotic Risk and Ischemic Stabilization, Management, and Avoidance (CHARISMA) trial randomly assigned 15,603 patients with either clinically evident cardiovascular disease (including ischemic stroke or TIA within the prior 5 years) or multiple risk factors to receive clopidogrel (75 mg per day) plus low-dose aspirin (75 to 162 mg per day) or placebo plus low-dose aspirin [25]. The primary efficacy end-point was a composite of myocardial infarction, stroke or death from cardiovascular causes. There was no reduction in the primary end-point (6.8% for aspirin plus clopidogrel vs. 7.2% for aspirin alone, RR = 0.93, 95% CI 0.83 to 1.05, p = 0.22).

The Management of Atherothrombosis With Clopidogrel in High-Risk Patients With TIA or Stroke (MATCH) trial randomized patients with ischemic stroke or TIA within the prior 3 months plus additional risk factors (n = 7599) to clopidogrel 75 mg plus placebo or to clopidogrel 75 mg plus aspirin 75 mg per day [26]. The primary outcome was a composite of ischemic stroke, myocardial infarction, vascular death or rehospitalization secondary to ischemic events. The combination was associated with a non-significant 6.4% (95% CI –4.6 to 16.3%, p = 0.224) relative reduction in the primary end-point, but a 26% (RR = 1.26, 95% CI 0.64 to 1.88, p < 0.0001) increase in life threatening bleeding. The combination of aspirin and clopidogrel is not indicated for secondary prevention in patients having had a TIA or stroke [27].

The European Stroke Prevention Study 2 (ESPS 2) compared the effects of aspirin (50 mg daily), sustained-release dipyridamole (400 mg daily), the same doses of aspirin and dipyridamole given in combination (ASA/DP), and placebo on the rates of stroke and death in patients with prior TIA or stroke [28]. Aspirin, dipyridamole and the combination each significantly reduced the risk of stroke or stroke and death compared to placebo. In pair-wise comparisons, ASA/DP reduced the risk of stroke compared to aspirin alone (RR = 23%, p = 0.006) and stroke or death (RR = 13%, p = 0.056).

The European/Australasian Stroke Prevention in Reversible Ischemia Trial (ESPRIT) randomized 2763 patients within 6 months of ischemic stroke or TIA of presumed arterial origin to open-label aspirin (30–325 mg/day) with or without dipyridamole (200 mg/day; 83% sustained release formulation) [29]. The primary outcome was a combination of non-fatal stroke, non-fatal MI, vascular death or major bleeding. Over a mean 3.5 years of follow-up, there was a 20% (HR = 0.80, 95% CI 0.66 to 0.98) reduction in the primary endpoint, supporting the results of the ESPS-2 trial.

Concern has been raised that dipyridamole might increase the risk of myocardial ischemia in patients with coronary heart disease. However, a *post hoc* analysis of the ESPS-2 trial found identical rates of myocardial infarction in patients who did and did not receive dipyridamole (2.5% in each group) [30]. Subgroup analysis of data from the ESPRIT found a non-significant reduction in first cardiac events in subjects receiving aspirin plus dipyridamole as compared to aspirin alone (HR = 0.73, 95% CI 0.49 to 1.08) [29]. Therefore, there is no evidence of an increase in cardiac risk in patients receiving dipyridamole.

The Blockade of the Glycoprotein IIb/IIIa Receptor to Avoid Vascular Occlusion (BRAVO) trial randomized to 9190 patients (41% with cerebrovascular disease and 59% with coronary artery disease) to lotrafiban or placebo in addition to aspirin [31]. The primary end-point was the composite of all-cause mortality, myocardial infarction, stroke, recurrent ischemia requiring hospitalization, and urgent revascularization. There was no difference in the primary end-point (17.5% compared with 16.4%, HR = 0.94, 95% CI 0.85 to 1.03, p = 0.19) but a 33% increase in vascular mortality (HR = 1.33, 95% CI 1.03 to 1.72, p = 0.026) with lotrafiban.

The efficacy of trifusal (n = 1058) as compared to aspirin (n = 1055) in the prevention of vascular events (non-fatal stroke, non-fatal myocardial infarction or vascular death) in patients having a stroke or TIA within the prior 6 months was evaluated in the Trifusal versus Aspirin in Cerebral Infarction Prevention (TACIP) trial [32]. There were no treatment associated differences for the primary end-point (HR = 1.09, 95% CI 0.85 to 1.38, p = 0.647). Trifusal is not available in the United States.

The TRITON-TIMI 38 trial compared prasugrel, a more potent, third-generation, thienopyridine to clopidogrel in patients with acute coronary syndromes undergoing PCI. Overall, the trial showed a 19% relative benefit for prasugrel (p < 0.001) for the primary end-point of cardiovascular death, non-fatal myocardial infarction or non-fatal stroke [33]. The subgroup of patients with stroke or TIA prior to entry into the trial had poorer outcomes than the overall population, with no reduction in the primary endpoint (19.1% for prasugrel vs. 14.4 for placebo, p = 0.15), a higher rate of major bleeding (5.0% vs. 2.9%, p = 0.06), and higher all cause mortality (23.0% vs. 16.0%, = 0.04). The p-values for statistical interactions based on a history of stroke or TIA were significant for the primary endpoint and all cause mortality, suggesting a different response to prasugrel in these patients as compared to those without known cerebrovascular disease [33]. Although the overall rate of intracranial hemorrhage was not different between the two therapies, there was a higher rate of ICH with prasugrel among patients with prior TIA or stroke.

The Prevention Regimen for Effectively avoiding Second Strokes (PRoFESS) trial directly compared clopidogrel (75 mg/day) with the combination of aspirin (25 mg) and sustained-release dipyridamole (200 mg) twice daily in over 20,000 subjects having an ischemic stroke within the prior 90 days. Presented at the 2008 European Stroke Conference, the study found no difference between the groups for the primary end-point (recurrent stroke) or any of a series of secondary end-points, including myocardial infarction, over approximately 2.5 years of average follow-up.

Secondary prevention with antiplatelet agents versus warfarin in specific conditions

Several randomized trials directly compare aspirin and warfarin in particular circumstances. In patients with atrial fibrillation, a history of prior stroke or TIA carries a high risk of recurrent stroke (~10% per year). The European Atrial Fibrillation Trial found a non-significant 17% reduction (HR = 0.83, 95% CI 0.65 60 1.05, p = 0.12) in the risk of non-fatal stroke, non-fatal MI, vascular death or systemic embolization (the study's primary end-point) and a non-significant 14% reduction (HR = 0.86, 95% CI 0.64 to 1.15, p = 0.31) in the risk of stroke in patients with non-valvular atrial fibrillation and prior stroke or TIA treated with aspirin [34]. Oral anticoagulation (target INR 3.0) was more effective than aspirin in preventing the primary outcome (HR = 0.60, 95% CI 0.41 to 0.87, p = 0.008), largely due to a 62% reduction in fatal and non-fatal stroke (HR = 0.38, 95% CI 0.23 to 0.64, p < 0.001). Oral anticoagulation (INR 2-3) is recommended over aspirin in patients with non-valvular atrial fibrillation and prior stroke or TIA unless contraindicated [27].

The Warfarin Aspirin Recurrent Stroke Study (WARSS) was a double-blind, randomized trial that directly compared warfarin (INR 2-3) with aspirin (325 mg/day) in patients (n = 2206) with non-cardioembolic ischemic stroke [35]. Over 2 years, there was a non-significant advantage associated with aspirin treatment (17.8% rate of recurrent stroke or death for warfarin vs. 16.0% for aspirin, HR = 1.13, 95% CI 0.92 to 1.38, p = 0.25). Although there was not a significant increase in bleeding complications, given the increased costs and monitoring associated with warfarin, there is no reason to use warfarin for this purpose.

Retrospective data suggested that warfarin might be of greater benefit than aspirin in reducing stroke in patients with symptomatic large-vessel intracranial disease [36]. The prospective Warfarin-Aspirin Symptomatic Intracranial Disease (WASID) trial subsequently compared warfarin (INR 2–3) with aspirin (1300 mg/day) [37]. The rate of recurrent ischemic strokes, intracerebral hemorrhage or non-stroke vascular death did not differ between warfarin and aspirin (22% with warfarin vs. 21% with aspirin; HR = 1.04; 95% CI 0.73 to 1.48, p = 0.83). There was a higher rate of major hemorrhages with warfarin (8.3% vs. 3.2%, p = 0.01). Because of a lack of efficacy and a higher rate of bleeding complications, warfarin should generally not be used for patients with symptomatic large-vessel intracranial steno-occlusive disease.

Table 14.2 gives relevant treatment recommendations as reflected in the current American Heart Association/American Stroke Association guidelines for the use of antiplatelet drugs for the secondary prevention of ischemic stroke [27].

Table 14.2 AHA/ASA guidelines for the use of antiplatelet agents for the secondary prevention of ischemic stroke [27]

1. For patients with ischemic stroke or TIA with persistent or paroxysmal (intermittent) atrial fibrillation, anticoagulation with adjusted-dose warfarin (target INR, 2.5; range, 2.0 to 3.0) is recommended. For patients unable to take oral anticoagulants, aspirin 325 mg/day is recommended.

2. For patients with non-cardioembolic ischemic stroke or TIA, antiplatelet agents rather than oral anticoagulation are recommended to reduce the risk of recurrent stroke and other cardiovascular events. Aspirin (50 to 325 mg/day), the combination of aspirin and extended release dipyridamole, and clopidogrel are all acceptable options for initial therapy.

3. Compared with aspirin alone, both the combination of aspirin and extended-release dipyridamole and clopidogrel are safe. The combination of aspirin and extended-release dipyridamole is suggested instead of aspirin alone, and clopidogrel may be considered instead of aspirin alone on the basis of direct-comparison trials. Insufficient data are available to make evidence-based recommendations about choices between antiplatelet options other than aspirin. The selection of an antiplatelet agent should be individualized on the basis of patient risk factor profiles, tolerance, and other clinical characteristics.

4. The addition of aspirin to clopidogrel increases the risk of hemorrhage and is not routinely recommended for ischemic stroke or TIA patients.

5. For patients allergic to aspirin, clopidogrel is reasonable.

6. For patients who have an ischemic stroke while taking aspirin, there is no evidence that increasing the dose of aspirin provides additional benefit. Although alternative antiplatelet agents are often considered for non-cardioembolic patients, no single agent or combination has been studied in patients who have had an event while receiving aspirin.

Antiplatelet agents in acute ischemic stroke

The Multicenter Acute Stroke Trial-Italy tested the effect of aspirin alone and in combination with streptokinase in patients with acute ischemic stroke [38]. The trial was stopped because of increased mortality and intracranial hemorrhages among the patients who received the combination of aspirin and streptokinase. Too few patients were enrolled to detect an effect of aspirin alone.

In a factorial design, the International Stroke Trial compared placebo, aspirin (300 mg/day) or aspirin in combination with one of two doses of subcutaneously administered heparin in patients with acute ischemic stroke [39]. Treatment was started within 48 hours of symptom onset. There was a significant reduction in recurrent events with aspirin over the first 2 weeks with no effect on mortality. Patients assigned to receive aspirin had a significantly lower incidence of death and dependency after 6 months. The Chinese Acute Stroke Trial found a reduction in mortality and recurrent stroke during the 28 days of treatment [40]. Mortality was reduced with aspirin, but the long-term rates of death and disability were not improved.

A preplanned combined analysis of the 40,000 subjects randomized in the International Stroke Trial and the Chinese Acute Stroke Trial showed that early administration of aspirin was effective in reducing recurrent ischemic stroke, death or dependency that included a small, but significant, increase in hemorrhage risk [40]. As calculated from the data in the report, the risk of any recurrent stroke is reduced by 18% (RR = 0.18, 95% CI 0.07 to 0.28, p = 0.002) and the risk of stroke or death is reduced by 17% (RR = 0.17, 95% CI 0.06 to 0.27, p = 0.004).

Glycoprotein IIb/IIIa receptor antagonists have been used as adjuvant therapy in patients receiving endovascular therapy for acute ischemic stroke, but data from prospective, randomized trials are not available [41–43]. An open-label, uncontrolled MRI-guided study suggested possible benefit in patients treated with intravenous abciximab between 3 and 24 hours after symptom onset [44]. A randomized Phase II trial evaluating intravenous abciximab enrolled 400 patients within 6 hours of onset of ischemic stroke and suggested that treatment might be associated with an increased risk of brain hemorrhage (OR = 3.7, 95% CI 0.7 to 25.9, p = 0.09), but an overall improvement in favorable outcomes assessed after 3 months (OR = 1.20, 95% CI 0.84 to 1.70, p = 0.33) [45]. A subsequent Phase III trial was halted prematurely due to an unfavorable risk/benefit profile as assessed by the trial's independent data safety monitoring committee [46]. No other antiplatelet agent has been proven to be efficacious when given in the acute setting in patients with ischemic stroke.

Based in part on these results, it is recommended to start aspirin within the first 48 hours of ischemic stroke (unless the patient had been treated with intravenous rt-PA in which case antithrombotics are prohibited for the first 24 hours; Table 14.3) [47].

Table 14.3 AHA/ASA guidelines for the use of antiplatelet agents for acute ischemic stroke [46]

1. The oral administration of aspirin (initial dose is 325 mg) within 24 to 48 hours after stroke onset is recommended for treatment of most patients.

2. Aspirin should not be considered a substitute for other acute interventions for treatment of stroke, including the intravenous administration of rt-PA.

3. The administration of aspirin as an adjunctive therapy within 24 hours of thrombolytic therapy is not recommended.

4. The administration of clopidogrel alone or in combination with aspirin is not recommended for the treatment of acute ischemic stroke (the panel supported research testing the usefulness of emergency administration of clopidogrel in the treatment of patients with acute stroke).

5. Outside the setting of clinical trials, the intravenous administration of antiplatelet agents that inhibit the glycoprotein IIb/IIIa receptor is not recommended.

Summary

Treatment with platelet antiaggregants is associated with a reduced risk of stroke and vascular events in patients in whom the risk of these events is sufficiently high to outweigh the risk of bleeding complications. Although aspirin treatment is associated with a reduction in stroke in patients with non-valvular atrial fibrillation, there is additional benefit with warfarin for those at more than low risk (which includes those with a history of stroke or TIA). Platelet antiaggregants are also efficacious for the prevention of stroke and other vascular events in patients with a prior history of non-cardioembolic stroke or TIA with the choice of a specific drug or regimen individualized. There is no evidence for a difference in benefit in doses of aspirin ranging between 50 and 1300 mg/day. The combination of aspirin and sustained release dipyridamole is more efficacious than either drug alone. The combination of clopidogrel and aspirin is associated with an increase in bleeding complications but no reduction in vascular events in patients with prior stroke. There is no evidence that warfarin is superior to aspirin in patients with either non-cardioembolic stroke or symptomatic, large-vessel intracranial stenosis. Aspirin treatment is associated with a reduction in stroke and vascular events in patients with acute ischemic stroke. Controlled trials of other platelet antiaggregants in this setting are not currently available. The tables summarize relevant AHA/ASA guideline recommendations.

References

1 Antiplatelet Trialists' Collaboration. Collaborative overview of randomized trials of antiplatelet therapy – I: Prevention of death, myocardial infarction, and stroke by prolonged antiplatelet therapy in various categories of patients. *BMJ* 1994; **308**: 81–106.

2 Hayden M, Pigone M, Phillips C, Mulrow C. Aspirin for the primary prevention of cardiovascular events: a summary of the evidence for the US Preventive Services Task Force. *Ann Intern Med* 2002; **136**: 161–172.

3 Pearson TA, Blair SN, Daniels SR, Eckel RH, Fair JM, Fortmann SP, Franklin BA, Goldstein LB, Greenland P, Grundy SM, Hong Y, Miller NH, Lauer RM, Ockne IS, Sacco R, Sallis JF, Smith SC, Stone NJ, Taubert KA. AHA guidelines for primary prevention of cardiovascular disease and stroke: 2002 update. *Circulation* 2002; **106**: 388–391.

4 Ridker PM, Cannon CP, Morrow D, Rifai N, Rose LM, McCabe CH, Pfeffer MA, Braunwald E. C-reactive protein levels and outcomes after statin therapy. *New Engl J Med* 2005; **352**: 20–28.

5 ISIS-2 Collaborative Group. Randomized trial of intravenous streptokinase, oral aspirin, both, or neither among 17,187 cases of suspected acute myocardial infarction: ISIS-2. *Lancet* 1988; **2**: 349–360.

6 Yusuf S, Zhao F, Mehta SR, Chrolavicius S, Tognoni G, Fox KK. Effects of clopidogrel in addition to aspirin in patients with acute coronary syndromes without ST-segment elevation. *New Engl J Med* 2001; **345**: 494–502.

7 Chen ZM, Jiang LX, Chen YP, Xie JX, Pan HC, Peto R, Collins R, Liu LS. Addition of clopidogrel to aspirin in 45,852 patients with acute myocardial infarction: randomised placebo-controlled trial.[see comment]. *Lancet* 2005; **366**: 1607–1621.

8 Hart RG, Benavente O, McBride R, Pearce LA. Antithrombotic therapy to prevent stroke in patients with atrial fibrillation: a meta-analysis. *Ann Intern Med* 1999; **131**: 492–501.

9 Goldstein LB, Adams R, Alberts MJ, Appel LJ, Brass LM, Bushnell CD, Culebras A, Degraba TJ, Gorelick PB, Guyton JR, Hart RG, Howard G, Kelly-Hayes M, Nixon JV, Sacco RL. Primary prevention of ischemic stroke: a guideline from the American Heart Association/American Stroke Association Stroke Council. *Stroke* 2006; **37**: 1583–1633.

10 Halliday A, Mansfield A, Marro J, Peto C, Peto R, Potter J, Thomas D. Prevention of disabling and fatal strokes by successful carotid endarterectomy in patients without recent neurological symptoms: randomised controlled trial. *Lancet* 2004; **363**: 1491–1502.

11 Executive Committee for the Asymptomatic Carotid Atherosclerosis Study. Endarterectomy for asymptomatic carotid artery stenosis. *JAMA* 1995; **273**: 1421–1428.

12 Hobson RWI, Weiss DG, Fields WS, Goldstone J, Moore WS, Towne JB, Wright CB. Efficacy of carotid endarterectomy for asymptomatic carotid stenosis. *New Engl J Med* 1993; **328**: 221–227.

13 Mayo Asymptomatic Carotid Endarterectomy Study Group. Results of a randomized controlled trial of carotid endarterectomy for asymptomatic carotid stenosis. *Mayo Clin Proceed* 1992; **67**: 513–518.

14 Antithrombotic Trialists' Collaboration. Collaborative meta-analysis of randomized trials of antiplatelet therapy for the prevention of death, myocardial infarction, and stroke in high risk patients. *BMJ* 2002; **324**: 71–86.

15 Dutch TIA Trial Study Group. A comparison of two doses of aspirin (30 mg vs. 283 mg a day) in patients after a transient ischemic attack or minor ischemic stroke. *New Engl J Med* 1991; **325**: 1261–1266.

16 Farrell B, Godwin J, Richards S, Warlow C. The United Kingdom transient ischaemic attack (UK-TIA) aspirin trial: final results. *J Neurol Neurosurg Psych* 1991; **54**: 1044–1054.

17 Taylor DW, Barnett HJM, Haynes RB, Ferguson GG, Sackett DL, Thorpe KE, Simard D, Silver FL, Hachinski V, Clagett GP, Barnes R, Spence JD. Low-dose and high-dose acetylsalicylic acid for patients undergoing carotid endarterectomy: a randomised controlled trial. *Lancet* 1999; **353**: 2179–2184.

18 Derry S, Loke YK. Risk of gastrointestinal hemorrhage with long term use of aspirin: meta-analysis. *BMJ* 2000; **321**: 1183–1187.

19 Hass WK, Easton JD, Adams HPJ, Pryse-Phillips W, Molony BA, Anderson S, Kamm B, Ticlopidine Aspirin Study Group. A randomized trial comparing ticlopidine hydrochloride with aspirin for the prevention of stroke in high-risk patients. *New Engl J Med* 1989; **321**: 501–507.

20 Bennett CL, Davidson CJ, Raisch DW, Weinberg PD, Bennett RH, Feldman MD. Thrombotic thrombocytopenic purpura associated with ticlopidine in the setting of coronary artery stents and stroke prevention. *Arch Intern Med* 1999; **159**: 2524–2528.

21 Hankey GJ. Clopidogrel and thrombotic thrombocytopenic purpura. *Lancet* 2000; **356**: 269–270.

22 Weisberg LA. The efficacy and safety of ticlopidine and aspirin in non-whites: Analysis of a patient subgroup from the Ticlopidine Aspirin Stroke Study. *Neurology* 1993; **43**: 27–31.

23 Gorelick PB, Richardson D, Kelly M, Ruland S, Hung E, Harris Y, Kittner S, Leurgans S. Aspirin and ticlopidine for prevention of recurrent stroke in Black patients. *JAMA* 2003; **289**: 2947–2957.

24 CAPRIE Steering Committee. A randomised, blinded, trial of clopidogrel versus aspirin in patients at risk of ischaemic events (CAPRIE). *Lancet* 1996; **348**: 1329–1339.

25 Bhatt DL, Fox KA, Hacke W, Berger PB, Black HR, Boden WE, Cacoub P, Cohen EA, Creager MA, Easton JD, Flather MD, Haffner SM, Hamm CW, Hankey GJ, Johnston SC, Mak KH, Mas JL, Montalescot G, Pearson TA, Steg PG, Steinhubl SR, Weber MA, Brennan DM, Fabry-Ribaudo L, Booth J, Topol EJ. Clopidogrel and aspirin versus aspirin alone for the prevention of atherothrombotic events. *New Engl J Med* 2006; **354**: 1706–1717.

26 Diener H-C, Bogousslavsky J, Brass LM, Cimminiello C, Csiba L, Kaste M, Leys D, Matias-Guiu J, Rupprecht H-J. Aspirin and clopidogrel compared with clopidogrel alone after recent ischaemic stroke or transient ischaemic attack in high-risk patients (MATCH): randomised, double-blind, placebo-controlled trial. *Lancet* 2004; **364**: 331–337.

27 Sacco RL, Adams R, Albers G, Alberts MJ, Benavente O, Furie KL, Goldstein LB, Gorelick P, Halperin J, Harbaugh RE, Johnston SC, Katzan I, Kelly-Hayes M, Kenton EJ, Marks M, Schwamm LH, Tomsick T. Guidelines for prevention of stroke in patients

with ischemic stroke or transient ischemic attack. A statement for healthcare professionals from the American Heart Association/American Stroke Association Council on Stroke. *Stroke* 2006; **37**: 577–617.

28 Diener H, Cunha L, Forbes C, Sivenius J, Smets P, Lowenthal A. European Stroke Prevention Study 2. Dipyridamole and acetylsalicylic acid in the secondary prevention of stroke. *J Neurolog Sci* 1996; **143**: 1–13.

29 ESPRIT Study Group. Aspirin plus dipyridamole versus aspirin alone after cerebral ischaemia of arterial origin (ESPRIT): randomised controlled trial. *Lancet* 2006; **367**: 1665–1673.

30 Diener HC, Darius H, Bertrand-Hardy JM, Humphreys M. Cardiac safety in the European Stroke Prevention Study 2 (ESPS2). *Int J Clin Prac* 2001; **55**: 162–163.

31 Topol EJ, Easton D, Harrington RA, Amarenco P, Califf RM, Graffagnino C, Davis S, Diener HC, Ferguson J, Fitzgerald D, Granett J, Shuaib A, Koudstaal PJ, Theroux P, Van de Werf F, Sigmon K, Pieper K, Vallee M, Willerson JT. Randomized, double-blind, placebo-controlled, international trial of the oral IIb/IIIa antagonist lotrafiban in coronary and cerebrovascular disease. *Circulation* 2003; **108**: 399–406.

32 Matiás-Guiu J, Ferro JM, Alvarez-Sabin J, Torres F, Jiménez MD, Lago A, Melo TP. Comparison of triflusal and aspirin for prevention of vascular events in patients after cerebral infarction: the TACIP Study – a randomized, double-blind, multicenter trial. *Stroke* 2003; **34**: 840–848.

33 Wiviott SD, Braunwald E, McCabe CH, Montalescot G, Ruzyllo W, Gottlieb S, Neumann FJ, Ardissino D, De Servi S, Murphy SA, Riesmeyer J, Weerakkody G, Gibson CM, Antman EM. Prasugrel versus clopidogrel in patients with acute coronary syndromes. *New England Journal of Medicine* 2007; **357**: 2001–2015.

34 EAFT Study Group. Secondary prevention in non-rheumatic atrial fibrillation after transient ischaemic attack or minor stroke. *Lancet* 1993; **342**: 1255–1262.

35 Mohr JP, Thompson JLP, Lazar RM, Levin B, Sacco RL, Furie KL, Kistler JP, Albers GW, Pettigrew LC, Adams HPJ, Jackson CM, Pullicino P. A comparison of warfarin and aspirin for the prevention of recurrent ischemic stroke. *New Engl J Med* 2001; **345**: 1444–1451.

36 Chimowitz MI, Kokkinos J, Strong J, Brown MB, Levine SR, Silliman S, Pessin MS, Weichel E, Sila CA, Furlan AJ, Kargman DE, Sacco RL, Wityk RJ, Ford G, Fayad PB. The Warfarin-Aspirin Symptomatic Intracranial Disease study. *Neurology* 1995; **45**: 1488–1493.

37 Chimowitz MI, Lynn MJ, Howlett-Smith H, Stern BJ, Hertzberg VS, Frankel MR, Levine SR, Chaturvedi S, Kasner SE, Benesch CG, Sila CA, Jovin TG, Romano JG. Comparison of warfarin and aspirin for symptomatic intracranial arterial stenosis. *New Engl J Med* 2005; **352**: 1305–1316.

38 The Multicenter Acute Stroke Trial – Europe Study Group. Thrombolytic therapy with streptokinase in acute ischemic stroke. *New Engl J Med* 1996; **335**: 145–150.

39 International Stroke Trial Collaborative Group. The International Stroke Trial (IST): a randomised trial of aspirin, subcutaneous heparin, both, or neither among 19,435 patients with acute ischaemic stroke. *Lancet* 1997; **349**: 1569–1581.

40 Chen ZM, Sandercock P, Pan HC, Counsell C, Collins R, Liu LS, Xie JX, Warlow C, Peto R. Indications for early aspirin use in acute ischemic stroke. A combined analysis of 40 000 randomized patients from the Chinese Acute Stroke Trial and the International Stroke Trial. *Stroke* 2000; **31**: 1240–1249.

41 Lee KY, Heo JH, Lee SI, Yoon PH. Rescue treatment with abciximab in acute ischemic stroke. *Neurology* 2001; **56**: 1585–1587.

42 Eckert B, Koch C, Thomalla G, Roether J, Zeumer H. Acute basilar artery occlusion treated with combined intravenous abciximab and intra-arterial tissue plasminogen activator: report of 3 cases. *Stroke* 2002; **33**: 1424–1427.

43 Eckert B, Koch C, Thomalla G, Kucinski T, Grzyska U, Roether J, Alfke K, Jansen O, Zeumer H. Aggressive therapy with intravenous abciximab and intra-arterial rtPA and additional PTA/stenting improves clinical outcome in acute vertebrobasilar occlusion: combined local fibrinolysis and intravenous abciximab in acute verte-brobasilar stroke treatment (FAST): results of a multicenter study. *Stroke* 2005; **36**: 1160–1165.

44 Mitsias PD, Lu M, Silver B, Morris D, Ewing JR, Daley S, Lewandowski C, Katramados A, Papamitsakis NI, Ebadian HB, Zhao Q, Soltanian-Zadeh H, Hearshen D, Patel SC, Chopp M. MRI-guided, open trial of abciximab for ischemic stroke within a 3- to 24-hour window. *Neurology* 2005; **65**: 612–615.

45 Adams HP, Jr., Hacke W, Oemar B, Dávalos A, Cook RA, Trouillas P, Fazekas F, Bogousslavsky J, Hilburn J, Torner J, Leclerc J, Shuaib A, Reid P. Emergency administration of abciximab for treatment of patients with acute ischemic stroke – Results of a randomized phase 2 trial. *Stroke* 2005; **36**: 880–890.

46 The AbESTT-II Investigators. Abciximab in Emergent Stroke Treatment Trial-II (AbESTT-II): results of a randomized, double-blind placebo-control Phase 3 study. *Cerebrovasc Dis* 2006; **21** (Suppl. 4): 59.

47 Adams HP, Jr., del Zoppo G, Alberts MJ, Bhatt DL, Brass L, Furlan A, Grubb RL, Higashida RT, Jauch EC, Kidwell C, Lyden PD, Morgenstern LB, Qureshi AI, Rosenwasser RH, Scott PA, Wijdicks EF. Guidelines for the early management of adults with ischemic stroke. *Stroke* 2007; **38**: 1655–1711.

PART V

Special Circumstances

Chapter 15

Antiplatelet therapy and coronary bypass surgery: risks and benefits

A. Burdess, N.L. Cruden and K.A. Fox

Introduction

First pioneered in the 1960s [1,2], coronary artery bypass grafting (CABG) is an effective treatment for patients with ischemic heart disease. The major benefits afforded by CABG include a reduction in anginal symptoms and, in selected patients groups including those with left main stem or triple vessel disease, prognostic benefit [3,4].

Coronary artery bypass grafting, however, is not without risk. In the short term, like any major surgical procedure, CABG is associated with a pro-inflammatory, prothrombotic state, particularly when cardiopulmonary bypass is employed. Platelet activation and dysfunction is thought to play a key role in this process, which can lead to vascular occlusion, tissue ischemia and, ultimately, organ failure or infarction. Periprocedural myocardial infarction or necrosis occur in ~5–10% of patients and stroke in 1–2%. In the longer term, CABG does nothing to modify the underlying disease pathophysiology and, in some cases, may even accelerate atherosclerotic disease progression and hyperplasia in the native circulation. Based upon individual trials and meta-analysis, it appears that antiplatelet therapy improves mortality and reduces ischemic vascular events in patients with, or at risk of, vascular disease, including patients undergoing CABG [5,6]. However, antiplatelet therapy also increases the risks of bleeding.

Patients presenting with acute coronary syndromes (ACS) frequently undergo early invasive investigation with a view to urgent coronary revascularization Fast Revascularization During Instability in Coronary Artery Disease (FRISC),

Antiplatelet Therapy in Ischemic Heart Disease, 1st edition. Edited by Stephen D. Wiviott.
© 2009 American Heart Association, ISBN: 9-781-4051-7626-2

Randomized Intervention Trial of Unstable Angina (RITA), Treat Angina with Aggrastat and Determine Cost of Therapy with an Invasive or Conservative Strategy (TACTICS-TIMI 18), Can Rapid Risk Stratification of Unstable Angina Patients Suppress ADverse Outcomes with Early Implementation of the ACC/ AHA Guidelines (CRUSADE), Global Registry of Acute Coronary Events (GRACE) [7–11]. This strategy is supported in higher risk patients in American Heart Association and European Society of Cardiology guidelines [12,13]. Up to 14% of these patients currently undergo CABG during the index hospitalization, leading to a significant increase overall, in the number of patients undergoing CABG in the urgent setting [7,8,9]. Current guidelines on the management of patients with non-ST elevation ACS recommend that both aspirin and clopidogrel be administered on hospital admission and continued for 12 months [12,13]. In addition, these patients often receive treatment with intravenous glycoprotein IIb/IIIa inhibitors, further potentiating platelet inhibition. Within the trials of combined antiplatelet therapy in ACS, patients were predominantly managed by either medical means alone or in combination with percutaneous coronary revascularization. It remains unclear, therefore, whether the benefits of dual antiplatelet therapy extend to patients with ACS undergoing CABG, where the potential for thrombotic complications must be balanced against a significantly greater bleeding risk.

In this chapter, we will review the evidence for and against antiplatelet therapy in patients undergoing CABG, both in the setting of stable coronary artery disease and following an ACS.

CABG in patients with stable coronary artery disease

Aspirin

The clinical benefits of aspirin in patients with atherosclerotic coronary artery disease are firmly established [5,6]. In two large meta-analysis performed by the Antiplatelet and Antithrombotic Trialists' Collaborations, administration of aspirin to high-risk patients reduced vascular events by approximately 25% when compared to control [5,6]. In the setting of elective CABG, perioperative aspirin administration appears to reduce overall mortality and ischemic vascular events. In a multicenter, prospective observational study of 5436 patients, administration of aspirin within 48 hours of CABG reduced in-hospital mortality, ischemic vascular events (MI, stroke, bowel infarction) and renal failure by 68%, 58% and 60% respectively when compared to no aspirin [14]. This impressive mortality benefit was not seen in patients commencing aspirin therapy more than 48 hours after surgery. The benefits of aspirin in the immediate postoperative period were evident despite 42% of patients in the control group being treated with aspirin prior to the index admission and 17% receiving aspirin until the day of surgery [14]. Discontinuation of aspirin preoperatively was associated with a significant increase in the risk of death or ischemic vascular complications [14].

Two additional, large-scale studies provide further evidence of a reduction in mortality with preoperative aspirin administration. In a case – control study from a registry of 8641 patients undergoing CABG, Dacey *et al.* demonstrated a 27% reduction in in-hospital mortality associated with preoperative aspirin [15]. More recently, in a retrospective cohort study of 1636 consecutive patients undergoing CABG predominantly for stable coronary heart disease, preoperative aspirin administration was associated with a relative reduction in the risk of death of approximately 60% [16]. Although retrospective and non-randomized, these data lend further support for a treatment benefit with preoperative aspirin administration in patients undergoing CABG.

Only 75% of saphenous vein grafts remain patent at 10 years compared to 90% of arterial conduits [22] (AHA). Graft occlusion has important implications for recurrence of symptoms and event-free survival; one in five patients will develop a recurrence of angina within 1 year and a similar proportion will require further coronary revascularization within 10 years [17]. Aspirin has been demonstrated to improve short- and medium-term graft patency when administered in the immediate postoperative period and continued long term [6,18–22]. Preoperative administration of aspirin may reduce graft occlusion rates further [21,23] although this finding has not been universal [24].

Clopidogrel

The thienopyridines are an appropriate alternative to aspirin in patients with stable coronary artery disease undergoing CABG. Compared to placebo, ticlopidine improves early- and medium-term graft patency [25,26] but its widespread use is associated with a significant risk of blood dyscrasia. Clopidogrel has similar efficacy to ticlopidine in patients undergoing percutaneous coronary intervention [27], and a better hematological safety profile. When compared to aspirin in a large, randomized, controlled trial of patients with stable vascular disease, clopidogrel was marginally superior at preventing combined end-point of ischemic stroke, MI or vascular death [28]. *Post hoc* analysis suggested that in patients undergoing CABG, greater benefit was seen in the clopidogrel group [28]. Although there have been no randomized, controlled trials comparing clopidogrel with aspirin in the setting of CABG, there is sufficient evidence to support the use of clopidogrel as an appropriate alternative in patients intolerant of aspirin who are undergoing CABG.

Combined antiplatelet therapy

In contrast to patients with an ACS [29], the CHARISMA trial failed to demonstrate a significant benefit with combined aspirin and clopidogrel therapy when compared to aspirin alone in patients with stable vascular disease [30]. Although subgroup analysis suggested a possible benefit in symptomatic patients, this did not appear to extend to patients with a history of prior CABG [30].

Data comparing the efficacy of dual and single antiplatelet therapy in patients with stable coronary artery disease undergoing CABG are limited. In a non-randomized, single center, single surgeon, observational study of 591 patients undergoing off-pump CABG, postoperative clopidogrel use, in addition to aspirin, was associated with a reduction in angina, adverse cardiac events and mortality at 33 months [31].

Novel potential strategies

One disadvantage of both aspirin and clopidogrel is the irreversible nature of platelet inhibition. Indobufen is a reversible platelet cycolo-oxygenase inhibitor that permits recovery of platelet function within 24 hours of discontinuing therapy. When used in the setting of CABG it appears to be as effective as aspirin at maintaining saphenous vein graft patency at 1 year postoperatively [32,33]. An alternative potential strategy during cardiopulmonary bypass is the administration of inhaled nitric oxide and the prostacyclin analogue, iloprost. In a small, randomized, controlled trial, intraoperative treatment with this combination resulted in reduced circulating markers of platelet activation and less postoperative bleeding [34]. Further evaluation on a larger scale is required before this treatment can be recommended routinely for patients undergoing CABG.

CABG in patients with unstable coronary artery disease

Whilst the benefits of combined antiplatelet regimens in patients with ACS managed medically or undergoing urgent percutaneous coronary revascularization are clear, there have been no large-scale, randomized trials specifically examining the role of combined antiplatelet therapy in patients undergoing urgent surgical revascularization. In patients with ACS, the median time from hospitalization to surgery varies between 4 [35] and 26 days [36]. Delaying surgery to reverse the effect of antiplatelet therapy, with the associated risk of thrombotic complications, needs to be carefully balanced against the risk of bleeding if antiplatelet therapy is continued perioperatively. It also remains to be clarified whether patients undergoing CABG in the setting of an ACS would also benefit from *post*operative dual antiplatelet therapy as well as in the run up to surgery.

Aspirin

In patients with ACS, aspirin reduces the risk of future cardiovascular events by 30–50% [12]. Evidence of a benefit with aspirin therapy in patients with ACS undergoing CABG is based largely on extrapolation of older data from heterogeneous populations comprised largely of patients with stable coronary heart disease discussed earlier [5,6,14–16,70].

Aspirin and clopidogrel

Dual antiplatelet therapy with aspirin and clopidogrel reduces the rate of adverse cardiac outcomes when compared to aspirin alone among patients with non-ST segment elevation (NSTE) ACS [36], ST elevation myocardial infarction (STE) ACS or undergoing percutaneous coronary intervention (PCI) [37,38].

The Clopidogrel in Unstable Angina to Prevent Recurrent Events (CURE) trial demonstrated that addition of clopidogrel to aspirin in patients presenting with NSTE ACS, reduced the subsequent risk of death, myocardial infarction or stroke by 20% [36]. To date, this randomized trial provides the most robust data for antiplatelet therapy in patients with ACS in whom CABG is performed.

Subgroup analysis of the 2072 patients undergoing CABG revealed an overall relative reduction in adverse events similar to the entire study population (16.2% placebo, 14.5% clopidogrel, RR 0.89 for all CABG subjects, compared to 11.4% placebo, 9.3% clopidogrel, RR 0.80 for all CURE patients). However, this reduction was only significant for presurgical events in patients progressing to early CABG at the index hospitalization (n = 1013; placebo 4.7% clopidogrel 2.9%, RR 0.56). Postoperative clopidogrel use was not associated with a significant reduction in cardiovascular events, irrespective of the duration of time to CABG. This may in part be explained by the fact that clopidogrel was discontinued for a median of 10 days postsurgery and only re-started in 75% of cases.

Further data for patients with NSTE ACS undergoing urgent CABG are available from the observational CRUSADE Initiative 2004 (Can Rapid Risk Stratification of Unstable Angina Patients Suppress Adverse Outcomes With Early Implementation of the ACC/AHA Guidelines) [39]. Within this Registry, 3977 (9.4%) of 42,156 patients admitted with NSTE ACS underwent CABG, with detailed antiplatelet data available for 2858 patients. Clopidogrel was administered within 24 hours of admission in 852 (30%) patients undergoing CABG and surgery was performed within 5 days of the last dose of clopidogrel in 739 (87%) patients. In contrast to data from the CURE trial [36], subgroup analysis demonstrated no difference in in-hospital mortality, non-fatal myocardial infarction or shock for patients undergoing CABG within 5 days of catheterization with or without clopidogrel treatment. It should be noted, however, that the CRUSADE Registry, in contrast to CURE was observational and systematic assessment of postprocedural cardiac enzymes or clinical events was not mandatory.

The Clopidogrel as Adjunctive Reperfusion Therapy - Thrombolysis in Myocardial Infarction 28 (CLARITY-TIMI 28) trial (2005) demonstrated increased patency of the infarct-related artery and reduced mortality with combined aspirin and clopidogrel therapy compared with aspirin alone in patients with

STE ACS receiving fibrinolysis [40]. Of the 3491 patients randomized to the study, 136 (3.9%) underwent early CABG (66 receiving clopidogrel and 70 placebo). Although the composite end-point of cardiovascular death, recurrent myocardial infarction or ischemia (10 events (15.2%) in clopidogrel-treated patients and 15 events (21.4%) in placebo-treated patients (OR 0.66, 95% CI 0.27–1.63; P = 0.37) was consistent with the treatment effect in the overall CLARITY-TIMI 28 population (OR 0.80, CI 0.65–0.97; P = 0.03), the size of the CABG subgroup limits interpretation of these data. Moreover, only eight patients restarted clopidogrel following CABG. As in the CURE trial, the suggestion of benefit with clopidogrel was largely restricted to the preprocedure period, with 9.1% of those in the clopidogrel group experiencing a primary outcome event compared to 17.1% in the placebo group (OR 0.46, CI 0.16–1.36).

Glycoprotein (GP) IIb/IIIa antagonists

The use of glycoprotein IIb/IIIa inhibitors is associated with a reduction in thrombotic cardiovascular events in patients with an ACS undergoing PCI Evaluation of c7E3 to Prevent Ischemic Complications (EPIC), c7E3 Anti Platelet Therapy in Unstable Refractory angina (CAPTURE), Evaluation in PTCA to Improve Long-Term Outcome with Abciximab GP IIb/IIIa Blockade (EPILOG), Evaluation of Platelet IIb/IIIa Inhibitor for Stenting (EPISTENT) [41–44]. For those patients with ACS not undergoing coronary revascularization, meta-analysis of several large randomized, placebo-controlled trials involving 31,402 patients (including GUSTO IV-ACS) suggests that these agents may improve outcome only in high-risk patient subgroups [45]. These data also favor upstream administration of GP IIb/IIIa inhibitors (i.e. prior to PCI) in preference to deferred use (i.e. administration in the catheterization laboratory once an intervention is planned). Despite these data, evidence of a treatment benefit with GP IIb/IIIa inhibition in patients with ACS undergoing CABG is limited.

Pooled analysis of the 82 patients in the EPILOG and EPISTENT trials undergoing CABG during hospitalization for ACS suggested a trend towards a reduction in ischemic end-points in patients treated with the monoclonal antibody to the GP IIb/IIIa inhibitor, abciximab (14% vs. 24%, P >0.2) [43,44]. Almost two-thirds of these patients were operated on within 6 hours of discontinuing abciximab. A similar benefit has been demonstrated with the shorter acting reversible glycoprotein inhibitor, eptifibatide. In the PURSUIT trial, 78 patients underwent emergency CABG within 2 hours of eptifibatide cessation [46]. Perioperative myocardial infarction was significantly reduced in patients who received eptifibatide (46% vs. 22%, p <0.05). There was no difference in perioperative stroke (2.2% vs. 6.3%) or mortality (6.3% vs. 6.5%).

Interestingly, several studies have reported a platelet-sparing effect of glycoprotein IIb/IIIa inhibitors during cardiopulmonary bypass [46,47]. Whilst this has the potential to reduce the need for blood-related products, and in a particular platelet transfusion during CABG, the clinical benefits remain to be determined.

Combination of heparin, oral and intravenous antiplatelet agents: "quadruple therapy"

Evidenced-based guidelines on the management of ACS recommend treatment with low molecular weight or unfractionated heparin (or other antithrombotics, bivalirudin or fondaparinux), in addition to dual antiplatelet therapy [13]. Data from the Stenting and Antithrombotic Regimen (ISAR) trials, using the glycoprotein IIb/IIIa inhibitor, abciximab, suggest that in patients undergoing contemporary PCI for ACS, there is an additional benefit with abciximab therapy over and above that of dual aspirin and clopidogrel alone, but it is limited to higher-risk patients (those with an elevated troponin concentration) [48–51]. Whilst the administration of a glycoprotein IIb/IIIa inhibitor to patients in the CURE trial receiving aspirin, clopidogrel and heparin appeared to be well tolerated [36], there has been no specific study examining the safety and efficacy of this "quadruple therapy" in patients with ACS undergoing CABG. It is likely that emerging guidelines will base choice of antithrombotic regime, doses and timings on patient risk stratification and bleeding risk.

Bleeding and antiplatelet therapy in CABG

An obvious concern with platelet inhibition in patients undergoing CABG is the risk of perioperative bleeding complications. Whilst some factors, such as identification of patients with abnormal bleeding diatheses and improvements in surgical technique can be addressed, the extent of platelet inhibition remains a major determinant of bleeding risk.

The importance of major bleeding must not be underestimated. It is an independent predictor of death (Figure 15.1), is associated with a significant increased risk of recurrent ischemia (MI and stroke) regardless of baseline characteristics [52–54], and exposes patients to the need for blood and blood product transfusion and the risks of reoperation.

Aspirin

An increased risk of perioperative bleeding with aspirin use has been reported in many older studies [55,56–58]. More recent data suggests that the bleeding risk with perioperative aspirin administration is unlikely to exceed the expected clinical benefit [14–16]. In these latter studies, neither preoperative [15,16], nor postoperative aspirin administration [14] was associated with an increase in the risk of bleeding or bleeding-related morbidities. In many of the original trials of a routine, early invasive strategy in patients with ACS,

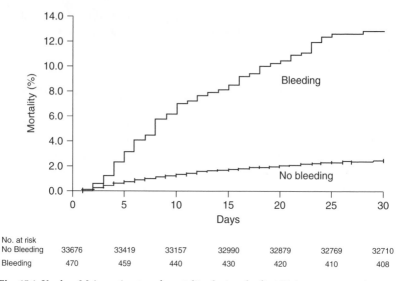

Fig. 15.1 Kaplan–Meier estimates of mortality during the first 30 days among patients who developed and those who did not develop major bleeding. Reproduced with permission from: Eikelboom, *et al. Circulation* 2006; **114**: 774–772.

patients were treated with aspirin and heparin with or without intravenous glycoprotein IIb/IIIa inhibition (TACTICS-TIMI 18, FRISC, RITA). Although these studies reported no significant increase in adverse bleeding, the timing of aspirin discontinuation was often not clear.

Aspirin and clopidogrel

Several small-scale trials and observational studies of combination therapy have produced conflicting evidence, with either no difference [59–61] or an increased risk of bleeding and bleeding-related complications [62–64] being reported. These studies have been confounded by lack of randomization, small sample size and variation in defined end-points. In addition, often no distinction is made between patients undergoing CABG in the setting of an ACS (where presurgical antiplatelet therapy is an essential part of medical therapy) and those undergoing CABG for stable coronary vascular disease. Given the differences in the extent of platelet inhibition, the bleeding risk could be expected to differ greatly between these two patient populations.

The most robust data for bleeding risk with dual antiplatelet therapy comes from the CURE study, which demonstrated a 1% absolute excess of major bleeding complications with the additional use of clopidogrel when compared to placebo in patients with ACS. There was no significant increase in life-threatening bleeding [36]. In the subgroup undergoing CABG, there was no excess of major (RR 1.27, P = 0.095 NS) or life-threatening bleeding (RR 1.24, P = 0.2 NS). However, where the clopidogrel was discontinued within 5 days of

CABG, the risk of bleeding (RR 1.53) outweighed any reduction in adverse events (RR 1.24) and if clopidogrel was discontinued on the day of, rather than 5 days prior to, surgery bleeding complications almost doubled. In contrast, there was no increase in bleeding risk (RR 0.83) in patients in whom clopidogrel was discontinued more than 5 days prior to surgery whilst the significant reduction in adverse events remained (RR 0.73). A *post hoc* analysis of the CURE data demonstrated that higher doses of aspirin increased bleeding risks irrespective of clopidogrel use without any reduction in primary end-points [65].

The CRUSADE registry demonstrated a 10% increase in the need for major red blood cell transfusion (4 or more units) with clopidogrel treatment in patients with ACS who underwent CABG [39]. This trend was still present even when patients receiving glycoprotein IIb/IIIa inhibitors were excluded. The rate of transfusion requirement returned to normal if surgery was performed more than 5 days after clopidogrel cessation.

In the subset of patients in CLARITY-TIMI 28 undergoing CABG, there were no significant differences in TIMI defined major bleeding events between CABG patients receiving clopidogrel or placebo (ARD 0.4%, P = 1.00), even when the medication was stopped less than 5 days before surgery (Absolute Risk Difference (ARD) 0.9%, P = 1.00) [40]. There was no excess in the need for reoperation for bleeding in the clopidogrel group. Significantly more CABG patients receiving clopidogrel required transfusion of 4 or more units compared to placebo (50% vs. 14%, P = 0.049). As in the CURE trial [36], there was a trend toward increased risk of TIMI major bleeding after CABG with increasing aspirin dose.

The TRITON-TIMI 38 trial compared prasugrel, a potent, third generation thienopyridine, to clopidogrel in patients with ACS undergoing planned PCI [66]. By design, coronary anatomy was to be known to be suitable for PCI, therefore a small number of subjects (approximately 3%) underwent CABG during the trial. However, among these patients a higher rate of TIMI major bleeding (13.4% vs. 3.2%, P <0.001) was observed with prasugrel.

Glycoprotein IIb/IIIa inhibition

Pooled data from the EPILOG and EPISTENT trials in patients with ACS demonstrated no increase in major bleeding and a trend towards a greater need for platelet transfusion (67% vs. 43% P = 0.09) in patients receiving abciximab [43,44]. A similar negative finding was reported in the EPIC trial, also using abciximab [41], although this may simply reflect the duration from abciximab administration to CABG (median >24 hours), allowing platelet function to recover. In the PURSUIT trial, 78 patients underwent CABG within 2 hours of eptifibatide cessation and no increase in bleeding complications was reported [46].

Summary

There is a clear role for antiplatelet agents in reducing the risk of ischemic thrombotic events in patients undergoing CABG.

Elective CABG, stable disease – low risk

Patients undergoing "elective" CABG (defined as stable on medical therapy and able to perform >5 metabolic equivalents by a standard BRUCE protocol) have previously had prolonged waiting times in some centers and some countries (at least 100 days in some centers), although waiting times are now very short in many countries. If patients were to wait for up to 100 days, it is estimated that 2–8 % will suffer a non-fatal ACS and 0.4–4% will die from a cardiovascular cause [67,68].

Urgent CABG – high risk

Not surprisingly, the risks of cardiovascular events are higher in patients requiring CABG in the setting of a recent ACS, although the waiting time is shorter [36,69]. The median time from hospitalization to surgery can range between 4 [36] and 26 days [11], with US centers having earlier operations. The mortality at 30 days in this population is estimated at 4–6% and the incidence of recurrent ischemia may be as high as 23–35% (GUSTO IIb). Whilst trial data are often criticized for not reflecting "real life", large-scale registries in ACS (GRACE, CRUSADE, CURE) report a similar 30 day in-hospital composite of death and re-infarction of ~5% (Table 15.1). The addition of clopidogrel

Table 15.1 Time course of outcome events occurring in the Clopidogrel in Unstable Angina to Prevent Recurrent Events (CURE) study. Reproduced with permission from: Yusuf S, *et al. Circulation* 2003; **107**: 966–972.

Time point/ outcome	% of events			
	Clopidogrel (n = 6259)	Placebo (n = 6303)	Relative risk (95% CI)	p
0 to 30 days				
Primary outcome (combined end-point of death from CV causes, non-fatal MI and stroke)	4.3	5.4	0.76 (0.67–0.92)	<0.004
Primary outcome and refractory ischemia	7.7	9.2	0.83 (0.73–0.93)	<0.002
30 days to 1 year				
Primary outcome	5.2	6.3	0.82 (0.70–0.95)	<0.01
Primary outcome and refractory ischemia	9.6	10.6	0.90 (0.80–1.01)	NS

(Continued)

Table 15.1 (Continued)

Time point/ outcome	% of events		Relative risk (95% CI)	P
	Clopidogrel (n = 6259)	Placebo (n = 6303)		
First 24 hours				
Primary outcome	0.4	0.5	0.80 (0.48–1.32)	NS
Primary outcome and severe ischemia (including refractory ischemia)	1.4	2.1	0.66 (0.51–0.86)	<0.003
0 to 7 days				
Primary outcome	2.1	2.5	0.82 (0.65–1.04)	NS
Primary outcome and refractory ischemia	3.5	4.2	0.82 (0.69–0.98)	<0.05
8 to 30 days				
Primary outcome	2.3	3.0	0.76 (0.61–0.94)	<0.05
Primary outcome and refractory ischemia	4.4	5.2	0.83 (0.71–0.98)	<0.05

CV = cardiovascular; MI = myocardial infarction.

to standard therapy, including aspirin and heparin, in patients with an ACS reduced the combined cardiovascular event rate in patients awaiting CABG from 4.7 to 2.9% when compared to placebo [36]. Thus antiplatelet therapy has a key role to play in protecting patients awaiting CABG from thrombotic cardiovascular events.

The benefits afforded by these regimens, however, must be balanced against a potential increase in the risk of bleeding and associated complications. The incidence of major bleeding during hospitalization for an ACS can be as high as 5% in high-risk groups (low-risk groups ~1%), with subsequent CABG surgery carrying its own additional 5% risk. Thus, in some patient populations, the risk of bleeding may approach or even exceed that of refractory ischemia, myocardial infarction or death. *In patients with stable ischemic heart disease*

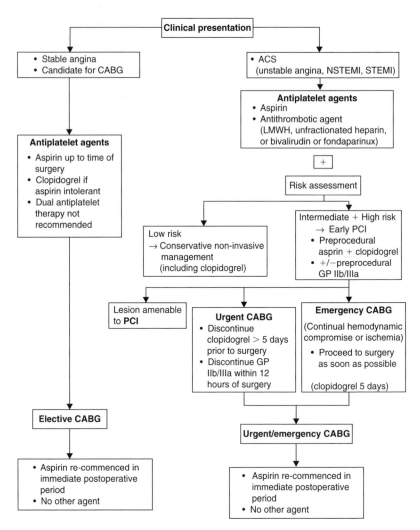

Fig. 15.2 Management algorithm. Reproduced with permission from Salim Yusuf, Shamir R. Mehta, Feng Zhao *et al*. Early and late Effect of Clopidogrel in Patients with Acute Coronary Syndromes. *Circulation* 2003; **107**: 966–972.

undergoing CABG, aspirin alone would appear the most appropriate antiplatelet regimen (Figure 15.2 and Table 15.2). Whilst, in patients undergoing CABG in the setting of a recent ACS, careful consideration must be given to the thrombotic and bleeding risks, duration and type of antiplatelet therapy, as well as the timing of bypass surgery (Figure 15.2 and Table 15.2). Current guidelines recommend that both aspirin and clopidogrel be administered to patients with ACS from admission. In those subsequently referred for CABG, current data

Table 15.2 Recommendations

1. Aspirin administered perioperatively and continued indefinitely improves saphenous vein graft patency, reduces subsequent ischemic vascular events and improves survival.

2. The best protection and bleeding profile is associated with a 75 mg to 100 mg dose of aspirin.

3. Where patients are intolerant to aspirin, clopidogrel is an appropriate alternative.

4. The routine use of combined antiplatelet therapy in patients undergoing coronary artery bypass grafting in the setting of stable coronary artery disease is not recommended.

5. In patients undergoing URGENT coronary artery bypass grafting in the setting of a recent acute coronary syndrome clopidogrel, in addition to aspirin, appears to be of benefit pre-operatively, but where possible should be discontinued at least 5 days prior to operation. The routine use of clopidogrel post-operatively, in addition to aspirin, is not recommended.

would suggest that clopidogrel should be discontinued at least 5 days prior to surgery. In patients deemed at high risk of further ischemic events, "bridging therapy" with a short-acting intravenous glycoprotein IIb/IIIa inhibitor (in place of clopidogrel) and discontinued at least 12 hours before CABG would seem a logical alternative, although this strategy remains, as yet, unproven.

Emergency CABG – very high risk

There are a small proportion of patients presenting with an ACS with refractory ischemia or with continuing hemodynamic compromise that are referred for "emergency" CABG, and will undergo surgery within 5 days of clopidogrel therapy. In the CURE trial, 66 patients (3.2%) underwent "emergency" CABG [36]. These high-risk patients face a significant thrombotic threat in addition to an increased bleeding risk. There is no evidence to support a role for routine administration of dual antiplatelet therapy following CABG in patients suffering a recent ACS.

References

1 Garrett HE, Dennis EW, DeBakey ME. Aortocoronary bypass with saphenous vein graft. Seven-year follow-up. *JAMA* 1973; **223**: 792–794.
2 Favaloro RG. Saphenous vein graft in the surgical treatment of coronary artery disease. Operative technique. *J Thorac Cardiovasc Surg* 1969; **58**: 178–185.

3 Yusuf S, Zucker D, Peduzzi P, *et al*. Effect of coronary artery bypass graft surgery on survival: overview of 10-year results from randomised trials by the Coronary Artery Bypass Graft Surgery Trialists Collaboration. *Lancet* 1994; **344**: 563–670.

4 Davis KB, Chaitman B, Ryan T, Bittner V, Kennedy JW. Comparison of 15-year survival for men and women after initial medical or surgical treatment for coronary artery disease: a CASS registry study. Coronary Artery Surgery Study. *J Am Coll Cardiol* 1995; **25**: 1000–1009.

5 Collaborative meta-analysis of randomised trials of antiplatelet therapy for prevention of death, myocardial infarction, and stroke in high risk patients. *BMJ* 2002; **324**: 71–86.

6 Antiplatelet Trialists' Collaboration. Collaborative overview of randomised trials of antiplatelet therapy – II: Maintenance of vascular graft or arterial patency by antiplatelet therapy. *BMJ* 1994; **308**: 159–168.

7 Largerqvist B, *et al*. 5-year outcomes in the FRISC-II randomised trial of an invasive versus a non-invasive strategy in non-ST-elevation acute coronary syndrome: a follow-up study. *Lancet* 2006; **368**: 998–1004.

8 Fox KA, *et al*. 5-year outcome of an interventional strategy in non-ST-elevation acute coronary syndrome: the British Heart Foundation RITA 3 randomised trial. *Lancet* 2005; **366**: 914–920.

9 Cannon CP *et al*. Invasive versus conservative strategies in unstable angina and non-Q-wave myocardial infarction following treatment with tirofiban: rationale and study design of the international TACTICS-TIMI 18 Trial. Treat Angina with Aggrastat and determine Cost of Therapy with an Invasive or Conservative Strategy. Thrombolysis In Myocardial Infarction. *Am J Cardiol* 1998; **82**: 731–736.

10 Bhatt DL, *et al*. Utilization of early invasive management strategies for high-risk patients with non-ST-segment elevation acute coronary syndromes: results from the CRUSADE Quality Improvement Initiative. *JAMA* 2004; **292**: 2096–2104.

11 Fox KA, *et al*. Intervention in acute coronary syndromes: do patients undergo intervention on the basis of their risk characteristics? The Global Registry of Acute Coronary Events (GRACE). *Heart* 2007; **93**: 177–182.

12 Anderson JL, Adams CD, Antman EM, et al. ACC/AHA 2007 guidelines for the management of patients with unstable angina/non–ST-elevation myocardial infarction: a report of the American College of Cardiology/American Heart Association Task Force on Practice Guidelines (Writing Committee to Revise the 2002 Guidelines for the Management of Patients With Unstable Angina/Non–ST-Elevation Myocardial Infarction). *Circulation*. 2007; **116**: e148–e304.

13 Bassand JP, Hamm CW, Ardissino D, Boersma E, Budaj A, Fernandez-Aviles F, *et al*. Guidelines for the diagnosis and treatment of non-ST-segment elevation acute coronary syndromes: The Task Force for the Diagnosis and Treatment of Non-ST-Segment Elevation Acute Coronary Syndromes of the European Society of Cardiology. *Eur Heart J* 2007; **28**: 1598–1660.

14 Mangano DT. Aspirin and mortality from coronary bypass surgery. *New Engl J Med* 2002; **347**: 1309–1317.

15 Dacey LJ, Munoz JJ, Johnson ER, *et al*. Effect of preoperative aspirin use on mortality in coronary artery bypass grafting patients. *Ann Thorac Surg* 2000; **70**: 1986–1990.

16 Bybee KA, Powell BD, Valeti U, *et al*. Preoperative aspirin therapy is associated with improved postoperative outcomes in patients undergoing coronary artery bypass grafting. *Circulation* 2005; **112**: 1286–1292.

17 Motwani JG, Topol EJ. Aortocoronary saphenous vein graft disease: pathogenesis, predisposition, and prevention. *Circulation* 1998; **97**: 916–931.

18 Chesebro JH, Fuster V, Elveback LR, *et al.* Effect of dipyridamole and aspirin on late vein-graft patency after coronary bypass operations. *New Engl J Med* 1984; **310**: 209–214.

19 Brown BG, Cukingnan RA, DeRouen T, *et al.* Improved graft patency in patients treated with platelet-inhibiting therapy after coronary bypass surgery. *Circulation* 1985; **72**: 138–146.

20 Gavaghan TP, Gebski V, Baron DW. Immediate postoperative aspirin improves vein graft patency early and late after coronary artery bypass graft surgery. A placebo-controlled, randomized study. *Circulation* 1991; **83**: 1526–1533.

21 Goldman S, Copeland J, Moritz T, *et al.* Improvement in early saphenous vein graft patency after coronary artery bypass surgery with antiplatelet therapy: results of a Veterans Administration Cooperative Study. *Circulation* 1988; **77**: 1324–1332.

22 Goldman S, Zadina K, Moritz T, *et al.* Long-term patency of saphenous vein and left internal mammary artery grafts after coronary artery bypass surgery: results from a Department of Veterans Affairs Cooperative Study. *J Am Coll Cardiol* 2004; **44**: 2149–2156.

23 Goldman S, Copeland J, Moritz T, *et al.* Saphenous vein graft patency 1 year after coronary artery bypass surgery and effects of antiplatelet therapy. Results of a Veterans Administration Cooperative Study. *Circulation* 1989; **80**: 1190–1197.

24 Goldman S, Copeland J, Moritz T, *et al.* Starting aspirin therapy after operation. Effects on early graft patency. Department of Veterans Affairs Cooperative Study Group. *Circulation* 1991; **84**: 520–526.

25 Chevigne M, David JL, Rigo P, Limet R. Effect of ticlopidine on saphenous vein bypass patency rates: a double-blind study. *Ann Thorac Surg* 1984; **37**: 371–378.

26 Limet R, David JL, Magotteaux P, Larock MP, Rigo P. Prevention of aorta-coronary bypass graft occlusion. Beneficial effect of ticlopidine on early and late patency rates of venous coronary bypass grafts: a double-blind study. *J Thorac Cardiovasc Surg* 1987; **94**: 773–783.

27 Muller C, Buttner HJ, Petersen J, Roskamm H. A randomized comparison of clopidogrel and aspirin versus ticlopidine and aspirin after the placement of coronary-artery stents. *Circulation* 2000; **101**: 590–593.

28 A randomised, blinded, trial of clopidogrel versus aspirin in patients at risk of ischaemic events (CAPRIE). CAPRIE Steering Committee. *Lancet* 1996; **348**: 1329–1339.

29 Yusuf S, Zhao F, Mehta SR, Chrolavicius S, Tognoni G, Fox KK. Effects of clopidogrel in addition to aspirin in patients with acute coronary syndromes without ST-segment elevation. *New Engl J Med* 2001; **345**: 494–502.

30 Bhatt DL, Fox KA, Hacke W, *et al.* Clopidogrel and aspirin versus aspirin alone for the prevention of atherothrombotic events. *New Engl J Med* 2006; **354**: 1706–1717.

31 Gurbuz AT, Zia AA, Vuran AC, Cui H, Aytac A. Postoperative clopidogrel improves mid-term outcome after off-pump coronary artery bypass graft surgery: a prospective study. *Eur J Cardiothorac Surg* 2006; **29**: 190–195.

32 Rajah SM, Nair U, Rees M, *et al.* Effects of antiplatelet therapy with indobufen or aspirin-dipyridamole on graft patency one year after coronary artery bypass grafting. *J Thorac Cardiovasc Surg* 1994; **107**: 1146–1153.

33 Cataldo G, Heiman F, Lavezzari M, Marubini E. Indobufen compared with aspirin and dipyridamole on graft patency after coronary artery bypass surgery: results of a combined analysis. *Coron Artery Dis* 1998; **9**: 217–222.

34 Chung A, Wildhirt SM, Wang S, Koshal A, Radomski MW. Combined administration of nitric oxide gas and iloprost during cardiopulmonary bypass reduces platelet dysfunction: a pilot clinical study. *J Thorac Cardiovasc Surg* 2005; **129**: 782–790.

35 Boersma E, Pieper KS, Steyerberg EW, *et al*. Predictors of outcome in patients with acute coronary syndromes without persistent ST-segment elevation. *Circulation* 2000; **101**: 2557–2567.

36 Fox KA, *et al*. Benefits and risks of the combination of clopidogrel and aspirin in patients undergoing surgical revascularization for non-ST-elevation acute coronary syndrome: the Clopidogrel in Unstable angina to prevent Recurrent ischemic Events (CURE) Trial. *Circulation* 2004; **110**: 1202–1208.

37 Steinhubl SR, *et al*. Early and sustained dual oral antiplatelet therapy following percutaneous coronary intervention: a randomized controlled trial. *JAMA* 2002; **288**: 2411–2420.

38 Mehta SR, *et al*. Effects of pretreatment with clopidogrel and aspirin followed by long-term therapy in patients undergoing percutaneous coronary intervention: the PCI-CURE study. *Lancet* 2001; **358**: 527–533.

39 Mehta RH, *et al*. Acute clopidogrel use and outcomes in patients with non-ST segment elevation acute coronary syndromes undergoing coronary artery bypass surgery. *J Am Coll Cardiol.* 2006; **48**: 281–286.

40 McLean DS, *et al*. Benefits and risks of clopidogrel pretreatment before coronary artery bypass grafting in patients with ST-elevation myocardial infarction treated with fibrinolytics in CLARITY-TIMI 28. *J Thromb Thrombolysis* 2007; **24**: 85–91.

41 EPIC Investigation, , Use of a monoclonal antibody directed against the platelet glycoprotein IIb/IIIa receptor in high-risk coronary angioplasty. *New Engl J Med* 1994; **330**: 956–961.

42 CAPTURE Investigators. Randomized placebo-controlled trial of abciximab before and during coronary intervention in refractory unstable angina: the CAPTURE Study. *Lancet* 1997; **349**: 1429–1435.

43 EPILOG Investigators, Platelet glycoprotein IIb/IIIa receptor blockade and low-dose heparin during percutaneous coronary revascularization. *New Engl J Med* 1997; **336**: 1689–1696.

44 EPISTENT Investigators (Evaluation of Platelet IIb/IIIa Inhibitor for Stenting). Randomized placebo-controlled and balloon-angioplasty-controlled trial to assess safety of coronary stenting with use of platelet glycoprotein-IIb/IIIa blockade. *Lancet* 1998; **352**: 87–92.

45 Boersma E, Harrington RA, Moliterno DJ, White H, Theroux P, Van de Werf F, *et al*. Platelet glycoprotein IIb/IIIa inhibitors in acute coronary syndromes: a meta-analysis of all major randomised clinical trials. *Lancet* 2002; **359**, 189–198.

46 Dyke CM, Bhatia D, Lorenz TJ, *et al*. Immediate coronary artery bypass surgery after platelet inhibition with eptifibatide: results from PURSUIT. Platelet Glycoprotein IIb/IIIa in unstable Angina: Receptor Suppression Using Integrelin Therapy. *Ann Thorac Surg* 2000; **70**: 866–871.

47 Bizzari F, Scolletta S, Tucci E, *et al*. Perioperative use of tirofiban hydrochloride (Aggrastat) does not increase surgical bleeding after emergency or urgent coronary artery bypass grafting. *J Thorac Cardiovasc Surg* 2001; **122**: 1181–1185.

48 Bromberg-Marin G, *et al*. Effectiveness and safety of glycoprotein IIb/IIIa inhibitors and clopidogrel alone and in combination in non-ST-segment elevation myocardial infarction (from the National Registry of Myocardial Infarction-4). *Am J Cardiol* 2006; **98**: 1125–1131.

49 Silva MA, *et al*. Platelet inhibitors in non-ST-segment elevation acute coronary syndromes and percutaneous coronary intervention: glycoprotein IIb/IIIa inhibitors, clopidogrel, or both? *Vasc Health Risk Manag* 2006; **2**: 39–48.

50 Kastrati A, Mehilli J, Neumann FJ, Dotzer F, ten Berg J, Bollwein H, Graf I, Ibrahim M, Pache J, Seyfarth M, Schühlen H, Dirschinger J, Berger PB, Schömig A; Intracoronary Stenting and Antithrombotic: Regimen Rapid Early Action for Coronary Treatment 2 (ISAR-REACT 2) Trial Investigators. Abciximab in patients with acute coronary syndromes undergoing percutaneous coronary intervention after clopidogrel pretreatment: the ISAR-REACT 2 randomized trial. *JAMA*. 2006; **295**: 1531-1538.

51 Mehilli J, *et al*. Randomized clinical trial of abciximab in diabetic patients undergoing elective percutaneous coronary interventions after treatment with a high loading dose of clopidogrel. *Circulation* 2004; **110**: 3627–3635.

52 Eikelboom JW, Mehta SR, Anand SS, Xie C, Fox KAA, Yusuf S. Adverse impact of bleeding on prognosis in patients with acute coronary syndromes. *Circulation* 2006; **114**: 774–782.

53 Moscucci M, Fox KAA, Cannon CP, *et al*. Predictors of major bleeding in acute coronary syndromes: the Global Registry of Acute Coronary Events (GRACE). *Eur Heart J* 2003; **24**: 1815–1823.

54 Yang X, Alexander KP, Chen AY, Roe MT, Brindis RG, Rao SV, Gibler WB, Ohman EM, Peterson ED; CRUSADE Investigators. The implications of blood transfusions for patients with non-ST-segment elevation acute coronary syndromes: results from the CRUSADE National Quality Improvement Initiative. *J Am Coll Cardiol* 2005; **46**: 1490–1495.

55 Goldman S, Copeland J, Moritz T, *et al*. Starting aspirin therapy after operation. Effects on early graft patency. Department of Veterans Affairs Cooperative Study Group. *Circulation* 1991; **84**: 520–526.

56 Ferraris VA, Ferraris SP. 1988: Preoperative aspirin ingestion increase in operative blood loss after coronary artery bypass grafting. Updated in 1995. *Ann Thorac Surg* 1995; **59**: 1036–1037.

57 Ferraris VA, Ferraris SP, Joseph O, Wehner P, Mentzer RM, Jr. Aspirin and postoperative bleeding after coronary artery bypass grafting. *Ann Surg* 2002; **235**: 820–827.

58 Sethi GK, Copeland JG, Goldman S, Moritz T, Zadina K, Henderson WG. Implications of preoperative administration of aspirin in patients undergoing coronary artery bypass grafting. Department of Veterans Affairs Cooperative Study on Antiplatelet Therapy.*J Am Coll Cardiol* 1990; **15**: 15–20.

59 Cannon CP, Shamir MR, Aranki SF. Balancing the benefit and risk of oral antiplatelet agents in coronary artery bypass surgery. *Ann Thorac Surg* 2005; **80**: 768–779.

60 Karabulut H, Toraman F, Evrenkaya S, Goksel O, Tarcan S, Alhan C. Clopidogrel does not increase bleeding and allogenic blood transfusion in coronary artery surgery. *Eur J Cardiothorac Surg* 2004; **25**: 419–423.

61 Carpino PA, Bojar RM, Khabbaz KR, Rastegar H, Warner KG. Clopidogrel therapy prior to coronary artery bypass surgery does not increase bleeding complications or use of blood products. (Abstract S120). *Crit Care Med* 2001; **29** (Suppl.): 314.

62 Chu MWA, Wilson SR, Novick RJ, Stitt LW, Quantz MA. Does clopidogrel increase blood loss following coronary artery bypass surgery? *Ann Thorac Surg* 2004; **78**: 1536–1541.

63 Hongo RH, Ley J, Dick SE, Yee RR. The effect of clopidogrel in combination with aspirin when given before coronary artery bypass grafting. *J Am Coll Cardiol* 2002; **40**: 231–237.

64 Kapetanakis EI, Medlam DA, Boyce SW, Haile E, Hill PC, Dullum MKC, Bafi AS, Petro KR, Corso PJ. Clopidogrel administration prior to coronary artery bypass grafting surgery: the cardiologist's panacea or the surgeon's headache? *Eur Heart J* 2005; **26**: 576–583.

65 Peters RJ, *et al*. Effects of aspirin dose when used alone or in combination with clopidogrel in patients with acute coronary syndromes: observations from the Clopidogrel in Unstable angina to prevent Recurrent Events (CURE) study. *Circulation* 2003; **108**: 1682–1687.

66 Wiviott SD, Braunwald E, McCabe CH, *et al*. Prasugrel versus clopidogrel in patients with acute coronary syndromes. *New Engl J Med* 2007; **357**: 2001–2015.

67 Cesena FH, Favarato D, *et al*. Cardiac complications during waiting for elective coronary artery bypass graft surgery: incidence, temporal distribution and predictive factors. *Eur J Cardio-thorac* 2004; **25**: 196–202.

68 Ray AA, Buth KJ, *et al*. Waiting for cardiac surgery: results of a risk-stratified queuing process. *Circulation* 2001: **104** (Suppl. 1): 192–198.

69 Solodky A, *et al*. The outcome of coronary artery bypass grafting surgery among patients hospitalized with acute coronary syndrome: the Euro Heart Survey of acute coronary syndrome experience. *Cardiology* 2005; **103**: 44–47.

70 Eagle KA, Guyton RA, Davidoff R, et al. ACC/AHA 2004 guideline update for coronary artery bypass graft surgery: a report of the American College of Cardiology/American Heart Association Task Force on Practice Guidelines (Committee to Update the 1999 Guidelines for Coronary Artery Bypass Graft Surgery). *Circulation*. 2004; **110**: e340–e438.

Chapter 16

Management of antiplatelet therapy for non-cardiac surgery

Nisheeth Goel, John F. Canales and James J. Ferguson

Introduction

Antiplatelet therapy has been shown to be extremely effective in reducing adverse cardiovascular events in a variety of cardiovascular disease patient populations. While antiplatelet therapy may also frequently be discontinued prior to non-cardiac surgery to decrease the risk of intra- or postoperative bleeding, several studies suggest that discontinuing antiplatelet therapy in certain populations can also be associated with adverse clinical outcomes. The perioperative management of antiplatelet therapy is a complex problem which requires clinicians to balance the inherent risk of bleeding that comes along with the use of antiplatelet drugs with the risk of adverse cardiovascular events that can be associated with their discontinuation (Table 16.1, Figure 16.1). This chapter will review the rationale for antiplatelet therapy, cover issues surrounding continuing and discontinuing antiplatelet therapy in the perioperative period, and present a risk/ benefit-based strategy for approaching the perioperative management of patients on antiplatelet therapy.

Rationale for antiplatelet therapy

The role of aspirin in the treatment of cardiovascular disease is well established. A comprehensive meta-analysis has demonstrated that aspirin reduces the outcome of non-fatal myocardial infarction by one-third, non-fatal stroke by one-quarter and vascular mortality by one-sixth in patients with high annual risk of a vascular event [1]. Dual antiplatelet therapy with aspirin and

Antiplatelet Therapy in Ischemic Heart Disease, 1st edition. Edited by Stephen D. Wiviott.
© 2009 American Heart Association, ISBN: 9-781-4051-7626-2

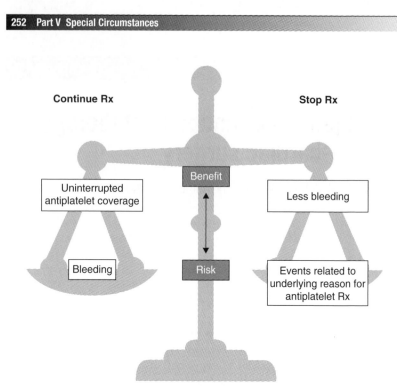

Fig. 16.1 Balance of the benefits (uninterrupted coverage versus less bleeding) and the risks (bleeding versus clinical events related to the underlying pathology), respectively.

Table 16.1 Issues with antiplatelet therapy in non-cardiac surgery

Surgery in patients on chronic antiplatelet therapy
Patients with drug-eluting stents
Patients with bare-metal stents
Patients with atherosclerosis
Coronary disease
Cerebrovascular disease
Peripheral vascular disease
Other indications for chronic antiplatelet therapy

thienopyridines has been shown to be superior to aspirin monotherapy in patients with a history of symptomatic atherothrombosis (myocardial infarction, stroke or peripheral vascular disease) [2], acute coronary syndromes [3,4], and in patients undergoing percutaneous coronary intervention (PCI) [5].

In the modern era, PCI with stent implantation has become the dominant revascularization strategy for patients with occlusive coronary artery disease.

Stent thrombosis is a rare but catastrophic complication of stent implantation that usually presents with ST-elevation myocardial infarction or death. Stent thrombosis can occur within 24 hours of stent implantation (early), within 30 days (subacute), within 1 year (late), or after 1 year (very late) of stent placement. Early trials evaluating stent implantation demonstrated a 20% incidence of stent thrombosis [6]. Adoption of dual antiplatelet therapy with aspirin and thienopyridines for 4 weeks after bare-metal stent (BMS) implantation dramatically reduced the incidence of early and subacute stent thrombosis as compared to aspirin plus warfarin or aspirin alone [5,7,8]. A pooled analysis of 6186 patients receiving BMS and dual antiplatelet therapy demonstrated an incidence of 0.9% of subacute stent thrombosis [9].

Randomized, controlled trials have also demonstrated the efficacy of long-term dual antiplatelet therapy in patients undergoing percutaneous coronary intervention (PCI). In Clopidogrel for the Reduction of Events During Observation (CREDO) trial, 2116 patients were randomly assigned to either pretreatment with 300-mg dose of clopidogrel or placebo 3 to 24 hours prior to PCI. All patients received clopidogrel, 75 mg daily, for 28 days. Thereafter, patients in the loading dose group received clopidogrel for 12 months and those in the control group received placebo. All patients received standard therapy with aspirin. At 1 year, long-term clopidogrel therapy was associated with a 27% relative risk reduction in the combined risk of death, MI or stroke [10]. Similar results of long-term dual antiplatelet therapy after PCI were reported in PCI-CURE study. Patients on both aspirin and clopidogrel had a 31% relative risk reduction in cardiovascular death or myocardial infarction at 1 year [11]. Based on the above observations, there is a compelling argument for dual antiplatelet therapy in patients receiving BMS for at least 1 month and up to 1 year.

Drug-eluting stents (DES) have largely replaced bare-metal stents in modern clinical practice after randomized controlled trials demonstrated decreased rates of in-stent stenosis and target lesion revascularization [12–14]. However, late thrombosis has been noted in DES months to years after implantation [15–17]. DES are associated with incomplete neointimal coverage [18] and hypersensitivity reactions [19,20], which may predispose them to late thrombosis. In an angioscopic study of 37 consecutively stented coronary artery lesions at 3 to 6 months after stent implantation, only 2/15 lesions treated with sirolimus-eluting stents demonstrated complete neointimal coverage. In contrast, all lesions treated with BMS demonstrated complete coverage at follow-up. Thrombi were more common in patients with incomplete coverage of stent struts [18]. In addition, several studies have reported increased incidence of stent thrombosis in DES once protocol-mandated dual antiplatelet therapy has been discontinued. This was illustrated in a study of 746 patients randomized to DES or BMS for 18 months. All patients received 6 months of aspirin and clopidogrel after which only aspirin was continued. After discontinuation of clopidogrel, stent thrombosis occurred more frequently in the DES group compared to BMS group (2.6% vs. 1.3%) [21]. Bavry *et al.* conducted a meta-analysis of 14 trials comparing DES to BMS, involving 6675 patients. The duration of dual antiplatelet therapy ranged from 2 to 6 months in all but one of the included trials. The incidence of late thrombosis (>6 months) was noted to be 4.4 events per 1000 DES patients compared to 0.6 events per 1000 patients implanted with BMS. The incidence of very-late thrombosis (>1 year) was 5 events per 1000 DES with no events in patients implanted with BMS [22].

These observations, along with the demonstrated benefit of prolonged dual antiplatelet therapy in preventing late stent thrombosis in patients treated with BMS and brachytherapy [23], raise the possibility that prolonged dual antiplatelet therapy in patients implanted with DES may be beneficial. This point was further emphasized in an observational study of 4666 patients undergoing percutaneous coronary intervention with either DES (n = 1501) or BMS (n = 3165). In patients implanted with DES, continued clopidogrel use up to 24 months after implantation was associated with significantly lower adjusted risk of death and myocardial infarction. There was no difference in mortality or myocardial infarction based on clopidogrel use or non-use in patients implanted with BMS [24].

A 2007 AHA/ACC/SCAI/ACS/ADA Science Advisory has recommended that dual antiplatelet therapy should be prescribed for at least 1 month, and ideally up to 1 year, after bare-metal stent implantation. In addition, dual antiplatelet therapy with aspirin and clopidogrel has been recommended for 12 months after implantation of DES [25]. Although observational data suggests benefit of dual antiplatelet therapy beyond 12 months [24], optimal duration of dual antiplatelet therapy after DES implantation in not known and requires further investigation.

Risks associated with discontinuation of antiplatelet therapy

Despite proven efficacy, antiplatelet therapy is frequently discontinued due to adverse side effects, patient non-compliance or perioperatively to avoid intra- or postoperative bleeding complications. Several studies have demonstrated the adverse cardiovascular consequences of discontinuing antiplatelet therapy in various patient populations.

In a prospective study of 1358 patients presenting with acute coronary syndromes and followed for 30 days, 73 (5.4%) patients had discontinued aspirin within 3 weeks before presentation. The reason for withdrawal was scheduled surgery in the majority (64%) of the patients. Patients who had discontinued aspirin therapy had a twofold increase in death or myocardial infarction at 1 month compared to patients who were on aspirin therapy. A multivariate analysis demonstrated aspirin cessation was independently associated with mortality at 30 days [26].

In a similar study, Ferrari *et al.* reported on 1236 patients presenting with acute coronary syndromes; 51 (4.1%) patients had stopped taking aspirin prior to presentation with a mean delay between aspirin cessation and acute coronary syndrome of 10 ± 1.9 days. The reason for aspirin cessation was an anticipated invasive procedure in approximately 55% of the cases. Patients who had withdrawn from aspirin were much more likely to present with a ST-elevation myocardial infarction (39% vs. 18%, p < 0.001). Of the patients presenting with ST-elevation MI after aspirin cessation, stent thrombosis was demonstrated in approximately 20% of the patients in bare-metal stents that had been implanted a mean 15.5 ± 6.5 months previously [27].

These findings were further corroborated by Biondi-Zoccaie *et al.* in their meta-analysis of six studies involving 50,279 patients with established coronary artery disease which showed that withdrawal or non-compliance with aspirin therapy was associated with approximately threefold increased risk of adverse events (HR −3.14 (1.75–5.61), p = 0.0001) [28]. Additional studies have reported cases of cerebrovascular events and acute limb ischemia after discontinuation of aspirin [29,30].

Premature discontinuation of dual antiplatelet therapy has been associated with stent thrombosis. A prospective, observational cohort of 2229 patients who underwent successful implantation of either a sirolimus-eluting stent (SES) or a paclitaxel-eluting stent (PES) demonstrated a 29% incidence of stent thrombosis in patients who prematurely discontinued dual antiplatelet therapy. In multivariate analysis, premature discontinuation of antiplatelet therapy was an independent predictor of both subacute (HR –161.2; p < 0.001) and late (>30 days) stent thrombosis (HR –57.13; p < .001) [31].

Similar results were reported in a study of 1911 consecutive patients who underwent DES implantation with either a SES or PES. During long-term follow-up (median 19.4 months), the incidence of stent thrombosis was 7.8% in patients with premature interruption of dual antiplatelet therapy as compared to 0.5% in the control group (HR –15.28; p < 0.001). Premature discontinuation of antiplatelet therapy was an independent predictor of both total and late stent thrombosis in multivariate analysis [32].

Another recent retrospective study was conducted in a cohort of 3137 ACS patients who received post-hospital treatment with clopidogrel. Rates of all-cause death and acute MI were documented following cessation of clopidogrel therapy in both medically managed patients (n = 1568; mean duration of therapy 302 days; mean duration of follow-up 196 days) and patients receiving stents (n = 1569; mean duration of therapy 278 days; mean duration of follow-up 203 days). In medically-treated patients, death or MI following cessation of clopidogrel occurred in 17.1%, and 60.8% of these were within 90 days of stopping clopidogrel. In patients receiving stents, death or MI following cessation of therapy occurred in 7.9%, and 58.9% of these were within 90 days of stopping clopidogrel. In both groups the first 90 days were independently associated with a higher rate of adverse events – this was especially notewor-thy in medically treated patients [33].

Antiplatelet therapy in the perioperative period

Surgery is associated with platelet activation, increased levels of circulating procoagulant factors and reduced fibrinolysis [34]. This prothrombotic state may increase the risk of atherothrombotic events in patients with athero-sclerotic vascular disease. Effective antiplatelet therapy mitigates the risk of such events and reduces adverse cardiovascular outcomes. Several studies have reported improved cardiovascular outcomes with perioperative use of antiplatelet therapy [35,36].

Although the exact incidence of adverse cardiovascular events after peri-operative discontinuation of either aspirin monotherapy or dual antiplatelet therapy is not known, retrospective data suggests increased cardiovascular risk with perioperative aspirin cessation [26–27]. Similarly, discontinua-tion of dual antiplatelet therapy perioperatively increases the risk of adverse cardiovascular events in patients implanted with coronary stents. Kaluza et al. reported on 40 patients undergoing surgery less than 6 weeks after BMS implantation. Seven patients suffered myocardial infarctions, all of which were presumed to be secondary to stent thrombosis. All cases of stent thrombosis occurred in patients who had discontinued dual antiplatelet therapy within 2 weeks of BMS implantation [37]. In another report of 192 patients implanted with either BMS or DES, perioperative cessation of dual antiplatelet therapy was associated with a significantly higher incidence of adverse cardiovascular events [38].

However, antiplatelet therapy does increase the risk of bleeding complica-tions. In patients undergoing CABG, use of aspirin therapy is associated with an increased risk of perioperative bleeding [39–40]. Several reports have also shown an increased risk of perioperative bleeding in those taking aspirin before non-cardiac surgeries, including general and gynecologic surgery [41], urologic surgery [42], dermatologic procedures [43], and orthopedic surgery [44]. A pooled analysis of 41 studies including 49,590 patients demonstrated that aspirin therapy increased the risk of bleeding complications by 50%. However, with the exception of intracranial surgery and transurethral prostate-ctomy, aspirin use did not increase the severity of bleeding complications [45].

Dual antiplatelet therapy is associated with increased risk of bleeding beyond what is seen with aspirin alone [4–5,11]. Several studies have noted increased risk of bleeding complications with dual antiplatelet therapy in patients undergoing coronary artery bypass surgery [4,46–47]. Moreover, several studies evaluating patients implanted with coronary stents and sub-sequently undergoing non-cardiac surgery have noted increased bleeding complications in patients receiving dual antiplatelet therapy [37,48].

Despite the overall risk of increased bleeding complications noted with aspirin therapy, certain procedures may be performed safely without perioperative aspirin cessation. For instance, in patients undergoing spinal or epidural anesthesia, aspirin did not increase the risk of periprocedural hematoma formation [49]. Preoperative aspirin use did not increase bleeding complications in patients who underwent emergent appendectomy or cholecystectomy [50]. Similarly, ophthalmologic procedures including vitreoretinal surgery and cataract removal did not increase hemorrhagic complications or risk of sight-threatening bleeding in patients on preoperative aspirin therapy [51–52]. A prospective study of single tooth extractions in patients randomized to aspirin or placebo did not demonstrate a statistically significant difference in postoperative bleeding [53]. Similar data on the perioperative use of aspirin combined with a thienopyridine is not available and the safety of continuing dual antiplatelet therapy perioperatively remains uncertain.

In the future, another option may be the use of newer intravenous antiplatelet agents such as AZD6140 (oral; Astra Zeneca, Wilmington, DE) and Cangrelor (intravenous; The Medicines Company, Parsippany, NJ). These drugs are a newer generation of short-acting, reversible ATP analogues that compete reversibly for the $P2Y_{12}$ platelet ADP receptor, the same one targeted by the thienopyridines ticlopidine and clopidogrel [54]. While they remain, as yet, experimental, in the future they may offer an alternative for reversible, potent bridging antiplatelet therapy in thienopyridine-treated patients who require surgery.

Perioperative management of antiplatelet therapy in patients with coronary stents

Perioperative management goals for patients implanted with coronary stents include optimization of antiplatelet therapy to minimize the risk of stent thrombosis and bleeding complications (Figures 16.2, 16.3). Three management pathways exist: (1) continuing antiplatelet therapy through surgery; (2) stopping antiplatelet therapy (or at least stopping dual therapy and continuing aspirin) and initiating some sort of "bridging" strategy using antithrombin therapy or shorter-acting antiplatelet agents; and (3) stopping dual antiplatelet therapy a few days before the procedure and restarting it as soon as possible afterwards. At the present time there are no consensus, evidence-based guidelines; there is a paucity of controlled trials evaluating antiplatelet therapy in the perioperative period, and the general approach has to balance the clinical risks and benefits of stopping or continuing therapy.

Dual antiplatelet therapy is mandatory for the prevention of stent thrombosis and advised for at least 1 month, and ideally up to 12 months, in patients with BMS and 12 months in patients implanted with DES. Continuing dual antiplatelet therapy perioperatively is the preferred strategy in patients who

Continue Rx	D/C-bridge	D/C-restart
Continue antiplatelet therapy through surgery	Stop antiplatelet therapy-bridge with antithrombin or short-acting intravenous small molecule IIb/IIIa antagonist	Stop antiplatelet therapy. Restart as soon as possible after surgery
Carries the lowest clinical risk	Carries intermediate clinical risk	Carries the highest clinical risk
Carries the highest bleeding risk	Carries intermediate bleeding risk	Carries the lowest bleeding risk

Fig. 16.2 Three potential strategies for managing patients on chronic antiplatelet therapy that require surgery and their associated clinical and bleeding risk. Continuing therapy carries the lowest clinical risk but the highest perioperative bleeding risk. Stopping dual therapy and restating after surgery carries the highest clinical risk, but the lowest perioperative bleeding risk. A bridging strategy carries an intermediate risk for both.

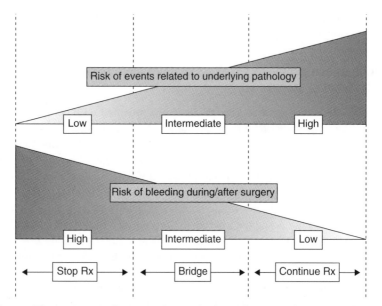

Fig. 16.3 The continuum of stopping therapy, bridging therapy and continuing therapy. The risk of events related to the underlying pathology increases, while the risk of perioperative bleeding decreases.

have had PCI with stent implantation and have not yet completed an appropriate course of dual antiplatelet therapy. Since dual antiplatelet therapy can be associated with a significantly increased risk of perioperative bleeding, a careful assessment of bleeding risk associated with the anticipated procedure should be made in consultation with the surgeon. Procedures associated with minor bleeding risk or procedures like dental extractions where excessive bleeding can be controlled with local measures can likely be performed while on dual antiplatelet therapy [25]. This strategy, however, is not appropriate for surgery associated with high risk of hemorrhagic complications like prostate surgery or neurosurgery. Therefore, all elective procedures requiring discontinuation of dual antiplatelet therapy should be deferred for at least 4 weeks in patients implanted with BMS and 12 months in patients receiving DES [25].

If a procedure cannot be delayed and dual antiplatelet therapy needs to be discontinued, clopidogrel can be stopped 5–7 days prior to surgery and restarted as soon as possible postoperatively [4]. A loading dose of 300 or 600 mg can be given when clopidogrel is reinitiated to minimize the time required for maximal inhibition of platelet aggregation. Alternatively, clopidogrel can be stopped prior to surgery and the patients can be "bridged" to surgery with intravenous glycoprotein IIb/IIIa inhibitors or an antithrombin. There is little data supporting this strategy, and this approach may not provide complete protection as the risk of stent thrombosis is greatest during or immediately after surgery [55]. However, this approach might be desirable for patients who are at a high risk of stent thrombosis (Figure 16.4) [21,31–32].

Aspirin therapy should be continued perioperatively in these patients to minimize the risk of stent thrombosis. This was well illustrated in a study that demonstrated the median time to stent thrombosis was 7 days when both aspirin and clopidogrel were discontinued as compared to 30 days when only clopidogrel was discontinued [56]. If both aspirin and clopidogrel need to be discontinued, these agents can be stopped 5–7 days prior to surgery and should be started as soon as possible postoperatively. This strategy is likely associated with the highest risk of stent thrombosis and should be reserved for procedures associated with very high risk of bleeding complications.

Perioperative management of antiplatelet therapy in patients without coronary stents

Perioperative management of antiplatelet therapy in patients without coronary stents generally follows the same principles as previously described. Aspirin should be continued perioperatively if at all possible to reduce the risk of atherothrombotic events. If bleeding risk associated with the anticipated surgical procedure mandates discontinuation of aspirin, it can be stopped 5–7 days prior to surgery and restarted as soon as possible to minimize the risk of adverse cardiovascular events. No data exists regarding perioperative

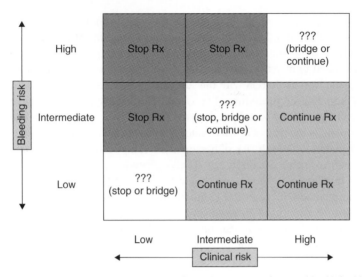

Fig. 16.4 A two-dimensional matrix of risk (low, intermediate and high) for bleeding and clinical events, and within each cell specify an appropriate strategy.

management of dual antiplatelet therapy in patients without coronary stents. However, procedures associated with minor bleeding risk can likely be performed without discontinuation of dual antiplatelet therapy. For other procedures, clopidogrel can be discontinued prior to surgery and restarted, when feasible, postoperatively. Since these patients are not at risk for stent thrombosis, "bridging" them to surgery with an antithrombin or glycoprotein IIb/IIIa inhibitor is generally not warranted.

Delaying surgery in recently stented patients

A related, specific area of clinical concern is exactly how long to delay surgery following the implantation of a coronary stent and a required time period of obligatory dual antiplatelet therapy. If future elective surgery is already planned prior to stenting, the choice of a DES or BMS will influence the timing of any such delay. In the clinical situation where surgery needs to be performed within 12 months, a BMS has been recommended as the preferable alternative [55]. Conversely, if the surgery can be delayed for more than 12 months, the use of a DES is not inappropriate, but the risk of very late stent thrombosis if dual antiplatelet therapy is withdrawn needs to be considered.

There has been a well-demonstrated association between the risk of stent thrombosis and shorter intervals between stenting and surgery [37,48,57,58]. The ACC/AHA Practice Guidelines recommend that non-cardiac surgery should be delayed for at least 2 weeks – and preferably 4 weeks – following the implantation of a BMS, although more recent data suggest that a period of 6 weeks may be even better [59]. For DES, the optimal delay remains problematic and unknown, but in the absence of any hard data the consensus is that the appropriate delay is at least 12 months, and may be longer in higher-risk individuals. Unfortunately, the exact specifics of just what constitutes "higher-risk" remains somewhat poorly characterized at present, and while discontinuation of dual antiplatelet therapy is a known (and modifiable) risk factor, the rest of the clinical picture is much murkier. Hence, again, appropriate stent selection is critical when a need for subsequent surgery is known at the time of stent implantation.

Conclusion

Antiplatelet therapy is an important component of therapy for various cardiovascular diseases. Adverse effects of discontinuing antiplatelet therapy have been well documented and can be catastrophic, particularly in patients implanted with coronary stents. Unfortunately, antiplatelet therapy is not without risk and is associated with an increase in bleeding complications. Perioperative management of antiplatelet therapy is a complex medical problem that requires a careful assessment of individual risk factors for thrombotic complications and bleeding risk associated with the anticipated procedure.

Antiplatelet therapy should only be discontinued if the bleeding risks clearly exceed the potential adverse cardiovascular consequences. Routine discontinuation of antiplatelet therapy prior to all non-cardiac surgery is unnecessary and should be discouraged, particularly in patients implanted with coronary stents.

References

1 Antithrombotic Trialists' Collaboration. Collaborative meta-analysis of randomized trials of antiplatelet therapy for prevention of death, myocardial infarction, and stroke in high-risk patients. *BMJ* 2002; **324**: 71–86.

2 Bhatt DL, Fox KAA, Hacke W *et al.* Clopidogrel and aspirin versus aspirin alone for the prevention of atherothrombotic events. *New Engl J Med* 2006; **354**: 1706–1717.

3 Sabatine MS, Cannon CP, Gibson CM *et al.* Addition of clopidogrel to aspirin and fibrinolytic therapy for myocardial infarction with ST-segment elevation. *New Engl J Med* 2005; **352**: 1179–1189.

4 Yusuf, S, Zhao, F, Mehta, SR, *et al.* Effects of clopidogrel in addition to aspirin in patients with acute coronary syndromes without ST-segment elevation. *New Engl J Med* 2001; **345**: 494–502.

5 Leon MB, Baim DS, Popma JJ, *et al.*, for the Stent Anticoagulation Restenosis Study Investigators. A clinical trial comparing three antithrombotic-drug regimens after coronary-artery stenting. *New Engl J Med* 1998; **339**: 1665–1671.

6 Serruys PW, Strauss BH, Beatt KJ, *et al.* Angiographic follow-up after placement of a self-expanding coronary-artery stent. *New Engl J Med* 1991; **324**: 13–17.

7 Urban P, Macaya C, Rupprecht H-J, *et al.*, for the MATTIS Investigators. Randomized evaluation of anticoagulant versus antiplatelet therapy after coronary stent implantation in high-risk patients: the multicenter aspirin and ticlopidine trial after coronary stenting (MATTIS). *Circulation* 1998; **98**: 2126–2132.

8 Schomig A, Neumann F-J, Kastrati A, *et al.* A randomized comparison of antiplatelet and anticoagulant therapy after the placement of coronary-artery stents. *New Engl J Med* 1996; **334**: 1084–1089.

9 Cutlip DE, Baim DS, Ho KK, *et al.* Stent thrombosis in the modern era: a pooled analysis of multicenter coronary stent clinical trials. *Circulation* 2001; **103**: 1967–1971.

10 Steinhubl SR, Berger PB, Mann JT, III, *et al.* Early and sustained dual oral antiplatelet therapy following percutaneous coronary intervention: a randomized controlled trial. *JAMA* 2002; **288**: 2411–2420.

11 Mehta SR, Yusuf S, Peters RJ, *et al.* Effects of pretreatment with clopidogrel and aspirin followed by long-term therapy in patients undergoing percutaneous coronary intervention: the PCI-CURE study. *Lancet* 2001; **358**: 527–533.

12 Morice MC, Serruys PW, Sousa JE, *et al.* A randomized comparison of a sirolimus-eluting stent with a standard stent for coronary revascularization. *New Engl J Med* 2002; **346**: 1773–1780.

13 Moses JW, Leon MB, Popma JJ, *et al.* Sirolimus-eluting stents versus standard stents in patients with stenosis in a native coronary artery. *New Engl J Med* 2003: **349**: 1315–1323.

14 Stone GW, Ellis SG, Cox DA, *et al.* A polymer-based paclitaxel-eluting stent in patients with coronary artery disease. *New Engl J Med* 2004; **350**: 221–231.

15 McFadden EP, Stabile E, Regar E, *et al.* Late thrombosis in drug-eluting coronary stents after discontinuation of antiplatelet therapy. *Lancet* 2004; **364**: 1519–1521.

16 Ong ATL, McFadden EP, Regar E, *et al.* Late angiographic stent thrombosis (LAST) events with drug-eluting stents. *J Am Coll Cardiol* 2005; **45**: 2088–2092.

17 Daemen J, Wenaweser P, Tsuchida K, *et al.* Early and late coronary stent thrombosis of sirolimus-eluting and paclitaxel-eluting stents in routine clinical practice: data from a larger two-institutional cohort study. *Lancet* 2007; **369**: 667–678.

18 Kotani J, Awata M, Nanto S, *et al.* Incomplete neointimal coverage of sirolimus-eluting stents: angioscopic findings. *J Am Coll Cardiol* 2006; **47**: 2108–2111.

19 Nebeker JR, Virmani R, Bennett CL, *et al.* Hypersensitivity cases associated with drug-eluting coronary stents: a review of available cases from the Research on Adverse Drug Events and Reports (RADAR) project. *J Am Coll Cardiol* 2006; **47**: 175–181.

20 Virmani R, Guagliumi G, Farb A, *et al.* Localized hypersensitivity and late coronary thrombosis secondary to a sirolimus-eluting stent: should we be cautious? *Circulation* 2004; **109**: 701–705.

21 Pfisterer M, Brunner-La Rocca HP, Buser PT, *et al.*, for the BASKET-LATE Investigators. Late clinical events after clopidogreal discontinuation may limit the benefit of drug-eluting stents: An observational study of drug-eluting vs bare-metal stents. *J Am Coll Cardiol* 2006; **48**: 2584–2591.

22 Bavry AA, Kumbhani DJ, Helton TJ, *et al.* Late thrombosis of drug-eluting stents: A meta-analysis of randomized clinical trials. *Am J Med* 2006; **119**: 1056–1061.

23 Waksman R, Ajani AE, Pinnow E, *et al.* Twelve versus six months of clopidogrel to reduce major cardiac events in patients undergoing γ-radiation therapy for in-stent

restenosis. Washington Radiation for In-Stent restenosis Trial (WRIST) 12 vs WRIST PLUS. *Circulation* 2002; **106**: 776–778.

24 Eisenstein EL, Anstrom KJ, Kong DF, *et al*. Clopidogrel use and long-term clinical outcomes after drug-eluting stent implantation. *JAMA* 2007; **297**: 159–168.

25 Grines CL, Bonow RO, Casey DE, Jr, *et al*. Prevention of premature discontinuation of dual antiplatelet therapy in patients with coronary artery stents. A Science Advisory from the American Heart Association, American College of Cardiology, Society of Cardiovascular Angiography and Interventions, American College of Surgeons, and American Dental Association, with representation from the American College of Physicians. *J Am Coll Cardiol* 2007; **49**: 734–739.

26 Collet JP, Montalescot G, Blanchet B, *et al*. Impact of prior use or recent withdrawal of oral antiplatelet agents on acute coronary syndromes. *Circulation* 2004; **110**: 2361–2367.

27 Ferrari E, Benhamou M, Cerboni P, *et al*. Coronary syndromes following aspirin withdrawal. *J Am Coll Cardiol* 2005; **45**: 456–459.

28 Biondi-Zoccai GGL, Lotrionte M, Agostoni P, *et al*. A systematic review and meta-analysis on the hazards of discontinuing or not adhering to aspirin among 50279 patients at risk for coronary artery disease. *Eur Heart J* 2006; **27**: 2667–2674.

29 Bachman DS. Discontinuing chronic aspirin therapy: another risk factor for stroke? *Ann Neurol* 2002; **51**: 137–138.

30 Albaladejo P, Geeraerts T, Francis F, *et al*. Aspirin withdrawal and acute limb ischemia. *Anesth Analg* 2004; **99**: 440–443.

31 Iakovou I, Schmidt T, Bonizzoni E, *et al*. Incidence, predictors and outcome of thrombosis after successful implantation of drug-eluting stents. *JAMA* 2005; **293**: 2126–2130.

32 Park DW, Park SW, Park KH, *et al*. Frequency of and risk factors for stent thrombosis after drug-eluting stent implantation during long-term follow-up. *Am J Cardiol* 2006; **98**: 352–356.

33 Ho PM, Peterson ED, Wang L, *et al*. Incidence of death and acute myocardial infarction associated with stopping clopidogrel after acute coronary syndromes. *JAMA* 2008; **299**: 532–539.

34 Bradbury A, Adam D, Garrioch M, *et al*. Changes in platelet count, coagulation and fibrinogen associated with elective repair of asymptomatic abdominal aortic aneurysm and aortic reconstruction for occlusive disease. *Eur J Vasc Endovasc Surg* 1997; **13**: 375–380.

35 Goldman S, Copeland J, Moritz T, *et al*. Improvement in early saphenous graft patency after coronary artery bypass surgery with antiplatelet therapy: Results of a veterans administration cooperative study. *Circulation* 1988; **77**: 1324–1332.

36 Lindblad B, Persson NH, Takolander R, *et al*. Does low-dose acetylsalicylic acid prevent stroke after carotid surgery? A double-blind, placebo-controlled randomized trial. *Stroke* 1993; **24**: 1125–1128.

37 Kaluza GL, Jospeh J, Lee JR, Raizner ME, Raizner AE. Catastrophic outcomes of non-cardiac surgery soon after coronary stenting. *J Am Coll Cardiol* 2000; **35**: 1288–1294.

38 Schouten O, van Domburg RT, Bax JJ, *et al*. Noncardiac surgery after coronary stenting: Early surgery and interruption of antiplatelet therapy are associated with an increase in major adverse cardiac events.*J Am Coll Cardiol* 2007; **49**: 122–124.

39 Michelson EL, Morganroth J, Torosian M, MacVaugh III H. Relation of preoperative use of aspirin to increased mediastinal blood loss after coronary artery bypass graft surgery. *J Thoracic Cardiovasc Surg* 1978; **76**: 694–697.

40 Torosian M, Michelson EL, Morganroth J, MacVaugh III H. Aspirin and coumadin-related bleeding after coronary artery bypass surgery. *Ann Intern Med* 1978; **89**: 325–328.

41 Kitchen L, Erichson RB, Sideropoulos H. Effect of drug-induced platelet dysfunction on surgical bleeding. *Am J Surg* 1982; **143**: 215–215.

42 Watson CJE, Deane AM, Doyle PT, Bullock KN. Identifiable factors in post-prostatectomy haemorrhage: the role of aspirin. *Br J Urol* 1990; **66**: 85–87.

43 Lawrence C, Sakuntabhai A, Tiling-Grosse S. Effect of aspirin and non-steroidal anti-inflammatory drug therapy on bleeding complications in dermatologic surgical patients. *J Am Acad Dermatol* 1994; **31**: 988–992.

44 Nuttall GA, Santrach PJ, Oliver WC, *et al.* The predictors of red cell transfusions in total hip arthroplasties. *Transfusion* 1996; **36**: 144–149.

45 Burger W, Chemnitius JM, Kneissl GD, Rucker G. Low-dose aspirin for secondary cardiovascular risks after its perioperative withdrawal versus bleeding risks with it continuation – review and meta-analysis. *J Intern Med* 2005; **257**: 399–414.

46 Kang W, Theman TE, Reed JF, Stoltzfus J, Weger N. The effect of preoperative clopidogrel on bleeding after coronary artery bypass surgery. *J Surg Educat* 2007; **64**: 88–92.

47 Hongo RH, Ley J, Dick SE, Yee RR. The effect of clopidogrel in combination with aspirin when given before coronary artery bypass grafting. *J Am Coll Cardiol* 2002; **40**: 231–237.

48 Reddy PR, Vaitkus PT. Risks of noncardiac surgery after coronary stenting. *Am J Cardiol* 2005; **95**: 755–757.

49 Horlocker TT, Wedel DJ, Schroeder DR, *et al.* Preoperative antiplatelet therapy does not increase the risk of spinal hematoma associated with regional anesthesia. *Anesth Analg* 1995; **80**: 303–309.

50 Ferraris VA, Swanson E. Aspirin usage and perioperative blood loss in patients undergoing unexpected operations. *Surg Gynecol Obstet* 1983; **156**: 439–442.

51 Assia EI, Raskin T, Kaiserman I, Rotenstreich Y, Segev F. Effect of aspirin intake on bleeding during cataract sugery. *J Cataract Refract Surg* 1998; **24**: 1243–1246.

52 Narendran N, Williamson TH. The effects of aspirin and warfarin on haemorrhage in vitreoretinal surgery. *Acta Opthalm Scand* 2003; **81**: 38–40.

53 Valerin MA, Brennan MT, Noll JL, *et al.* Relationship between aspirin use and post-operative bleeding from dental extractions in a healthy population. *Oral Surg Oral Med* 2006; **102**; 326.

54 Steinhubl S, Roe MT. Optimizing platelet $P2Y_{12}$ inhibition for patients undergoing PCI. *Cardiovasc Drug Rev* 2007; **25**: 188–203

55 Brilakis ES, Banerjee S, Berger PB. Perioperative management of patients with coronary stents. *J Am Coll Cardiol* 2007; **49**: 2145–2150.

56 Artang R, Dieter RS. Analysis of 36 reported cases of late thrombosis in drug-eluting stents placed in coronary arteries. *Am J Cardiol* 2007; **99**: 1039–1043.

57 Wilson SH, Fasseas P, Orford, JL, *et al.* Clinical outcome of patients undergoing non-cardiac surgery in the two months following coronary stenting. *J Am Coll Cardiol* 2003; **42**: 234–240.

58 Sharma AK, Ajani AE, Hamwi SM, *et al.* Major noncardiac surgery following coronary stenting: When is it safe to operate? *Catheter Cardiovasc Interv* 2004; **63**: 141–145.

59 Eagle KA, Berger PB, Calkins H, *et al.* ACC/AHA guideline update for perioperative cardiovascular evaluation for noncardiac surgery – Executive summary: A report of the American College of Cardiology/American Heart Association Task Force on Practice Guidelines (Committee to Update the 1996 Guidelines on Perioperative Cardiovascular Evaluation for Noncardiac Surgery). *Circulation* 2002; **105**: 1257–1267.

Chapter 17

Antiplatelet therapy and coronary stents

Alanna Coolong and Laura Mauri

Introduction

With the widespread adoption of coronary stenting to prevent abrupt vessel closure and restenosis following balloon angioplasty came the recognition of an infrequent but devastating complication, stent thrombosis (ST). Initial attempts at preventing this complication involved systemic anticoagulation with heparin, aspirin, dipyridamole and low molecular weight dextran, resulting in ST rates of 16–24% [1–3]. Warfarin was subsequently added to the above regimen (Stent Restenosis Study (STRESS) [4], The Benestent Study [5]) and, while effective at reducing the rates of ST to approximately 3.5%, this more aggressive regimen resulted in high rates of major bleeding and vascular complications (~7–14%) [6]. The Stent Anticoagulation Restenosis Study (STARS) and Intracoronary Stenting and Antithrombotic Regimen Trial (ISAR) studies established the efficacy of dual antiplatelet therapy (aspirin and ticlopidine) in reducing the frequency of ST from 3–5% to approximately 1% while reducing major bleeding complications associated with systemic anticoagulation [6,7]. Ticlopidine has been replaced by clopidogrel as the thienopyridine of choice, due to improved tolerability. Dual antiplatelet therapy with aspirin and clopidogrel is now recommended for a minimum of 1, 3 and 6 months post procedure depending on the type of stent implanted, with the longer durations of use associated with implantation of drug-eluting stents (DES), and for patients receiving stents for acute coronary syndromes. If dual antiplatelet therapy is well-tolerated, current recommendations are to continue aspirin indefinitely and clopidogrel for 12 months [8].

In addition to reducing the frequency of ST, antiplatelet therapy has the additional benefit of reducing periprocedural, 30-day and late (12 months) myocardial infarction and mortality. Adjunctive use of glycoprotein IIb/IIIa

Antiplatelet Therapy in Ischemic Heart Disease, 1st edition. Edited by Stephen D. Wiviott.
© 2009 American Heart Association, ISBN: 9-781-4051-7626-2

inhibition, combined with aspirin and thienopyridine therapy, has been shown to be efficacious in both low- and high-risk patients undergoing percutaneous coronary intervention (PCI). Despite the large number of randomized, controlled trials of these agents involving patients, spanning a wide range of periprocedural risk, the most efficacious therapy, resulting in the optimal degree of platelet inhibition and resultant reduction in periprocedural and long-term outcomes, has not been established. This chapter reviews the evidence supporting the use of the available antiplatelet agents at the various time points surrounding stent placement and to highlight remaining questions surrounding this adjunctive therapy.

Periprocedural antiplatelet therapy

Aspirin pretreatment

While the value of combination therapy with aspirin and dipyridamole given prior to PCI in reducing acute thrombosis [9] and periprocedural myocardial infarction (MI) [10] was recognized early in the era of percutaneous transluminal angioplasty (PTCA), the minimal effective dose of aspirin has not been established [11]. Based on recommended doses used in randomized trials of patients undergoing elective to emergent PCI for acute coronary syndrome (ACS) [12–15], the present recommendation is to give aspirin 75–325 mg to patients on chronic aspirin therapy before PCI [8] and 300–325 mg of aspirin a minimum of 2 hours before PCI to aspirin-naïve patients [8], as lower doses may not completely block thromboxane A_2 production [16].

Clopidogrel pretreatment

When possible, a loading dose of clopidogrel prior to PCI should be given (Class I, Level of Evidence: A) [8]. The optimal dose and timing of the clopidogrel load has been evaluated in several randomized trials in both low- and high-risk patients undergoing PCI. The Clopidogrel in Unstable Angina to Prevent Recurrent Events (CURE) trial [13] evaluated the benefit of a clopidogrel load of 300 mg followed by long-term clopidogrel therapy (mean of 9 months) versus placebo in 12,562 patients presenting with non-ST-segment elevation myocardial infarction (NSTEMI). The relative risk of the composite primary outcome of death, MI, and stroke at 1 year was reduced by 20% (9.3% vs. 11.4%, $p < 0.001$) in the group of patients treated with clopidogrel. This risk reduction was driven by a decrease in the rate of MIs. The PCI-CURE study [14] examined the subset of patients enrolled in the CURE trial [13] who underwent PCI. PCI-CURE demonstrated a 30% relative risk reduction (RRR) (4.5% vs. 6.4%, $p = 0.03$) in the primary end-point of death, MI or target vessel revascularization (TVR) at 30 days in patients preloaded with clopidogrel a median of 6 days before the procedure [14].

The Clopidogrel for the Reduction of Events During Observation (CREDO) trial was the first randomized evaluation of the benefit of a clopidogrel loading dose prior to PCI. In the CREDO trial, 2116 patients undergoing elective PCI were assigned to either a clopidogrel load, 300 mg 3–24 hours before PCI, followed by chronic therapy for 1 year or a placebo load followed by clopidogrel for 1 month. A 26.9% RRR in the combined end-point of death, MI and stroke was observed in patients treated with long-term clopidogrel (8.5% vs. 11.5%; p = 0.02). In an effort to better characterize the relationship between the timing of the 300 mg load of clopidogrel and major adverse events (death, MI, TVR) at 28 days, a prespecified secondary analysis evaluated clinical outcomes in patients loaded with drug less than 6 hours versus greater than 6 hours before PCI. While there was a non-significant 18% RRR of the primary end-point at 28 days in the clopidogrel arm (6.8% vs. 8.3%, p = 0.23), the subgroup analysis revealed that patients treated greater than 6 hours before PCI experienced a borderline significant risk reduction of 38.6% compared with patients treated less than 6 hours before PCI (95% CI −1.6% to 62.9%; p = 0.051).

While PCI-CURE and CREDO support administration of 300 mg of clopidogrel 6 hours before PCI to reduce adverse cardiovascular events, significant variability of platelet reactivity and responsiveness to clopidogrel exists [17], the incremental benefit of glycoprotein IIb/IIIa inhibition in combination with clopidogrel was not investigated, and many patients undergoing PCI are not loaded prior to the procedure. The ISAR-REACT trial, which studied the incremental benefit of abciximab in 2159 patients undergoing elective PCI after receiving 600 mg of clopidogrel at least 2 hours beforehand, showed no difference in the frequency of the primary end-point (death, MI, TVR at 28 days) in the two groups (4% vs. 4%, p = 0.82) [18]. Additionally, a substudy of ISAR-REACT suggested no incremental benefit to the administration of high-dose clopidogrel any longer before PCI than 2 hours [19]. A smaller study, ARMYDA-2 (n = 255), comparing clopidogrel 300 mg versus 600 mg given 4–8 hours before PCI in a broad patient population (25% NSTEMI, 75% stable angina) suggested a significant reduction in the primary end-point of death, MI or TVR (predominantly MI) in favor of high-dose clopidogrel (4% vs. 12% at 30 days, p = 0.041) [20]. Of interest in this small study was the much higher rate of adverse events in the lower-dose clopidogrel arm than was seen in any of the previous studies. The ISAR-REACT 2 trial (n = 2022) evaluated the incremental benefit of abciximab to 600 mg of clopidogrel in a high-risk population (ACS, NSTEMI) undergoing PCI and found a 25% risk reduction in patients treated with abciximab (8.9% vs. 11.9%; p = 0.03). It appeared the benefit of abciximab administration was confined to the subgroup of patients who had elevated troponin levels (13.1% vs. 18.3% death, MI, or TVR at 30 days, p = 0.02) [21]. Lastly, the benefit of clopidogrel pretreatment has been shown in patients presenting with ST-segment elevation MI (STEMI); The PCI-Clopidogrel as Adjunctive Reperfusion Therapy (PCI-CLARITY) study randomized 1863 patients with STEMI treated with fibrinolytics to clopidogrel 300 mg or placebo with subsequent angiography and PCI 2 to 8 days later [15]. Clopidogrel pretreatment was associated with a significant reduction in death or ischemic complications both before and after PCI (death, MI or stroke after PCI to 30 days, 3.6% vs. 6.2%; p = 0.008; MI or stroke before PCI, 4.0% vs. 6.2%; p = 0.03).

In summary, while the strongest evidence supports a loading dose of 300 mg of clopidogrel at least 6 hours before the procedure (Class I indication), evidence is accumulating that a 600 mg dose may be preferred, ideally 2 hours before the procedure (Class IIa indication) if the former is not possible. Recent evidence suggests high dose clopidogrel given before PCI obviates the need for concomitant glycoprotein IIb/IIIa inhibition in elective PCI (ISAR-REACT), but in troponin-positive patients undergoing PCI, the relative risk of adverse events is further reduced with adjunctive abciximab (ISAR-REACT 2). A loading dose of clopidogrel reduces adverse cardiovascular events in the STEMI population treated with fibrinolytic therapy that subsequently undergo PCI.

Glycoprotein IIb/IIIa inhibitors

The glycoprotein IIb/IIIa inhibitors (abciximab, eptifibatide and tirofiban) block the "final common pathway" of platelet aggregation, with numerous, large randomized trials supporting their use in PCI. The glycoprotein IIb/IIIa inhibitor, abciximab, was shown to reduce the composite end-point of death, MI and repeat revascularization at 30 days in both high-risk [22] and low-risk [23] patients in the prestent era when used with heparin compared to heparin alone, with no increase in bleeding complications when weight-adjusted heparin was used. The benefit of abciximab and weight-adjusted heparin in the setting of PCI with stenting was demonstrated in the Evaluation of Platelet IIb/IIIa Inhibition in Stenting (EPISTENT) trial, where 2399 patients were randomized to stenting with heparin, stenting with heparin and abciximab, or PTCA with heparin and abciximab [24]. The composite end-point of death, MI and urgent revascularization at 30 days was 10.8% in the stenting with heparin group, 5.3% in the stenting with heparin and abciximab group (hazard ratio 0.48; p < 0.001), and 6.9% in the PTCA with heparin and abciximab group (hazard ratio 0.63; p = 0.007).

Eptifibatide for use in PCI has been best studied in three randomized trials. IMPACT-II [25] randomized 4010 patients undergoing PCI to treatment with low-dose bolus eptifibatide (135 µg/kg) followed by low dose infusion (0.5 µg/kg/min), and heparin versus low-dose bolus eptifibatide (135 µg/kg) followed by higher dose infusion (0.75 µg/kg/min) and heparin versus heparin plus placebo. No difference in the primary composite end-point of death, MI and repeat revascularization (CABG or PCI) at 30 days was found between the three groups. Subsequently, the PURSUIT trial [26] evaluated the use of higher dose eptifibatide versus placebo in 10,948 patients with unstable angina/NSTEMI undergoing PCI. Patients were assigned to heparin plus placebo versus heparin plus eptifibatide 180 µg/kg bolus followed by a 1.3 µg/kg/min infusion versus heparin plus eptifibatide 180 µg/kg bolus followed by a 2.0 µg/kg/min infusion. The 30-day end-point of death or MI was significantly lower in the patients assigned to eptifibatide 180 μg/kg bolus followed by a 2.0 μg/kg/min infusion (n = 4722) compared with placebo (n = 4739) (14.2% vs. 15.7%; p = 0.042). The efficacy of eptifibatide in low-risk patients undergoing PCI was evaluated in the Enhanced Suppression of the Platelet IIb/IIIa Receptor with Integrilin Therapy (ESPRIT) trial, which randomized 2064 patients to heparin plus placebo versus heparin plus double bolus eptifibatide (180 μg/kg 10 minutes apart) followed by a 2.0 μg/kg/min infusion. Eptifibatide was associated with a 35% reduction in the 30-day composite end-point of death, MI and TVR (6.8% vs. 10.4%; p = 0.0034) [27]. Dosing recommendations for eptifibatide in PCI are based on findings of the ESPRIT trial.

While the evidence for the glycoprotein IIb/IIIa inhibitor tirofiban supports its use upstream of PCI in patients with ACS for the reduction of ischemic events at 30 days [28], two randomized trials found no benefit to the periprocedural use of the drug in reducing adverse events. The Randomized Efficacy Study of Tirofiban for Outcomes and Restenosis (RESTORE) trial, which randomized 2139 patients undergoing PCI within 72 hours of presentation with ACS (unstable angina or NSTEMI) to tirofiban bolus plus infusion versus placebo, found no significant difference between the two groups with respect to the combined primary end-point of death, MI or TVR at 30 days [29] or at 6 months [30]. A study of 4809 patients undergoing PCI randomized to treatment with tirofiban versus abciximab found that treatment with abciximab resulted in a significantly lower frequency of the composite primary end-point of death, MI or TVR at 30 days (7.6% vs. 6.0%; p = 0.038) [31].

While the preponderance of evidence suggests the primary benefit of glycoprotein IIb/IIIa inhibitors is in the reduction of periprocedural and 30-day ischemic events, a meta-analysis of 12 trials involving 20,186 patients found a significant reduction in 30-day mortality with the use of glycoprotein IIb/IIIa inhibitors (odds ratio 0.73, 95% CI 0.55, 0.96; p = 0.024) [32]. The reduction in 6-month mortality with glycoprotein IIb/IIIa inhibition suggested benefit but failed to reach statistical significance (odds ratio 0.84, 95% CI 0.69, 1.03; p = 0.087). Another meta-analysis of 19 trials involving 20,137 patients found a significant reduction in the hard end-point of mortality at 30 days (risk ratio 0.69, 95% CI 0.53, 0.90) and 6 months (risk ratio 0.79, 95% CI 0.64, 0.97) in patients treated with glycoprotein IIb/IIIa inhibitors [33]. This analysis included all the trials of the preceding meta-analysis (excluding the 796 patients in the EPISTENT trial assigned to abciximab/PTCA arm) and included seven additional small studies enrolling a total of 747 patients.

Patients with diabetes undergoing PCI derive particular benefit from the use of glycoprotein IIb/IIIa inhibitors with reductions in mortality. A meta-analysis of diabetic patients enrolled in the EPIC, EPILOG and EPISTENT trials (n = 1462 diabetic patients) demonstrated a reduction in 1-year mortality associated with abciximab (4.5% vs. 2.5%, p = 0.031) [34]. Another meta-analysis of the diabetic populations of six trials of glycoprotein IIb/IIIa inhibitors in ACS (n = 6458 diabetic patients) demonstrated a reduction in 30-day mortality [35]. This reduction was maintained in the subgroup of diabetic patients undergoing PCI (n = 1279) where the mortality of patients treated with glycoprotein IIb/IIIa inhibitors at 30 days was 1.2% vs. 4.0% in patients treated with placebo (OR 0.30; 95% CI 0.14, 0.69; p = 0.002) [35].

In an effort to better define the most efficacious antiplatelet regimen in the periprocedural setting, Gurbel *et al.* studied platelet aggregation and cardiac biomarker release in 120 patients randomized to one of four treatment groups; 300 mg loading dose of clopidogrel +/− eptifibatide and 600 mg loading dose of clopidogrel +/− eptifibatide [36]. The clopidogrel loading dose was given *after* stent placement. They were able to demonstrate that inhibition of platelet aggregation was greatest with the combination of eptifibatide and clopidogrel and that CK-MB release was lowest in the groups treated with eptifibatide. These findings suggest glycoprotein IIb/IIIa administration should be considered in patients undergoing PCI who have not been pretreated with clopidogrel.

In summary, the randomized trials of glycoprotein IIb/IIIa inhibitors in PCI support their use in the setting of ACS where clopidogrel has not been used (unstable angina, NSTEMI) (Class I, Level of Evidence A) and in the setting of ACS (unstable angina, NSTEMI) where clopidogrel has been used (Class IIa, Level of Evidence B). All three agents have been given a Class IIa indication for use in elective PCI (Level of Evidence B). Abciximab has been given a Class IIa indication for use in the setting of STEMI (Level of Evidence B), with eptifibatide and tirofiban being given a Class IIb indication in this setting (Level of Evidence C) [8]. Further study is ongoing regarding whether there is incremental value of glycoprotein IIb/IIIa inhibition in conjunction with high-dose clopidogrel in low-risk patient populations.

Postprocedural antiplatelet therapy

Aspirin after stent implantation

Present recommendations for aspirin therapy immediately after PCI with stent placement are based on randomized trial protocols for the type of stent used. Aspirin, 325 mg daily, is recommended for 1 month after bare-metal stent (BMS) implantation, 3 months after sirolimus-eluting stent (SES) implantation, and 6 months after paclitaxel-eluting stent (PES) implantation [8]. Given the reductions in late cardiovascular death, MI and stroke associated with long-term aspirin therapy in patients with cardiovascular disease, lifelong therapy is recommended in the absence of contraindications. As extended dual antiplatelet therapy increases the risk of bleeding complications, the optimal dosage of aspirin is also of considerable import. An analysis of the CURE study by Peters *et al.* [37] evaluated the incidence of the combined end-point of cardiovascular death, MI or stroke at 12 months stratified by aspirin dose (≤100 mg, 101–199 mg, ≥200 mg) in 12,562 patients with ACS randomized to clopidogrel or placebo and found an increased risk in major bleeding with increasing aspirin dose without any gain in efficacy. This finding was also observed in the subgroup of patients undergoing PCI. The finding of no incremental benefit of aspirin doses higher than 75 mg daily by the Antithrombotic Trialists' Collaboration [38] supports a lower dose of daily aspirin for long-term therapy.

Clopidogrel after stent implantation

The current recommendation for the duration of clopidogrel therapy after stent placement is dependent upon the type of stent implanted. Based on the indications for use of approved stents, clopidogrel has been recommended for a minimum of 4 weeks after bare-metal stent placement [6], at least 3 months after sirolimus stent placement [39], and at least 6 months after paclitaxel stent placement [40]. It is clear that interruption of therapy (whether undertaken for medical reasons or due to non-compliance) is associated with an increased risk of stent thrombosis [41,42]. The morbidity and mortality (~20–45% mortality) associated with stent thrombosis [41–43] make these durations of antiplatelet therapy absolute requirements. Beyond the period of highest stent thrombosis risk, however, the results of the PCI-CURE and CREDO trials [12,14] have supported extending clopidogrel therapy for 12 months after stenting, as is currently recommended by the ACC/AHA/SCAI guidelines for percutaneous intervention in patients not at high risk for bleeding [8,44].

Long-term clopidogrel therapy

Evidence is accumulating to suggest that patients may derive incremental benefit in terms of reductions in the rates of death and MI with long-term (1-year) clopidogrel therapy. As described previously, patients enrolled in the clopidogrel arm of the CURE trial experienced a 20% relative reduction in death, MI or stroke at late follow-up, primarily due to a decreased incidence in MI. In PCI-CURE, while patients loaded with clopidogrel benefited from a reduction in the primary composite end-point of death, MI and urgent revascularization at 30 days, they also faired better when evaluated from immediately post-PCI to the end of follow-up. Patients treated with clopidogrel had lower rates of the combined end-point of death or MI (6.0% vs. 8.0%; p = 0.047), again driven by a reduction in the rate of MI.

The CREDO trial [12], which also assessed the efficacy of long-term clopidogrel in a lower-risk population than that enrolled in the CURE trial, supported the benefit of long-term therapy. Patients treated with long-term (1-year) clopidogrel experienced a 26.9% risk reduction in the combined end-point of death, MI or stroke (8.5% vs. 11.5%, p = 0.02). Together, these two studies would suggest that long-term clopidogrel therapy post PCI (9–12 months) reduces the risk of ischemic events. Finally, quantitative analysis suggests that treatment for up to 1 year with clopidogrel following acute coronary syndromes is relatively cost-effective [45].

An important limitation to this conclusion is that it is difficult to determine whether the benefit in reduced events is attributable to the duration of therapy or the upfront clopidogrel load. In PCI-CURE, while the overall rates of death or MI at 1-year follow-up were 6.0% and 8.0% for the clopidogrel preload and placebo groups respectively (p = 0.047), the comparable rates of death or MI from day 31 to long-term follow-up were 3.1% and 3.6% respectively (number needed to treat, 200). In looking at the hard events of death or myocardial infarction from day 29 to long-term follow-up in the CREDO trial, the rates of death for the clopidogrel preload group versus placebo group were 1.7% and 1.9%, with the respective rates of myocardial infarction being 1.7% and 2.8%. Given the low event rates in these trials, the fact that these trials were not designed to answer the question of whether long-term treatment is beneficial in patients who have been preloaded with clopidogrel (which is presently the standard of care for patients anticipated to undergo stent implantation) and the seemingly low absolute reduction in hard events for patients treated with long-term clopidogrel, it is difficult to definitively conclude that long-term therapy is beneficial in reducing death and MI in patients undergoing elective PCI. In individual cases, the risks of treatment (bleeding) must be weighed against the potential for benefit.

Long-term clopidogrel and very late ST

Whether clopidogrel therapy should be continued for longer than 1 year is also a matter of considerable debate. Longer-term (>1 year) therapy with clopidogrel has been proposed in the era of drug-eluting stenting to prevent very late ST. Case reports of late stent thrombosis in patients treated with DES [46,47] and the temporal correlation of these cases of ST with the discontinuation of clopidogrel therapy [42,47–50], raise questions regarding how long clopidogrel therapy should be continued, and whether certain subgroups merit prolonged therapy.

The incidence of ST in randomized trials of DES (either PES or SES) is comparable to that of BMS, and ranges from 0.4 to 0.6% at 12 months [51–54]. But the observed rate of ST in the "real world", where off-label use is commonplace, is almost double that observed in clinical trials [42]. Further complicating matters is that ST in patients treated with DES can occur outside the 30-day period post stent placement typically seen in patients treated with bare-metal stents. In a consecutive cohort of 2229 patients treated with either SES or PES, ST was observed in 29 patients (1.3%) at 9-month follow-up, with a mortality rate of 45% [42]; 15 of these patients developed ST greater than 30 days after stent placement.

In patients undergoing BMS implantation, persistent dissection, total stent length and final in-stent minimal luminal diameter have been identified as independent predictors of ST [43]. As has been recently demonstrated, premature discontinuation of clopidogrel therapy is the strongest predictor of ST in patients undergoing DES implantation [41,42]. In the cohort of patients studied by Iakovou and colleagues, premature discontinuation of antiplatelet therapy was associated with a hazard ratio for ST of 89.78 (95% CI 29.90–269.60; p < 0.001) [42]. Other independent predictors of ST were renal failure, bifurcation stenting, diabetes and reduced ejection fraction [42]. Given the pervasiveness of "off-label" use of DES, the low frequency of ST and the incomplete ascertainment of this outcome, it is possible that additional predictors will be determined as longer-term follow-up of patients undergoing DES implantation in large multicenter datasets is performed. In addition to attention to important procedural factors by the interventional cardiologist (complete stent expansion, avoidance of residual edge dissections) in patients undergoing DES implantation, when one or more of the above predictors of ST is present, or where the consequences of ST would be severe (left main, or extensive multivessel stenting), it may be prudent to treat with a longer course of clopidogrel.

Recent observational studies of "real-world" patients treated with DES, where off-label use approaches 60% [55,56] have suggested an increased incidence of late ST [57], death and MI [58–60] in patients treated with DES relative to BMS. Recent observational studies have suggested increased late events (death, MI) in patients treated with DES, and have implicated very late ST as the etiology for these events, raising the issue of whether clopidogrel therapy should be continued indefinitely. The largest observational study of DES is the Swedish Coronary Angiography and Angioplasty Registry (SCAAR) study [60], a Swedish registry which enrolled 13,738 patients treated with BMS and 6033 patients treated with DES evaluating the end-point of all-cause mortality and all-cause mortality or MI at 6 months and 3 years. The propensity-score adjusted analysis found a significantly increased risk of death from 6 months to 3 years (RR = 1.32; 95% CI 1.11, 1.57) and at 3 years (RR = 1.18; 95% CI 1.04, 1.35). These observational findings are not definitive as it is possible that selection bias remains and that the differences in the two treatment groups may not have been completed accounted for by the propensity score approach.

Another observational study raising concerns regarding late events in patients treated with DES was recently published by Eisenstein et al., evaluating the combined end-point of death and MI in patients treated with DES (n = 1501) versus BMS (n = 3165) at Duke between both 6 months and 24 months and 12 months and 24 months stratified by clopidogrel use [58]. They found that patients treated with DES who were maintained on clopidogrel had a significantly decreased rate of death compared with patients treated with DES who were not on clopidogrel, both between 6 and 24 months (2.0% vs. 5.3%; p = 0.03) and between 12 and 24 months (0% vs. 3.5%; p = 0.004). The mortality rate in patients treated with BMS maintained on clopidogrel was no different than the mortality rate in patients treated with BMS not on clopidogrel at either time point (3.7% vs. 4.5% between 6 and 24 months; p = 0.50; 3.3% vs. 2.7% between 12 and 24 months; p = 0.57). When looking at the combined end-point of death and MI, the DES patients treated with clopidogrel had lower event rates at both time-points compared with DES patients not treated with clopidogrel (3.1% vs. 7.2% at 6–24 months; p = 0.02, 0% vs. 4.5% at 12–24 months; p = 0.004), whereas the event rates in BMS patients treated with clopidogrel compared with BMS patients not on clopidogrel were not significantly different (5.5% vs. 6.0% at 6–24 months; p = 0.70, 4.7% vs. 3.6% at 12–24 months; p = 0.44). Given the observational nature of the study, clopidogrel therapy was not randomly assigned, and it is possible that confounding remains and that bias was introduced by excluding 0–6 month data. Before one can attribute a protective effect of long term clopidogrel (>1 year) in patients treated with DES, randomized controlled studies are warranted.

The Basel stent cost-effectiveness trial-LAte Thrombotic Events (BASKET-LATE) [59], an observational study involving the 746 patients enrolled in the BASKET trial [61] randomized to DES vs. BMS in 2:1 fashion, evaluated patients who were event-free at the end of a 6-month course of clopidogrel to determine if there was a difference in event rates between these two groups with respect to cardiac death and MI at 18 months. Patients treated with DES had a higher event rate at 18 months versus patients treated with BMS (4.9% vs. 1.3%). It is important to note that no significant difference between the two groups in the combined end-point of death and MI existed when the groups were compared from 0 to 18 months (8.4% vs. 7.5%; p = 0.63). The authors suggested the late events observed in this study are attributable to very late ST. However, it is not clear from this data whether continuation of clopidogrel would have reduced the event rates.

These observational studies have raised concerns regarding the late events of death and MI in patients treated with DES but have been limited by their non-randomized design. A pooled analysis of 4 years of follow-up data from the Randomized Study with the Sirolimus-Coated Bx-Velocity Balloon-Expandable Stent in the Treatment of Patients with de Novo Native Coronary Artery Lesions (RAVEL), Sirolimus-Eluting Stent in Coronary Lesions (SIRIUS), European Sirolimus-Eluting Stent in Coronary Lesions (E-SIRIUS), Canadian Sirolimus-Eluting Stent in Coronary Lesions (C-SIRIUS), Paclitaxel-Eluting Stent (TAXUS I), II, IV, and V trials was performed and found no significant difference in the incidence of ST at 4 years for either the SES or PES versus BMS [62]. Approximately half of the ST events in either the DES or BMS occurred in the setting of ongoing dual antiplatelet therapy. Overall, ST accounted for approximately 10% of the total mortality in follow-up.

When patients are followed for late outcomes and overall event rates are low, non-cardiac death and competing risks become an important issue. As the main concern in the use of DES is delayed endothelialization and predisposition to very late ST, it becomes critical to clearly identify whether late events can be attributed to ST. As the duration of follow-up extends beyond the periprocedural period (when the highest risks of stent thrombosis are present), the likelihood of the clinical events of death or MI become significantly more likely than very late ST. In regards to the protective effects of dual antiplatelet therapy, the beneficial effect due to prevention of death and myocardial infarction outside the stented segment grows proportionally larger over time.

In summary, the strongest evidence for long-term (1 year) therapy with clopidogrel is from the PCI-CURE and CREDO trials. The small but measurable benefits observed as reductions in postprocedural cardiovascular complications (primarily MI) in the PCI-CURE and CREDO trials must be weighed against risks of bleeding and cost. Further evidence is needed to determine which clinical factors determine the subgroups of patients most likely to benefit from longer-term (>1 year) clopidogrel use. Presently, no data exist to support routine clopidogrel administration longer than 1 year. Given the increased clinical event rate observed in patients treated with DES compared to BMS in some observational studies and the high frequency of off-label use of DES, careful scrutiny of DES is warranted. Until more data are available to determine which subgroup of patients undergoing stent placement would derive benefit from clopidogrel therapy beyond 1 year, routine extension of dual antiplatelet therapy cannot replace careful clinical assessment of the risk–benefit ratio for individual patients.

References

1 Baim DS, Carrozza JP Jr. Stent thrombosis. Closing in on the best preventive treatment. *Circulation* 1997; **95**: 1098–1100.
2 Serruys PW, *et al.* Angiographic follow-up after placement of a self-expanding coronary-artery stent. *New Engl J Med* 1991; **324**: 13–17.
3 Schatz RA, *et al.* Clinical experience with the Palmaz-Schatz coronary stent. Initial results of a multicenter study. *Circulation* 1991; **83**: 148–161.
4 Fischman DL, *et al.* A randomized comparison of coronary-stent placement and balloon angioplasty in the treatment of coronary artery disease. Stent Restenosis Study Investigators. *New Engl J Med* 1994; **331**: 496–501.
5 Serruys PW, *et al.* A comparison of balloon-expandable-stent implantation with balloon angioplasty in patients with coronary artery disease. Benestent Study Group. *New Engl J Med* 1994; **331**: 489–495.
6 Leon MB, *et al.* A clinical trial comparing three antithrombotic-drug regimens after coronary-artery stenting. Stent Anticoagulation Restenosis Study Investigators. *New Engl J Med* 1998; **339**: 1665–1671.
7 Schomig A, *et al.* A randomized comparison of antiplatelet and anticoagulant therapy after the placement of coronary-artery stents. *New Engl J Med* 1996; **334**: 1084–1089.
8 King SB, et al. 2007 focused update of the ACC/AHA/SCAI 2005 Guideline Update for Percutaneous Coronary Intervention: a report of the American College

of Cardiology/American Heart Association Task Force on Practice Guidelines: (2007 Writing Group to Review New Evidence and Update the 2005 ACC/AHA/SCAI Guideline Update for Percutaneous Coronary Intervention). *J Am Coll Cardiol* 2008; **51**: 172–209.

9 Barnathan ES, *et al.* Aspirin and dipyridamole in the prevention of acute coronary thrombosis complicating coronary angioplasty. *Circulation* 1987; **76**: 125–134.

10 Schwartz L, *et al.* Aspirin and dipyridamole in the prevention of restenosis after percutaneous transluminal coronary angioplasty. *New Engl J Med* 1988; **318**: 1714–1719.

11 Popma JJ, *et al.* Antithrombotic therapy during percutaneous coronary intervention: the Seventh ACCP Conference on Antithrombotic and Thrombolytic Therapy. *Chest* 2004; **126** (3 Suppl.): 576S–599S.

12 Steinhubl SR, *et al.* Early and sustained dual oral antiplatelet therapy following percutaneous coronary intervention: a randomized controlled trial. *JAMA* 2002; **288**: 2411–2420.

13 Yusuf S, *et al.* Effects of clopidogrel in addition to aspirin in patients with acute coronary syndromes without ST-segment elevation. *New Engl J Med* 2001; **345**: 494–502.

14 Mehta SR, *et al.* Effects of pretreatment with clopidogrel and aspirin followed by long-term therapy in patients undergoing percutaneous coronary intervention: the PCI-CURE study. *Lancet* 2001; **358**: 527–533.

15 Sabatine MS, *et al.* Effect of clopidogrel pretreatment before percutaneous coronary intervention in patients with ST-elevation myocardial infarction treated with fibrinolytics: the PCI-CLARITY study. *JAMA* 2005; **294**: 1224–1232.

16 Awtry EH, Loscalzo J. Aspirin. *Circulation* 2000; **101**: 1206–1218.

17 Gurbel PA, *et al.* Clopidogrel for coronary stenting: response variability drug resistance and the effect of pretreatment platelet reactivity. *Circulation* 2003; **107**: 2908–2913.

18 Kastrati A, *et al.* A clinical trial of abciximab in elective percutaneous coronary intervention after pretreatment with clopidogrel. *New Engl J Med* 2004; **350**: 232–238.

19 Kandzari DE, *et al.* Influence of treatment duration with a 600-mg dose of clopidogrel before percutaneous coronary revascularization. *J Am Coll Cardiol* 2004; **44**: 2133–2136.

20 Patti G, *et al.* Randomized trial of high loading dose of clopidogrel for reduction of periprocedural myocardial infarction in patients undergoing coronary intervention: results from the ARMYDA-2 (Antiplatelet therapy for Reduction of MYocardial Damage during Angioplasty) study. *Circulation* 2005; **111**: 2099–2106.

21 Kastrati A, *et al.* Abciximab in patients with acute coronary syndromes undergoing percutaneous coronary intervention after clopidogrel pretreatment: The ISAR-REACT 2 Randomized Trial. *JAMA* 2006.

22 Use of a monoclonal antibody directed against the platelet glycoprotein IIb/IIIa receptor in high-risk coronary angioplasty. The EPIC Investigation. *New Engl J Med* 1994; **330**: 956–961.

23 Platelet glycoprotein IIb/IIIa receptor blockade and low-dose heparin during percutaneous coronary revascularization. The EPILOG Investigators. *New Engl J Med* 1997; **336**: 1689–1696.

24 Lincoff AM, *et al.* Complementary clinical benefits of coronary-artery stenting and blockade of platelet glycoprotein IIb/IIIa receptors. Evaluation of Platelet IIb/IIIa Inhibition in Stenting Investigators. *New Engl J Med* 1999; **341**: 319–327.

25 Randomised placebo-controlled trial of effect of eptifibatide on complications of per-cutaneous coronary intervention: IMPACT-II. Integrilin to Minimise Platelet Aggregation and Coronary Thrombosis-II. *Lancet* 1997; **349**: 1422–1428.

26 PURSUIT Trial Investigators. Inhibition of platelet glycoprotein IIb/IIIa with eptifibatide in patients with acute coronary syndromes. Platelet glycoprotein IIb/IIIa in unstable angina: receptor suppression using integrilin therapy. *New Engl J Med* 1998; **339**: 436–443.

27 Novel dosing regimen of eptifibatide in planned coronary stent implantation (ESPRIT): a randomised placebo-controlled trial. *Lancet* 2000; **356**: 2037–2044.

28 Platelet Receptor Inhibition in Ischemic Syndrome Management in Patients Limited by Unstable Signs and Symptoms (PRISM-PLUS) Study Investigators. Inhibition of the platelet glycoprotein IIb/IIIa receptor with tirofiban in unstable angina and non-Q-wave myocardial infarction. *New Engl J Med* 1998; **338**: 1488–1497.

29 RESTORE Investigators. Effects of platelet glycoprotein IIb/IIIa blockade with tirofiban on adverse cardiac events in patients with unstable angina or acute myocardial infarction undergoing coronary angioplasty. Randomized Efficacy Study of Tirofiban for Outcomes and REstenosis. *Circulation* 1997; **96**: 1445–1453.

30 Gibson CM, *et al*. Six-month angiographic and clinical follow-up of patients prospectively randomized to receive either tirofiban or placebo during angioplasty in the RESTORE trial. Randomized Efficacy Study of Tirofiban for Outcomes and Restenosis. *J Am Coll Cardiol* 1998; **32**: 28–34.

31 Topol EJ, *et al*. Comparison of two platelet glycoprotein IIb/IIIa inhibitors tirofiban and abciximab for the prevention of ischemic events with percutaneous coronary revascularization. *New Engl J Med* 2001; **344**: 1888–1894.

32 Kong DF, *et al*. Meta-analysis of survival with platelet glycoprotein IIb/IIIa antagonists for percutaneous coronary interventions. *Am J Cardiol* 2003; **92**: 651–655.

33 Karvouni ED, Katritsis G, Ioannidis JP. Intravenous glycoprotein IIb/IIIa receptor antagonists reduce mortality after percutaneous coronary interventions. *J Am Coll Cardiol* 2003; **41**: 26–32.

34 Bhatt DL, *et al*. Abciximab reduces mortality in diabetics following percutaneous coronary intervention. *J Am Coll Cardiol* 2000; **35**: 922–928.

35 Roffi M, *et al*. Platelet glycoprotein IIb/IIIa inhibitors reduce mortality in diabetic patients with non-ST-segment-elevation acute coronary syndromes. *Circulation* 2001; **104**: 2767–2771.

36 Gurbel PA, *et al*. Clopidogrel loading with eptifibatide to arrest the reactivity of platelets: results of the Clopidogrel Loading With Eptifibatide to Arrest the Reactivity of Platelets (CLEAR PLATELETS) study. *Circulation* 2005; **111**: 1153–1159.

37 Peters RJ, *et al*. Effects of aspirin dose when used alone or in combination with clopidogrel in patients with acute coronary syndromes: observations from the Clopidogrel in Unstable angina to prevent Recurrent Events (CURE) study. *Circulation* 2003; **108**: 1682–1687.

38 Collaborative meta-analysis of randomised trials of antiplatelet therapy for prevention of death myocardial infarction and stroke in high risk patients. *BMJ* 2002; **324**: 71–86.

39 Moses JW, *et al*. Sirolimus-eluting stents versus standard stents in patients with stenosis in a native coronary artery. *New Engl J Med* 2003; **349**: 1315–1323.

40 Stone GW, *et al.* A polymer-based paclitaxel-eluting stent in patients with coronary artery disease. *New Engl J Med* 2004; **350**: 221–231.

41 Jeremias A, *et al.* Stent thrombosis after successful sirolimus-eluting stent implantation. *Circulation* 2004; **109**: 1930–1932.

42 Iakovou I, *et al.* Incidence predictors and outcome of thrombosis after successful implantation of drug-eluting stents. *JAMA* 2005; **293**: 2126–2130.

43 Cutlip DE, *et al.* Stent thrombosis in the modern era: a pooled analysis of multicenter coronary stent clinical trials. *Circulation* 2001; **103**: 1967–1971.

44 Grines CL, *et al.* Prevention of premature discontinuation of dual antiplatelet therapy in patients with coronary artery stents: a science advisory from the American Heart Association American College of Cardiology Society for Cardiovascular Angiography and Interventions American College of Surgeons and American Dental Association with representation from the American College of Physicians. *J Am Coll Cardiol* 2007; **49**: 734–739.

45 Weintraub WS, *et al.* Long-term cost-effectiveness of clopidogrel given for up to one year in patients with acute coronary syndromes without ST-segment elevation. *J Am Coll Cardiol* 2005; **45**: 838–845.

46 Virmani R, *et al.* Localized hypersensitivity and late coronary thrombosis secondary to a sirolimus-eluting stent: should we be cautious? *Circulation* 2004; **109**: 701–705.

47 Ong AT, *et al.* Late angiographic stent thrombosis (LAST) events with drug-eluting stents. *J Am Coll Cardiol* 2005; **45**: 2088–2092.

48 Kuchulakanti PK, *et al.* Correlates and long-term outcomes of angiographically proven stent thrombosis with sirolimus- and paclitaxel-eluting stents. *Circulation* 2006; **113**: 1108–1113.

49 McFadden EP, *et al.* Late thrombosis in drug-eluting coronary stents after discontinuation of antiplatelet therapy. *Lancet* 2004; **364**: 1519–1521.

50 Lemos PA, *et al.* Unrestricted utilization of sirolimus-eluting stents compared with conventional bare stent implantation in the "real world": the Rapamycin-Eluting Stent Evaluated At Rotterdam Cardiology Hospital (RESEARCH) registry. *Circulation* 2004; **109**: 190–195.

51 Holmes DR Jr. , *et al.* Analysis of 1-year clinical outcomes in the SIRIUS trial: a randomized trial of a sirolimus-eluting stent versus a standard stent in patients at high risk for coronary restenosis. *Circulation* 2004; **109**: 634–640.

52 Stone GW,*et al.*One-year clinical results with the slow-release polymer-based paclitaxel-eluting TAXUS stent: the TAXUS-IV trial. *Circulation* 2004; **109**: 1942–1947.

53 Moreno R, *et al.* Drug-eluting stent thrombosis: results from a pooled analysis including 10 randomized studies. *J Am Coll Cardiol* 2005; **45**: 954–959.

54 Bavry AA, *et al.* What is the risk of stent thrombosis associated with the use of paclitaxel-eluting stents for percutaneous coronary intervention?: a meta-analysis. *J Am Coll Cardiol* 2005; **45**: 941–946.

55 Urban P, *et al.* Safety of coronary sirolimus-eluting stents in daily clinical practice: one-year follow-up of the e-Cypher registry. *Circulation* 2006; **113**: 1434–1441.

56 Rao SV, *et al.* On- versus off-label use of drug-eluting coronary stents in clinical practice (report from the American College of Cardiology National Cardiovascular Data Registry [NCDR]). *Am J Cardiol* 2006; **97**: 1478–1481.

57 Daemen J, *et al*. Early and late coronary stent thrombosis of sirolimus-eluting and paclitaxel-eluting stents in routine clinical practice: data from a large two-institutional cohort study. *Lancet* 2007; **369**: 667–678.

58 Eisenstein EL, *et al*. Clopidogrel use and long-term clinical outcomes after drug-eluting stent implantation. *JAMA* 2007; **297**: 159–168.

59 Pfisterer M, *et al*. Late clinical events after clopidogrel discontinuation may limit the benefit of drug-eluting stents: an observational study of drug-eluting versus bare-metal stents. *J Am Coll Cardiol* 2006; **48**: 2584–2591.

60 Lagerqvist B, *et al*. Long-term outcomes with drug-eluting stents versus bare-metal stents in Sweden. *New Engl J Med* 2007; **356**: 1009–1019.

61 Kaiser C, *et al*. Incremental cost-effectiveness of drug-eluting stents compared with a third-generation bare-metal stent in a real-world setting: randomised Basel Stent Kosten Effektivitats Trial (BASKET). *Lancet* 2005; **366**: 921–929.

62 Mauri L, *et al*. Stent thrombosis in randomized clinical trials of drug-eluting stents. *New Engl J Med* 2007; **356**: 1020–1029.

Index

Working group member	Employment	Research grant	Other research support	Speakers bureau/honoraria	Expert witness	Ownership interest	Consultant/advisory board	Other
Aleil	EFS Alsace	None	None	None	None	None	None	None
Bhatt	Cleveland Clinic Abraxis, Alexion Pharma, Astra Zeneca, Atherogenics, Aventis, Biosense Webster, Biosite, Boehringer Ingelheim, Boston Scientific, Bristol Myers Squibb, Cardionet, Centocor, Converge Medical Inc, Cordis, Dr Reddy's, Edwards Lifesciences, Esperion, GE Medical, Genentech, Gilford, GSK, Guidant, J&J, Kensey Nash, Lilly, Medtronic, Merck, Mytogen, Novartis, Novo Nordisk, Orphan Therapeutics, P&G Pharma, Pfizer, Roche, Sankyo, Sanofi-Aventis, Schering – Plough, Scios, St Jude MEDICAL, Takeda, TMC, VasoGenix, Viacor+	Bristol Myers Squibb, Eisai, Sanofi Aventis, Heartscape, The Medicines Company, Ethicon, Heartscape+	None	Astra Zeneca, Bristol Myers Squibb, Centocor, Eisai, Eil Lilly, GlaxoSmithKlien, Millennium, Paringenix, PDL, Sanofi Aventis, Schering Plough, The Medicines Company, tns Healthcare*	Clopidogrel+	None	Astra Zeneca, Byser, Bristol Myers Squibb, Cardax, Centocor, Cognetus, Daiichi-Sankyo, Eisai, Eli Lilly, GlaxoSmithKline, Johnson & Johnson, McNeil, Medtronic, Millennium, Otsuka, Paringenix, PDL, Portola, Sanofi Aventis, Schering Plough, Scios, The Medicines Company, tns Healthcare, Vertex, Arena*	None

Working group member	Employment	Research grant	Other research support	Speakers bureau/honoraria	Expert witness	Ownership interest	Consultant/ advisory board	Other
Berger	Geisinger Health Systems	None	None	BMS, Sanofi-Aventis, Lilly/ Daiichi Sankyo, Sheering Plough*	None	Lumen Inc+	Boston Scientific, PlaCor, CV Therapeutics*	None
Blankenship	Geisinger Medical Center	None	None	None	None	None	None	None
Burdess	University of Edinburgh	Educational Grant from Sanofi Aventis, BMS+	None	None	None	None	None	None
Canales	Texas Heart Institution of St Luke's Episcopal Hospital, Baylor College of Medicine	None	None	None	None	None	None	None
Chen	JYA Co Ltd	None	None	None	None	None	None	None
Cohen	Newark Beth Israel Medical Center	Sanofi-Aventis, Schering, Merck*	None	Sanofi-Aventis, Schering, Merck*	None	None	None	None
Collet	Groupe Hospitalier Pitié-Salpêtrière	None	None	None	None	None	None	None
Coolong	Brigham and Women's Hospital	None	None	None	None	None	None	None
Cruden	University of Edinburgh	None	None	None	None	None	None	None

Dunn	University of Kentucky	None	None	None	None	None	None	None
Eikelboom	McMaster University	BMS, Sanofi Aventis, GlaxoSmithKlein+	None	BMS, Sanofi Aventis, GlaxoSmtihKlein*	None	BMS, Sanofi Aventis, GlaxoSmtihKlein*	None	BMS, Sanofi Aventis, GlaxoSmtihKlein*
Ferguson	Texas Heart Institute and Baylor College of Medicine	Eisai Pharmaceuticals, Sanofi-Aventis, The Medicines Company*	None	Astellas Pharmaceuticals, Astra Zeneca, Bristol Myers-Squibb, Daiichi-Sankyo, Eisai Pharmaceuticals, Eli Lilly, GlaxoSmithKlien, Johnson & Johnson, Sanofi-Aventis, Schering-Plough, Takeda Pharmaceuticals, The Medicines Company, Therox*	None	Astellas Pharmaceuticals, Astra Zeneca, Bristol Myers-Squibb, Daiichi-Sankyo, Eisai Pharmaceuticals, Eli Lilly, GlaxoSmithKlien, Johnson & Johnson, Sanofi-Aventis, Schering-Plough, Takeda Pharmaceuticals, The Medicines Company, Therox*	None	Astellas Pharmaceuticals, Astra Zeneca, Bristol Myers-Squibb, Daiichi-Sankyo, Eisai Pharmaceuticals, Eli Lilly, GlaxoSmithKlien, Johnson & Johnson, Sanofi-Aventis, Schering-Plough, Takeda Pharmaceuticals, The Medicines Company, Therox*
Frelinger III	University of Massachusetts Medical School	Eli Lilly, Daiichi Sankyo, GL Synthesis+	None	None	None	None	None	None
Fox	University of Edinburgh	Sanofi-Aventis, BMS, GSK+	None	Sanofi-Aventis, BMS, GSK*	None	Sanofi-Aventis*	None	Sanofi-Aventis*
Gachet	Etablissement Francais du Sang	Sanofi-Aventis / BMS*	None	Sanofi-Aventis, Eli-Lilly*	None	Sanofi-Aventis*	None	Sanofi-Aventis*

Working group member	Employment	Research grant	Other research support	Speakers bureau/honoraria	Expert witness	Ownership interest	Consultant/ advisory board	Other
Goldstein	Duke University	Boehringer Ingelheim*	None	None	None	None	Bayer, BMS*	None
Gornick	Cleveland Clinic	Summit Doppler Inc+ Sanofi-Aventis*	None	None	None	None	None	None
Hamm	None	None	None	Lilly, Merck, GlaxoSmithKlein, Nycomed, Medic Comp*	None	None	GlaxoSmithKlein, Merck, Nycomed*	None
Kamran	Cleveland Clinic	None	None	None	None	None	None	None
Kim	Cleveland Clinic	None	None	None	None	None	None	None
Mauri	Brigham and Women's Hospital	None	None	None	None	None	None	None
Mejevoi	Newark Beth Israel Medical Center	None	None	None	None	None	None	None
Michelson	University of Massachusetts Medical School	Accumetrics, Arena Pharmaceuticals, Biocytex, Dade Behring, Lilly/ Daiichi Sankyo, McNeil Consumer Healthcare, Sanofi-Aventis/ Bristol-Myers Squibb+	None	Sanofi-Aventis/ Bristol-Myers Squibb*	None	None	McNeil Consumer Healthcare*	None

Montalescot	Groupe Hospitalier Pitié-Salpêtrière	Sanofi, Eli Lilly+	None	Sanofi, Eli Lilly+	None	None	Sanofi, Eli Lilly+	None
O'Donoghue	None	None	None	None	None	None	None	None
Raju	McMaster University (Hamilton General Hospital)	Hamilton Health Sciences+	Hematology Society of Australia and New Zealand+	None	None	None	None	None
Simon	University Hospitals-Case Medical, Case Western Reserve University School of Medicine	Cordis/J & J Accumetrics, Schering-Plough+	None	Cordis, Schering-Plough+	None	None	Cordis+ Medtronic, Sanofi-Aventis*	None
Sabatine	Brigham and Women's Hospital	Sanofi-Aventis, Schering-Plough+	None	Sanofi-Aventis, Bristol-Myers Squibb*	None	None	None	None
Steinhubl	The Medicines Company+	None	None	Astra Zeneca, Sanofi Aventis, Eli Lilly, Diacchi Sankyo, Cardax*	None	None	None	None
Storey	University of Sheffield	Astra Zeneca, Eli Lilly+	None	Astra Zeneca, Eli Lilly, Schering Plough*	None	None	The Medicines Company*	None
Suarez	Sinai Hospital of Baltimore	None	None	None	None	None	None	None

Working group member	Employment	Research grant	Other research support	Speakers bureau/honoraria	Expert witness	Ownership interest	Consultant/ advisory board	Other
Tantry	Sinai Center for Thrombosis Research	None	None	None	None	None	None	None
Tanwir	Newark Beth Israel Medical Center	None	None	None	None	None	None	None
Wiviott	Brigham and Women's Hopsital	Eli Lilly, Daiichi Sankyo Co Ltd, Schering-Plough+	None	Pfizer, Eli Lilly, Daiichi Sankyo Co Ltd+ Accumetrics, Astra-Zeneca, Schering-Plough, Merck, Pfizer*	None	None	Sanofi-Aventis+ Abbott, Arena Pharmaceuticals, Biogen Idec, Forrest Laboratories, Inotek, Medicure, Portola, Transform Pharmaceuticals*	None
Wong	Stanford University Medical Center	None	None	None	None	None	None	None

*Modest

+Significant

This table represents the relationships of writing group members that may be perceived as actual or reasonably perceived conflicts of interest as reported on the Disclosure Questionnaire which all writing group members are required to complete and submit. A relationship is considered to be "Significant" if (a) the person receives $10,000 or more during any 12 month period, or 5% or more of the person's gross income; or (b) the person owns 5% or more of the voting stock or share of the entity, or owns $10,000 or more of the fair market value of the entity. A relationship is considered to be "Modest" if it is less than "Significant" under the preceding definition.

The AHA Clinical Series

SERIES EDITOR • ELLIOTT ANTMAN

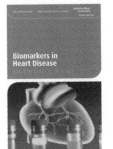

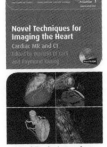

Biomarkers in Heart Disease
James A. de Lemos
9781405175715

Novel Techniques for Imaging the Heart
Marcelo Di Carli & Raymond Kwong
9781405175333

Pacing to Support the Failing Heart
Kenneth A. Ellenbogen
& Angelo Auricchio
9781405175340

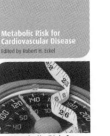

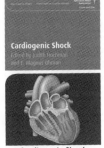

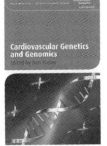

Metabolic Risk for Cardiovascular Disease
Robert H. Eckel
9781405181044

Cardiogenic Shock
Judith Hochman
& E. Magnus Ohman
9781405179263

Cardiovascular Genetics and Genomics
Dan Roden
9781405175401

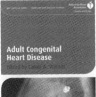

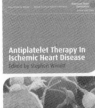

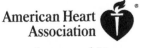

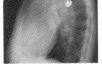

Adult Congenital Heart Disease
Carole A. Warnes
9781405178204

Antiplatelet Therapy In Ischemic Heart Disease
Stephen Wiviott
9781405176262